GRETCHEN DAHL REEVES

GRETCHEN DAHL REEVES
3750 EAST DRAHNER
OXFORD, MI 48370
(248) 628-9548

D1265969

Pain Management by Physical Therapy

Pain Management by Physical Therapy

Second Edition

Edited by

Peter E. Wells BA, FCSP, DipTP, SRP

Chartered Physiotherapist and Postgraduate Teacher,
The Physiotherapy Centre, London, UK

Victoria Frampton MCSP, SRP

Chartered Physiotherapist and Therapy Manager,
Thanet Health Care Trust, Margate, UK

David Bowsher MD, PhD, MRCP(Ed), FRCPath

Director of Research, Pain Research Institute;
Honorary Consultant Neurologist, Regional Centre for Pain Relief, Liverpool, UK

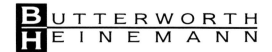

Butterworth-Heinemann Ltd
Linacre House, Jordan Hill, Oxford OX2 8DP

℞ A member of the Reed Elsevier plc group

OXFORD LONDON BOSTON
MUNICH NEW DELHI SINGAPORE SYDNEY
TOKYO TORONTO WELLINGTON

First published 1988
Reprinted 1988
Second edition 1994

British Library Cataloguing in Publication Data

Pain Management by Physical Therapy. –
2Rev.ed
  I. Wells, Peter E.
  616.0472

ISBN 0 7506 0569 3

Library of Congress Cataloguing in Publication Data

Pain management by physical therapy/edited by Peter E. Wells,
  Victoria Frampton, David Bowsher.—2nd ed.
  p.   cm.
  Includes bibliographical references and index.
  ISBN 0 7506 0569 3
  1. Pain—Physical therapy. I. Wells, Peter E. II. Frampton,
  Victoria. III. Bowsher, David.
  [DNLM: 1. Pain. 2. Pain—prevention & control. 3. Physical
  Therapy.   WL 704 P146593 1994]
  RB127.P33237 1994
  616′.0472—dc20
  DNLM/DLC
  for Library of Congress   93–46263
                                                CIP

Printed in Great Britain by Bath Press Ltd Avon.

Contents

List of contributors

Jon Alltree MSc, MCSP
Superintendent physiotherapist, The National Hospital for Neurology and Neurosurgery, London

David Bowsher MD, PhD, MRCP(Ed), FRCPath
Reader (Clinical), Department of Neurological Sciences, University of Liverpool; Director of Research, Pain Relief Foundation; Honorary Consultant in Pain Relief, Centre for Pain Relief, Walton Hospital, Liverpool

Jeffrey D. Boyling MSc, BPhty, MCSP, MErgS
Director, Jeffrey Boyling Associates
Chartered Physiotherapists and
Ergonomists, London

David Fitzgerald DipEng, MCSP, Grad Dip Manip Ther
Private Practitioner, The Physiotherapy Centre, London

Victoria Frampton MCSP, SRP
Chartered Physiotherapist and Therapy Manager, Thanet Health Care Trust, Margate, Kent

Sally French BSc, MSc(psych), MSc(soc), Grad Dip Phys, DipTP
Lecturer, School of Health, Welfare and Community Education, Open University, Milton Keynes

Jean Gifford MCSP, DipTP, SRP
Private Practitioner, Falmouth, Cornwall

Louis Gifford BSc, PGCE, MCSP, Grad Dip Adv Manip Ther
Private Practitioner, North Adelaide, South Australia; Part-time Tutor in Advanced Manipulative Therapy, School of Physiotherapy, South Australia Institute of Technology

A. J. Guymer FCSP, DipTP, SRP
Clinical Tutor in Physiotherapy, Chelsea and Westminster Hospitals, London

Alexandra Hough BA, MCSP, DipTP
Freelance Lecturer, London

Fiona Jones MCSP, SRP
Physiotherapy Department, Wolfson Medical Rehabilitation Centre, Copse Hill, London

John Low BA(Hons), MCSP, DipTP, SRP
Formerly Acting Principal, School of Physiotherapy, Guy's Hospital, London

Betty O'Gorman MCSP, SRP
Superintendent Physiotherapist, St Christopher's Hospice, Sydenham, London

Nigel Palastanga MA, BA, MCSP, DMS, DipTP
Principal, Cardiff School of Physiotherapy, I.H.C.S., University Hospital of Wales, Cardiff

Margaret Polden MCSP, SRP
Superintendent Obstetric Physiotherapist, Hammersmith Hospital, London

Alison T. Skinner BA, MCSP, HT, DipTP
Senior Teacher, University College London and the Middlesex School of Physiotherapy, The Middlesex Hospital, London

Carol Sweet MSc, Grad Dip Phys, MCSP, SRP, MBES
Research Fellow in Physiotherapy, Manchester and Salford Back Pain Centre, Ladywell Hospital, Salford

Gillian Thomas
Physiotherapy Department, Wolfson Medical Rehabilitation Centre, Copse Hill, London

John W. Thompson MB, BS, PhD, FRCP
Director of Studies and Honorary Physician, St Oswald's Hospice, Newcastle upon Tyne; Emeritus Consultant Clinical Pharmacologist, Newcastle Health Authority; Former Director, Pain Relief Clinic, Royal Victoria Infirmary, Newcastle upon Tyne; Emeritus Professor of Pharmacology, University of Newcastle upon Tyne

Ann M. Thomson MSc, BA, MCSP, DipTP
Head of School, University College London and Middlesex, School of Physiotherapy, The Middlesex Hospital, London

Peter E. Wells BA, FCSP, DipTP, SRP
Chartered physiotherapist and postgraduate teacher, The Physiotherapy Centre, London

Preface to the second edition

Since the first edition of this book, physiotherapy in the United Kingdom has attained the status of an all-degree profession. A greater emphasis in education and training is now placed upon the critical evaluation of the many assessment and treatment procedures which underpin professional practice. Post-graduate specialisation has continued to develop in recent years to the point where *consultant* physiotherapists operate in practice, if not yet by formal recognition, within the specialist areas of physiotherapy in the United Kingdom.

In Australia, specialist physiotherapy status has become formally recognised for those suitably highly qualified, reinforcing that the professions' priority is to foster and deliver the best possible skills and care.

As the provision of healthcare in general continues to be remodelled, sometimes drastically, to fit this or that priority as well as constrained budgets both in the public and private health fields, physiotherapy—along with all the other sectors—is increasingly being challenged to prove its worth. Research by physiotherapists is exploring many corners of theory and practice where previously empiricism alone was the norm.

Where clinical methods do not yet have convincing scientific evidence from suitable clinical trials to support their use, but nevertheless *are* used in view of their apparent efficacy, a convincing body of 'evidence' may be built up from related scientific texts to explain and justify such approaches. Many techniques used in physiotherapy related to pain control are of this sort, e.g. adverse neural tension techniques. However, because an approach or technique has not yet been proven to be effective does not mean it is ineffective. Whilst the dictum 'prove it or lose it' must be in the forefront of our thinking, yet there is no substitute, on the 'shop floor' of day by day clinical practice, for well-informed clinical experience. This second edition brings together such experience in the context of pain control from a wider field of physiotherapy theory and practice than was covered in the first edition.

Peter E. Wells BA, FCSP, DipTP, SRP

Preface to the first edition

Pain is a problem for the majority of patients managed by physiotherapists, and in many cases acute or chronic pain from a variety of sources can be relieved altogether by appropriate physiotherapy intervention. This book highlights the unique contribution of the physiotherapist in the management and control of pain, bringing together information on pain control using a wide range of modalities and special techniques, with critical discussion of the part each can play in the overall treatment of pain.

Physiotherapy must increasingly be seen as a first option. Frequently, patients referred for assessment and treatment have already received courses of analgesics or anti-inflammatory drugs, or have undergone surgery, yet report only partial relief, if any, from their pain. Such patients are often depressed, apprehensive and sceptical and it says much for the skills of the physiotherapist that success in pain control is frequently achieved in spite of such formidable physical and psychological odds.

The effective relief of pain not only improves the wellbeing of the individual patient, but may also have major financial implications for that person's family or dependants, and for the national economy. For example, in the United Kingdom in 1982, the total cost of low back pain to the National Health Service was estimated at over £150 million (1982 figures) and is calculated to have cost a further £1000 million in lost production.

It will be clear to readers of this book that physiotherapy, using relatively low-cost techniques, has a major part to play in both clinical and economic terms in the management of pain. The movement of more physiotherapists into primary health care signals still greater involvement of the profession in prevention, advice and early treatment and this too leads to greater cost-effectiveness in the management of many common pain problems (Hackett *et al.*, 1993).

Our aim in this book is to provide the physiotherapist, whether in training or in practice, with an up-to-date review of the anatomical and physiological basis of pain, some knowledge of the pharmacology of pain control, and an understanding of the contribution of various physiotherapy modalities to the overall treatment of pain. We conclude by reviewing a number of special areas where physiotherapy intervention has proved particularly effective.

It is our hope that both students and qualified physiotherapists, together with the medical practitioners who refer patients for their care, will find within these pages the information necessary to encourage good practice, provoke thought, and stimulate further investigation.

In order not to encumber the text with alternative pronouns, both physiotherapists and all patients are variously referred to as he or she throughout the book. It is hoped that a 50:50 distribution between the sexes has been achieved.

Finally, the editors would like to express their thanks to Caroline Makepeace of Heinemann Medical Books for all her dedicated hard work during the various stages of book development.

Peter E. Wells
Victoria Frampton
David Bowsher

Reference

Hackett, G. I., Bundred, P., Hutton, J. L., O'Brien, J. and Stanley, M. (1993) Management of joint and soft tissue injuries in three general practices: value of on-site physiotherapy. *Br. J. Gen. Pract.*, **43**, 61–4

1   *Introduction*

PETER E. WELLS

The public do not generally associate physiotherapists with the management and relief of pain. Ask anyone, even a doctor or nurse, what they understand a physiotherapist's role to be in the medical team and their answers will almost certainly revolve around concepts such as 'getting people going after illness or accident', 'mobilising patients who have had a fracture', 'teaching people to walk again' and so on. In turn, what is done in these situations will be related to strengthening, mobilizing and coordinating certain functions and activities. While not incorrect, this stereotyped and narrow view of the role of physiotherapy omits, for example, the great part played by physiotherapists in the management and control of pain. Part of the reason for this may well stem from the fact that the physiotherapy model of examination, assessment and treatment is related primarily to malfunction and disability and not to the medical model of disease processes and pathology.

Even when a patient's complaint includes a degree of pain, or is largely one of pain, he will often regard the pain relief gained as a result of specific physiotherapy procedures as a spin-off from something else, which it may be. Consider, for example, the patient with an acutely painful neck and grossly restricted movement. During the initial treatment, let us say by various manipulative procedures, the movement of his neck dramatically improves. He may well remark with surprise at this improvement in function ('I wasn't able to look behind me an hour ago!'), and then secondarily he will notice that the level of pain has dropped. His conclusion, and it will be at least in part correct, is that the physiotherapist was intent upon **mobilizing** his neck, getting him **moving**. On the other hand, it is likely that the physiotherapist was intent upon **directly altering the behaviour of the pain**, as a result of which movement has improved. Perhaps, within examples like this, lies the root of the lack of appreciation of a specific physiotherapeutic

role in the management of pain. Hence the various physical methods for pain relief employed by physiotherapists are often seen as peripheral and apart from the drugs, surgical procedures and counselling offered by doctors. They are, of course, not much different; after all pain relief is pain relief. Where acupuncture or manipulation or corrective exercise and advice has produced the relief of chronic, intermittent low back pain (which a variety of drugs have not been effective in relieving), then the worth and suitability of the approach in this case is clear.

Is all this important? The answer, for a number of reasons, must most definitely be yes! One example, the management of chronic headache, deserves a mention. This condition, frequently a distressing and disabling one, is among the most common if not *the* most common with which patients consult their general practitioners. A large proportion of such patients are women.

A great many of these headaches arise from mechanical disturbances in the cervical joints, often perpetuated by poor postural alignment of the head–neck and neck–trunk and long-standing muscle imbalance. These very commonly occurring problems, which may include disturbing symptoms affecting the eyes and ears and facial pain, are generally very responsive to judicious manual treatment of the offending joints, postural and muscle re-education and detailed advice about avoiding further episodes. How many of these problems are referred to physiotherapists for treatment? Very few, unless, of course, those in a position to refer them are made aware of what can be done by **physical agencies** and how complete and lasting such relief can be.

It is a prime example of a situation where a lack of understanding of the alternatives to drugs, surgery and 'learning to live with it', condemns the sufferers to years of chronic pain.

The potential for effective pain relief which

physiotherapy offers across a wide spectrum of medical care is only slowly becoming generally recognized. The reluctance of many people to take drugs for pain, unless these are highly effective and short-term, is increasingly evident and is an important factor motivating such sufferers to seek alternatives. Physiotherapists must inform the public of their important role in this field and educate medical practitioners, including those in primary health care, of the many safe, effective and inexpensive procedures available for the management of pain problems by physiotherapy.

2 *The role of the physiotherapist in the pain clinic*

CAROL SWEET

The treatment of pain as a specialty is relatively new. During the late 1960s and early 1970s there was a significant increase in the number of pain clinics being developed within the National Health Service (NHS). However, there is not only a need for more but also for improved facilities, according to a comprehensive report written by Wells in 1987. The demands upon pain clinics are increasing and the input of a multidisciplinary team is becoming more evident with the complexity of the referrals.

Many physiotherapists looked forward to the development of a specialized service which promised to offer a sympathetic forum and support for sufferers who could not be helped by conventional therapy. A clinic concerned exclusively in the management of intractable pain would address the difficulties associated with the interpretation and the measurement of this very unpredictable and complex symptom (see Chapters 1 and 2). However, representation in pain clinics by the physiotherapy profession, which has in the past often provided the only available treatment for some patients with persisting pain, is sadly small. Those privileged physiotherapists who are on the staff of a pain clinic have found an invaluable environment devoted to the care of patients with intractable pain and have given considerable help to their patients.

The services offered by a pain clinic to treat pain will vary according to the professions of the members of staff. The aims of treatment may, for example, be such as the following:

1. Global assessment of a patient from the combined efforts of some or all members of the pain clinic staff. A multidisciplinary assessment may reveal a new diagnosis or confirmation of a provisional diagnosis for a referring practitioner and provide advice on a patient's future management.

2. Treatment being initiated following discussion with each member of the pain clinic where the patient's physical dysfunction and psychosocial condition are considered.
3. Management of the patient's condition being carried out either individually or in a group by one or more members of the staff, drawing from a range of treatments from a specialized multidisciplinary team.

The pain clinic is designed to provide the facility to assess and treat the many components of a patient's pain problem.

In this chapter I will outline the development of pain clinics, the initial involvement of physiotherapists, and their role in differential diagnosis and treatment, with some case histories as illustration.

History of pain clinics

In about 1936 Rovenstine started the first pain clinic, a nerve block clinic, at Bellevue Hospital, New York. In 1961 Bonica established the first more broadly based pain relief clinics in Tacoma and Washington and Alexander developed a clinic in McKinney, Texas. The first pain relief clinics in Europe were established in Great Britain (Swerdlow, 1986).

Pain relief clinics that subsequently started in Europe followed the development pattern of those in Great Britain. In some European countries formal clinics have still to be established.

In the United Kingdom, as in the United States of America, the treatment provided was nerve blocks performed by anaesthetists. Clinics were set up in London in 1947 by Dr B.G.B. Lucas at University College Hospital, followed a year later by Dr E. Angel in Plymouth and soon after clinics were established in Liverpool and Bristol in 1950. The first multidisciplinary clinic was started in 1964 in Oxford by Dr Ritchie Russell, a noted neurologist. The other members of this clinic were a psychiatrist and an anaesthetist.

In 1967 the Intractable Pain Society of Great Britain was founded. There were 17 doctors at the inaugural meeting. By 1972 there were 42 members and by 1977 43 clinics were in existence acknowledged by the response to a questionnaire sent out in May of that year. Of these 43 clinics, 23 were multidisciplinary and 19 had been in existence for 19 years.

Involvement of physiotherapists with pain clinics

Physiotherapists became involved with care of patients attending pain clinics during the 1970s. At first this involvement was indirect where a patient was referred from the clinic with a request from the pain consultants to try a particular treatment. Treatments recommended for chronic pain patients would vary from ultrasound to transcutaneous electrical nerve stimulation (TENS), vibration therapy to relaxation, and back or neck school to hydrotherapy.

Soon physiotherapists themselves started a reverse referral system. Non-responders to physiotherapeutic interventions sent from orthopaedic and rheumatology clinics, were referred in turn to pain clinics. This may have been the trigger to initiate the actual involvement of physiotherapists in pain clinics. Considering the extent and nature of the physiotherapists' treatment of painful conditions, it is interesting that their inclusion as members of a pain clinic has come at such a late stage in the development of this service and is not universal.

At the same time that physiotherapists started becoming directly involved with patients attending pain clinics, nurses, occupational therapists and social workers were joining the multidisciplinary team. Initially clinics rarely had both physiotherapists and nurses because their role was often the same, for example in the provision and use of TENS machines.

Nurses have worked with anaesthetists in advising postoperative and oncology patients in the use of TENS for pain relief for some years. The occupational therapist's role is less well defined and may overlap with that of the physiotherapists in the

field of relaxation and goal-setting, although both offer valuable contributions to the patient and often work together. A social worker's involvement with the pain clinic extends to the patient's home life where a patient's ability to manage their day and effect the self-help approach to treatment can be monitored. Also social workers can offer guidance with social integration as patients suffering from chronic pain often become isolated from their family and friends.

In a few pain clinics in the UK the role of the physiotherapist has broadened to encompass the greater need for assessment in differential diagnosis and the appropriate use of a variety of treatment modalities.

Differential Diagnosis

The subject of diagnosis, or assessment – the term more often used by physiotherapists – is fundamental to the achievement of a successful outcome. In the management of musculoskeletal conditions, it is this author's belief that the physiotherapist's skills of assessment are superior. However, assessment of patients attending a pain clinic is a challenge, putting each assessor's skills to the ultimate test. As pain is a combination of physiological and psychological factors (**see Chapter 4**), a diagnosis is reached by a compilation of the assessments of some or all of the multidisciplinary team.

A pain clinic provides a unique environment where differential diagnosis can be achieved for the patient during one hospital visit, even for the most complex of conditions. The sensory, physiological and psychological components of pain can be fully explored by the members of the clinic. One or more assessments of the patient's pain are made. Depending on the outcome, the patient is treated either individually or in a group setting or referred to another department for further management.

The route to a diagnosis is seldom straightforward and trial treatments or further investigations often preclude the final conclusion.

Method of Assessment

Whichever format is used to elicit a history of the painful condition, the first essential is to gain the patient's confidence. At the time of the examination the patient will have already seen the pain consultant and possibly other members of staff in the clinic. The patient also may previously have had physiotherapy, the experience of which may have left negative associations towards further intervention. The treatment may have been of short-term benefit only, completely ineffective or even perhaps worsened their condition. The greater the number of visits to medical practitioners the worse a patient's pain will become. This is known as an 'iatrogenic' effect (Pither and Nicholas, 1991) and will also occur after a succession of unsuccessful or failed treatments.

One of the ways a physiotherapist can cope with starting from such a disadvantageous position is to be clear and decisive about what treatment **can** offer. If doubt is apparent in the physiotherapist's voice the patient will quickly resist in-depth examination and subsequently reject new advice or treatment and become uncooperative.

During the assessment it is reassuring for the patient to hear an explanation for the different examination procedures. For example, 'this machine will determine the strength of your leg muscles', 'this device measures the mobility of your spine', 'this test will show your tolerance to pain' etc. Explanation that tests do not always reveal information but may eliminate certain pathologies, as in a radiograph, may reduce the anxieties experienced by some patients. Rarely have reasons for tests been given or understood and yet patients allow the medical profession to look, move, probe and invade their bodies.

It is not surprising therefore that resistance to further examination may be evident. The patient may have been given a number of different clinical diagnoses or none at all. In the latter case, the patient may have been labelled as having a 'functional component' to their condition or been told that their pain is psychosomatic. The frustration and anger that either description induces adds tenfold to the severity of the pain the patient suffers and can make effective examination complex.

From the confused emotions, overreaction to examination and the very slow guarded movements performed by the patient, it is possible to identify information related to their present complaint. The Maitland concept of assessment (see Chapter 1) is particularly suitable for extricating the relevant details of examination and may help to eliminate a number of the 'labels' a patient may have been given. The attention to detail of the subjective and physical examination will demonstrate to the physical patient that their condition is being taken seriously and they may 'open up'

about other worries and fears regarding possible pathology. A common concern among patients with chronic pain is the fear of having a terminal illness.

Modalities of treatment practised by physiotherapists in pain clinics

Transcutaneous electrical nerve stimulation (TENS)

Initially the physiotherapist's input in a pain clinic was the assessment of the patient and their suitability for treatment with a TENS machine. Bending in 1989 described the use of TENS in the pain clinic at The National Hospital. During the assessment the area, extent and nature of their pain is recorded and its behaviour and relationship to activity and rest established. Explanation of and instruction in the use of the device is carried out and the application of electrodes practised until the exact site is located and the desired sensation experienced (See Chapter 14 for more details).

Patients are encouraged to use the device for long periods during the day to achieve successful control of their pain thus using TENS in a preventative manner prior to activities that may aggravate their condition. Long-term use for chronic pain is supported by Bending (1989) and also by Hyodo et al. (1990) who describes a novel cordless mini-TENS. Both authors advise that the benefits gained in the treatment of chronic pain are not as good as for acute pain.

If symptoms become more severe, patients are instructed either to increase the intensity or the frequency of the stimulation or change to an intermittent burst mode of stimulation of their choice. In a study by Nash et al. in 1990 patients with chronic pain found that higher frequencies effected a speedier recovery.

A follow-up appointment is made to check a patient's management of the TENS machine, appearance of any side effects, for example, adverse skin reactions to the tape or gel, and importantly, if pain reduction is being achieved. They are then given a trial of this treatment for a further period of, for example 3 weeks, after which the patients are recommended either to purchase their own machine or are offered a machine on loan from the pain clinic for an indefinite period.

The efficacy of TENS is constantly being challenged (Deyo et al., 1990). If TENS emerges solely as a strong placebo, its success in reducing pain and medication intake will maintain its role as a useful tool in the treatment of chronic pain. The efficacy of TENS is supported by the research of Frampton (1982), Eriksson et al. (1984), Fried et al. (1984), Wynn Parry and Girgis (1988), and Johnson et al. (1991) and is continuing to be prescribed for the treatment of pain (see Chapter 14).

Pain management

As part of the multidisciplinary team, physiotherapists have become involved in the physical rehabilitation of patients with chronic pain. The treatment can be managed individually or in groups. In the case of group therapy, small numbers of between four and six patients are seen together. The team may include an anaesthetist, neurologist or rheumatologist, i.e. the pain consultant of the clinic, a psychiatrist or psychologist, an occupational therapist, a social worker as well as a physiotherapist or nurse.

The concept is to provide:

1. Information, that is each discipline provides the group of patients with as much information as possible on treatments that are currently available to alleviate pain. The majority of patients will have previously received, and failed to respond to, conventional therapies, and various invasive and non-invasive procedures. The information provided by the different disciplines concentrates on the self-help approach to enable a patient to become more independent. Main and Parker in 1989 described how pain management programmes consider the person as well as their chronic pain and teach the patient skills to cope with their pain.
2. A self-help approach which may include the following components: the pain consultant providing advice to the patient on self-medication, the psychologist on stress-reducing techniques and cognitive-behavioural therapy, the psychiatrist on autohypnosis or imagery, the physiotherapist on automobilization, isometric muscle strengthening exercises and posture, the occupational therapist on relaxation methods, pacing and goal achievement and the social worker on distraction techniques, self-help groups and advice on domestic issues.

Evidence has favoured a multidisciplinary approach for a variety of chronic pain syndromes

(Parry, 1983; Crook et al., 1986; Mayer et al., 1987; Murphy, 1987; Neumann, 1988; Wynn Parry and Girgis, 1988; Hazard et al., 1989) using a variety of physical and psychological modalities. The rationale for group, as opposed to individual treatment is also supported by the literature (Toomey and Sanders, 1983; Moore et al., 1984; Main and Parker, 1989: 139). The benefits of group treatment are the support achieved by communication of the patients and the sharing of common symptoms, emotional experiences and fears with fellow sufferers. Undoubtedly there is also an economy on time for the staff of a busy pain clinic but evidence justifies the positive advantages of the group effect on patients with chronic pain. Moore et al. in 1984 studied 51 patients who completed small group multidisciplinary programmes and showed significant reductions in scores for pain, disability and hypochondriasis. Response to treatment depended in some part on the response of the other patients in the group. However, Moore concluded that as social factors play an important role in the aetiology of chronic pain, treatment programmes should be designed to capitalize on these influences.

It is apparent that patients suffering from a chronic pain syndrome need specific management and do less well when their treatment is combined with patients who have non-chronic conditions. In an attempt to advise a group of chronic back pain patients on activities of daily living (ADL), ergonomics at home and at work and information on the structure and function of their joints and muscles, they were invited to join a back school (Sweet 1988). The chronic sufferers became withdrawn, more negative and eventually disruptive to the group. The patients thought their conditions more disabling than the acute back pain patients and became impatient during the sessions. Isolating the same chronic group of patients permitted specific problems to be discussed. Where emphasis on rest was made for the acute patients, activity and frequent changes in posture were encouraged for the chronic patients. Klaber Moffett (1989) describes a back school run specifically for patients with long-term problems and supports the need for less emphasis to be put on rest, and the need to emphasize the non-threatening nature of a chronic pain problem.

Acupuncture

After physiotherapists had established their expertise in the management of patients with TENS machines, this led to their practising acupuncture in some pain clinics. As stated in the codes of practice, physiotherapists may treat patients by this means for pain relief.

This treatment has been available from anaesthetists in pain clinics for some time. An interesting combination of application practised by the anaesthetist was for the patient to receive acupuncture once or twice weekly for a course of 3–4 weeks and then to use a TENS machine at home thereafter. The TENS electrodes were placed over the same site used previously for needling. Another approach used was for the physiotherapist to treat the patient with TENS initially, the success of which would indicate the patient's greater suitability for a course of acupuncture, the TENS thus acting as a precursor to acupuncture. This use of a combined application of acupuncture and TENS may now be questioned. Further research has revealed that the effects of acupuncture and TENS on pain mechanisms are not identical, although agreement on the exact mechanisms involved has still to be reached.

Duffin (1985), supports the theory of chemical neurotransmitters producing the analgesic effects of acupuncture. Lundeberg et al. in 1991 showed that there were no significant differences in pain reduction with sham and actual acupuncture and that naloxone does not reduce the analgesia produced by acupuncture in patients with osteoarthritic pain. Nienhuis and Hoekstra (1984) support the theory of the endogenous production of beta-endorphins by TENS, and Mannheimer (1985), in the same publication as Duffin, explains the effects of TENS occurring in the substancia gelatinosa, which acts as a gate control system (Melzak and Wall, 1965) (see also Chapters 9 and 10).

Now physiotherapists are treating chronic pain patients with acupuncture either in the clinic as a member of the multidisciplinary staff or accepting patients referred from a pain clinic for individual treatment. Support for the acceptance of the role of acupuncture in the reduction of pain has grown with the publication of single case studies of the successful treatment of chronic pain conditions. Dr Chan Gunn in Canada and Dr George Lewith in England are two notable practitioners responsible for promoting the wider use of acupuncture within the health services of the western world and training physiotherapists in its use in the past 20 years.

Relaxation techniques

Stress, anxiety and increased muscle tension are factors associated with a rise in pain intensity and severity and a reduction in the patient's ability to cope with their symptoms. Relaxation therapies have been revived in recent years and are being taught to chronic pain sufferers to alleviate and minimize factors that exacerbate their symptoms. Through relaxation therapy patients learn to recognize increased tension in their muscles and to effect a reduction of this tension through mental and physical means. Practice of relaxation techniques may enhance a patient's control of their pain or, if practised regularly, can prevent a severe exacerbation of symptoms.

Methods of inducing relaxation take various forms:

Audiotaped training.
EMG biofeedback-assisted relaxation.
Using a patient's memory of peaceful events.
Muscle stretching.
Bernstein and Borkovec (1973) tense–release technique.
Yoga.
Deep breathing.

The above techniques have been recently described and reviewed, and their efficacy reported in the role of pain control by Achterberg *et al.* (1989), Grunert *et al.* (1990), McCaffery (1990), Middaugh *et al.* (1991) and Nespor (1991). Most benefit appears to be gained when relaxation techniques are combined with other therapies as a component of a multimodal pain programme (Grunert *et al.*, 1990; Middaugh *et al.*, 1991).

Methods of relaxation can be taught either individually or in groups and may enhance the effect of analgesia or improve a patient's ability to sleep.

Pacing

All patients with a chronic pain syndrome will benefit from pacing activities. Pacing means breaking up the day to balance rest or relaxation with activity to avoid severe exacerbations of a patient's symptoms (Sternbach, 1987). Initially the patient learns how much time can be spent at a task before the pain increases. Pacing will then help the patient achieve control over the symptoms by the stopping of an activity *before* the pain increases. The practice of changing the task or posture at regular intervals can also act as a break and help to prevent an increase of pain. Planning the day ahead to combine essential daily tasks with relaxation and exercise periods may help a patient to extend their physical ability or working capability without an increase of symptoms. Certain skills are required to practise effective pacing such as relaxation and exercise and patients can learn these techniques by attending a multimodal pain management programme (see Pain management above).

The patient who has learned relaxation techniques and has a suitable exercise regime can allocate times of the day for these activities to break up the day. The relaxation forces the patient to stop everything for a short time to slow down and be tranquil. The exercises, designed to improve physical condition, will reduce joint stiffness and muscle tension and increase muscle strength. Eventually the patient will be able to increase the time spent at a task or begin to extend time spent working or at leisure.

Case histories

Patient A

A woman in her early sixties, of slim build, agile but clearly having difficulty weight-bearing on one of her legs, complained of sharp penetrating pain in her groin. She had been referred direct to the pain clinic from her general practitioner having undergone 18 months of previous investigations. As the site of pain appeared deep in the perineal region, investigations had concentrated on her genitourinary and gynaecological state of health, extending ultimately to a D&C.

History revealed that the pain covered a small area, was intermittent in behaviour and frequently related to weight-bearing. The pain was worse on rising and eased by lying down which completely relieved the symptoms. Other symptoms of a movement similar to something slipping into her perineal area occurred on straining or climbing stairs. She had recently started holding on to walls for support as the condition was becoming worse. Major operations included a total hip replacement a few years earlier.

On examination the pain was reproduced by one-leg standing on the affected side, manual compression and passive flexion/adduction of the affected hip joint. A clinical diagnosis of a loosened hip prosthesis was made and was subsequently confirmed by the orthopaedic department.

Patient B

A man in his late fifties presented with extensive, unremitting pain down his right arm for approxi-

mately 6 months. The pain extended from the point of the right shoulder to the right thumb with proximal radiation to the ipsilateral side of his neck. The severity of the pain had prevented any movement of the upper limb from the elbow distally. The skin of the hand had a shiny appearance simulating reflex sympathetic dystrophy and the hyperthenar eminence was wasted.

After two sessions devoted to examination and assessment, the pain was related to any movement of the right arm. The patient was reluctant to actively move the limb or allow passive movements to be performed. The patient was unable to lie on the right side.

The history revealed the pain had started immediately following a heart transplant operation but because the pain was down the right arm there had been no concern shown by the medical team. He had been referred to the pain clinic by his general practitioner. He also revealed that he was soon to marry a nurse 25 years his junior, whom he had met while attending the heart clinic.

On examination there was stiffness and limitation of all the joints of the upper limb including the wrist and hand. There was associated muscle weakness and grip was weak and very painful. However, the total pain area was reproduced by anteroposterior accessory movement and compression of the right acromioclavicular (A/C) joint. Two sessions of mobilization of the right A/C joint completely cleared the neck and arm pain, leaving a residual soreness over the A/C joint itself. Use of the right arm and hand returned spontaneously. The patient cancelled the third treatment due to a complete resolution of symptoms and full use of the upper limb. A clinical diagnosis of A/C joint dysfunction following heart transplantation, complicated by anxiety over his forthcoming marriage, was made.

Patient C

A man in his early thirties presented with constant burning pain, acute tenderness and hypersensitivity in the lower leg. The history revealed the onset of symptoms related to non-union of a fractured tibia 5 years previously but that symptoms had persisted after satisfactory union. The patient used crutches and was non-weight-bearing on the affected leg. He had received numerous unsuccessful treatments to reduce pain and increase function in the lower leg.

Examination was difficult to complete, taking two sessions owing to the patient's obvious reluctance for any contact to be made with the lower leg. With gentle encouragement, all available movement and palpation, to identify the painful area, was performed by the patient himself. A provisional diagnosis of causalgia, otherwise known as reflex sympathetic dystrophy, was made in agreement with the diagnosis of the pain consultant and the psychiatrist in the clinic. Causalgia is the result of either proven peripheral neural damage or post-traumatic symptomatology without proven neural damage (Gutman *et al.*, 1986).

A TENS machine was prescribed and advice given in its use. The patient applied the electrodes himself right from the beginning of treatment thus initiating management of the treatment. The patient was also instructed to increase his activity gradually and was shown some mobilizing and strengthening exercises. After 2 months using the TENS daily for up to 8 hours, combined with help from the psychiatrist, he was almost fully weight-bearing with a stick and had allowed closer examination of the limb. Although still in pain he was able to be more active and independent. In conclusion, a diagnosis of causalgia complicated by fear that the lower leg would not support his weight was made.

Patient D

A woman in her fifties was referred with chronic low back pain and signs of illness behaviour (Waddell *et al.* 1984). Her symptoms started as a result of a car crash 5 years previously. She had received numerous unsuccessful physical treatments and pain relieving interventions. She had been to a psychiatrist and become angry at suggestions of 'inventing her pain'. The compensation claim for injuries from the accident had been settled the previous year. During the past 4 years she had become a recluse, had not seen her children and had separated from her husband.

The examination took two sessions to complete owing to frequent emotional outbursts and tears combined with constant unguarded movements of her arms and legs. Eventually it was established that there was hyperalgesia over her lumbar spine and severe restriction of spinal movement but no serious pathology. Individual treatment of graded exercise and back care using an operant approach where unguarded movements and emotional outbursts were ignored and praise given to controlled movement and completion of exercises was started. After 3 weeks of three times weekly attendance there was a noticeable reduction in unguarded movements, no emotional outbursts and she had made contact with her children. Her mobility had improved so that she was now taking short walks in her garden. A clinical diagnosis of chronic low back pain aggravated by severe distress as a result of the long compensation case and failed treatments was made.

Summary

The possible involvement of a physiotherapist in differential diagnosis, individual and group management in the pain clinic has been outlined and examples of conditions treated in a pain clinic have been described. The approach to the assessment and treatment of patients with chronic pain has radically changed in the past decade, particularly with an increase in emphasis on functional restoration. We now appreciate that pacing, increase in functional ability and recognition of distress can help a patient gain more control over their pain.

The pain consultant may now appreciate the small but significant changes achieved by a patient as a result of physiotherapy treatment, for example increased sitting, standing and walking tolerance, and is less concerned by symptoms such as pain intensity, severity or distribution that have remained unchanged by therapy. So physiotherapists can offer their many skills and varied experience for the benefit of this very severely disabled population: skills such as the restoring of physical function, and the teaching of methods to cope with pain.

References

Achterberg, J., Kenner, C. and Casey D. (1984) Behavioral strategies for the reduction of pain and anxiety associated with orthopedic trauma. *Biofeedback Self Regul.* **14** (2), 101–14.

Bending, J. (1989) TENS in a pain clinic. *Physiotherapy,* **75**(5), 292–4

Bernstein, D.A. and Borkovec, T.D. (1973) *Progressive Relaxation Training*, Research Press, Champaign, Ill.

Carlson, C.R., Collins, F.L., Nitz, A.J. *et al.* (1990) Muscle stretching as an alternative relaxation training procedure. *J. Behav. Ther. Psychiat.*, **21** (1), 29–38

Crook, J., Tunks, E., Rideot, E. and Browne, G. (1986) Epidemiologic comparison of persistent pain sufferers in a speciality pain clinic and in the community. *Arch Phys. Med. Rehabil.*, **67**(7), 451–5

Deyo, R.A., Walsh, N.E., Martin, D.C. *et al.* (1990) A controlled trial of transcutaneous electrical nerve stimulation (TENS) and exercise for chronic low back pain. *N. Engl. J. Med.*, **322**(23), 1627–34

Duffin, D. (1985) Acupuncture and acupressure. In *Pain* (ed. Theresa Hoskins Michel), Churchill Livingstone, Edinburgh, ch. 5, pp. 122–51

Eriksson, M.B., Sjolund, B.H. and Sundbarg, G. (1984) Pain relief from peripheral conditioning stimulation in patients with chronic facial pain. *J. Neurosurg.*, **61**(1), 149–55

Fay, M.F. (1985) Controlling pain. *Todays O.R. Nurse*, **5**(10), 10–13

Frampton, V.M. (1982) Pain control with the aid of

Transcutaneous Nerve Stimulation. *Physiotherapy*, **68**(3), 77–81

Fried, T., Johnson, R. and McCracken, W. (1984) Transcutaneous electrical nerve stimulation: its role in the control of chronic pain. *Arch Phys. Med. Rehabil.*, **65**(5), 228–31

Grunert, B.K., Devine C.A., Sanger J.R. *et al.* (1990) Thermal self-regulation for pain control in reflex sympathetic dystrophy syndrome. *J. Hand Surg. (Am)*, **15**, 615–18

Gutman, H. Zelikovski, A., Haddad, M. and Reiss, A. (1986) Causalgia – the syndrome, its causes, diagnosis and treatment. *The Pain Clinic*, **1**(2), 101–5

Hazard, R.G. Fenwick, J.W., Kalisch, S.M. *et al.* (1989) *Spine*, **14**(2), 157–61

Hyodo, M., Toyota, S. and Kawacki, A. (1990) *The Pain Clinic*, **3**(2), 103–7

Johnson, M.I., Ashton, C.H. and Thompson, J.W. (1991) An in-depth study of long-term users of transcutaneous electrical nerve stimulation (TENS). Implications for clinical use of TENS. *Pain*, **44**, 221–9.

Klaber Moffett, J.A. (1989) Back schools. In *Back Pain: New Approaches to Rehabilitation and Education* (eds M. Roland and J.R. Jenner), Manchester University Press, Manchester and New York

Lundeberg, T., Eriksson, S.V., Lundeberg, S. and Thomas, M. (1991) Effect of acupuncture and naloxone in patients with osteoarthritic pain. A sham acupuncture controlled study. *The Pain Clinic*, **4**(3), 155–61.

Main, C.J. and Parker, H. (1989) The evaluation and outcome of pain management programmes for chronic low back pain. In *Back Pain: New Approaches to Rehabilitation and Education*, (eds M. Roland and J.R. Jenner, Manchester University Press, Manchester and New York

Mannheimer, J.S. (1985) TENS: uses and effectiveness. In *Pain* (ed. Theresa Hoskins Michel, Churchill Livingstone, Edinburgh

Mayer, T.C., Gatchel, R.J., Mayer, H. and Kishino, J. (1987) A prospective 2-year study of functional restoration in industrial low back injury. An objective assessment procedure. *J. Am. Med. Assoc.*, **258**(13), 1763–7

McCaffery, M. (1990) Nursing approaches to nonpharmacological pain control. *Int. J. Nurs. Stud.*, **27**(1), 1–5

Melzak, R. and Wall, P.D. (1965) Pain mechanisms: a new theory. *Science*, **150**(3699), 971–9

Middaugh, S.J., Woods, S.E., Kee, W.G. *et al.* (1991) Biofeedback-assisted relaxation training for the aging chronic pain patient. *Biofeedback Self Regul. (US)*, **16**(4), 367–77.

Moore, M.E., Berk, S.N. and Nypaver A. (1984) Chronic pain: inpatient treatment with small group effects. *Arch Phys. Med. Rehabil.*, **65**(7), 356–61

Murphy, T.M. (1987) Treatment of intractable pain. *Ann. Acad. Med. Singapore*, **16**(2), 256–60

Nash, T.P., Williams, J.D. and Machin, D. (1990) TENS: does the type of stimulus really matter? *The Pain Clinic*, **3**(3), 161–8.

Nespor, K. (1991) Pain management and yoga. *Int. J. Psychosom. (US)*, **38**(1–4), 76–81.

Neumann, N.M. (1988) Nonsurgical management of pain secondary to peripheral nerve injuries. *Orthop. Clin. North Am.*, **19**(1), 165–74.

Nienhuis, R.L. and Hoekstra, A.J. (1984) Transcutaneous electronic nerve stimulation in ankylosing spondylitis. *Arth. Rheum.*, **27**(9), 1074–5

Parry, C.B. (1983) Principles of rehabilitation medicine as applied to lesions of the peripheral nerves. *Ann. Acad. Med. Singapore*, **12**(3), 449–53

Pither, C.E. and Nicholas, M.K. (1991) The identification of iatrogenic factors in the development of chronic pain syndromes: abnormal treatment behaviour? *Proceedings of the VIIth World Congress on Pain 1991*, Elsevier Science Publishers BV, Amsterdam/New York.

Souhrada, L. (1989) Pain programs offer opportunities for hospitals. *Hospitals*, **63**(23), 52

Sternbach, R.A. (1987) *Mastering Pain*, Arlington Books, London, ch. 6

Sweet, C.A. (1988) Comparison of two group treatments of chronic back pain patients (unpublished observations). Lecture at a PANG meeting, Charing Cross Hospital, London

Swerdlow, M. (1986) A preliminary history of pain relief clinics in Europe. *The Pain Clinic* **1**(2), 77–82

Waddell, G., Main, C.J., Morris, E.W., *et al.* (1984) Chronic low-back pain, psychologic distress, and illness behavior. *Spine*, **9**(2), 209–13.

Wall P.D. (1987) Recent advances in the knowledge of mechanisms of intractable pain. *Int. Disabil. Stud.*, **9**(1), 22–3.

Wells, J.C. (1987) The place of the pain clinic. *Bailleres Clin. Rheumatol.* **1**(1), 123–3.

Wynn Parry C.B. and Girgis F. (1988) The assessment and management of the failed back, Part II. *Int. Disabil. Stud.*, **10**(1), 25–8.

3 Clinical aspects of pain

PETER E. WELLS

Introduction: the selection of treatment

The diverse situations in which physiotherapists, as part of their daily round, are called upon to assist those in pain are reflected in the contents of this book. The response to their management will largely depend upon the cause of the symptoms and the matching of suitable modalities to the cause. Broadly speaking, it is those pains which have a mechanical origin (e.g. most low back pain, many degenerative joint conditions and certain types of headache) which are most likely to respond to mechanically based treatment, such as the manipulative procedures, corrective exercise and postural realignment. Conversely, those caused by the inflammatory response of certain 'disease' processes or trauma (e.g. acute tenosynovitis, pelvic inflammatory disease, sinusitis, recent haematomas and certain types of osteoarthritis) are more likely to respond to physical modalities which may alter aspects of this process, such as ultrasonics and pulsed or unpulsed shortwave diathermy. Many pain problems, of course, arise from a mixed cause, i.e. both mechanical and inflammatory (e.g. osteoarthritis, sprained ankle and surgical wounds) and may require a two-pronged approach. The specialized sensory techniques of transcutaneous electrical nerve stimulation (TENS) and acupuncture have a wide application across a spectrum of acute and chronic pain problems.

The balance between the mechanical and inflammatory causes of pain in a given situation are often impossible to decide, e.g. severe retropatellar pain in a young patient diagnosed as having chondromalacia patellae. It is only a retrospective assessment of the response to different modalities which may give some idea of which contributed more to the patient's symptoms. The response to anti-inflammatory drugs would be of great interest in such a case.

Frequently, as is made clear in a number of chapters throughout this book, the complex nature of the cause of many patients' symptoms demands a high degree of expertise from the physiotherapist in order to identify effective procedures which will bring benefit to the patient, e.g. as with brachial plexus lesions or in a case such as a painful hemiplegic shoulder (Davies, 1985). Similarly, as in some instances of terminal disease, in situations where physical modalities may not be able to alleviate pain to any appreciable extent, at least it should not be made worse by anything the physiotherapist does. In such situations, the physiotherapist has an invaluable role in monitoring the response to activities which he or she is attempting to maintain and will gather essential information in order to help make the administration of drugs maximally effective (see Chapter 22).

As with many other methods regularly in use for pain control, the selection of physiotherapy procedures entails a degree of empiricism. The difference between an informed and critical empirical approach and an unthinking, blunderbuss one is frequently the difference between success and failure. The informed and critical approach begins with a thorough recording of the patient's symptoms and the behaviour of those symptoms.

Recording the Subjective Findings

It is necessary to follow a clear and systematic line of questioning in order to elicit a very accurate and thorough picture of the patient's pain and other symptoms.

The format for such an examination and its recording recommended by Maitland (1986) is as good as any and better than most. It is particularly intended for the examination of musculoskeletal complaints, but the headings followed are suitable for helping define and assess the symptoms likely to fall within the sphere of management of any of the specialized areas of physiotherapy.

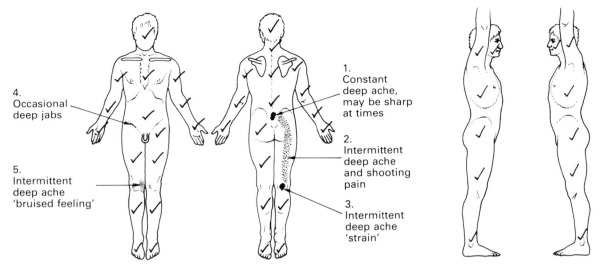

4.
Occasional
deep jabs

5.
Intermittent
deep ache
'bruised feeling'

1.
Constant
deep ache,
may be sharp
at times

2.
Intermittent
deep ache
and shooting
pain

3.
Intermittent
deep ache
'strain'

Fig. 3.1   Clear and concise recording on the body chart is essential to provide a quick and accurate check of the symptoms. New symptoms which appear after the recorded date must be added to the body chart and dated.

The more the physiotherapist knows of the many facets of the patient's pain (or other symptoms), the better position he or she is in to manage it effectively.

The main aim must be to gain control of the pain and in so doing to alter it, reduce it and, where possible, obliterate it. This depends upon the ability of the physiotherapist to assess accurately the many factors relating to the condition and its response throughout treatment. Assessment is discussed in more detail later.

The subjective examination

The following points must be clarified before any treatment is undertaken:

1. **What, at the time of examination, is the patient's main problem in his own opinion?** Is it pain or is it weakness, stiffness or something else?
2. **Where precisely does he feel the pain (and other symptoms, such as numbness, pins and needles)?** The patient, with the relevant areas uncovered, should demarcate clearly with his hand each area and whether these areas run together or are separate and clear-cut with their own boundaries. These areas *must* be entered on to a body chart, with heavier shading for the more intense symptoms (Figure 3.1).

Each area should be given a number 1, 2, 3, etc., and the relevant areas clear of symptoms ticked.
3. **Is the pain (each area separately) superficial (on the skin) or deep (below the skin) or deeper still (e.g. deep inside a joint or deep in the chest or pelvis)?**
4. **What type or kind of pain is it?** That is, how would they describe its **quality**, e.g. throbbing, burning, shooting etc.? Any other words of description, in addition, should be recorded, e.g. 'sickening', 'dreadful', 'punishing', 'frightening' (see Chapter 6). It is not uncommon to have different kinds of pain with one disorder.
5. **Is the pain (area by area) constant or intermittent?** If constant, is it varying?
6. **What is the characteristic behaviour of each area of pain?** In other words, what makes the pain worse and what makes it better? Both activities and postures must be explored, e.g. the activities which may make a specific pain worse might be walking, running, going up or down stairs/steps, coughing, deep breathing, lifting, turning suddenly, typing, etc. Postures causing or aggravating pain might include: sitting, kneeling, lying on the affected area, keeping the part in one position etc. A note should also be recorded if the patient reports the pain is worse when they are stressed or at the time of menstruation etc.

It is important, in addition, to know how much of the aggravating activity can be undertaken or for how long a posture can be maintained before the pains complained of are brought on or made worse. Furthermore, what must the patient then do? Must he move to another position, e.g. lie flat, stand up, or stop the activity because of the pain? When this is so, how quickly does the pain go or take to return to its previous level?

Finally, the physiotherapist must have clearly in their mind the daily, weekly and even monthly pattern of behaviour of the pain. A typical 24 h cycle of behaviour should have been elicited to answer the following questions:

(a) **Does pain interfere with sleeping?** If so, is it worse at night than in the daytime? Is it transient at night allowing the patient to go back to sleep quickly? Is it so bad that the patient must get up, walk around, take drugs etc at night? (Severe, intractable night pain may indicate serious pathology for which the patient will require a rapid referral back to his doctor.) How many times is the patient woken by pain?

(b) **Is pain present on waking or does it start when rising or once the patient** is up? When is it first felt and what position or activity precedes it?

(c) **In general, does** the **pain steadily worsen or improve as the day progresses?**

(d) **Is the pain activity-dependent?**

7. **What was the precise history of onset of this episode and have there been similar episodes in the past?** If similar pain has occurred in the past, did it require treatment? What treatment was received? What effect did it have? If any previous treatment did help, was the pain completely relieved?

It is possible to make some important deductions if all this information has been elicited. These conclusions do not primarily relate to an attempt to diagnose the problem, but are firstly related to the choice of a suitable initial treatment approach and secondly to the precise assessment of the effect of that treatment upon the patient's symptoms.

Analysing the Information from the Subjective Examination

The information gathered needs to be assessed critically before any form of objective examination ('looking, testing, feeling') is begun. Accepting that 'the vitally important physiotherapist's examination is less of a diagnostic sorting procedure than an "indications" examination' (Grieve, 1975), what are the 'indications' which may be gleaned from it so far?

The following should be decided:

1. **Which structures should be tested as possibly contributing to the symptoms?** This question will naturally be relevant only in cases where the musculoskeletal structures are thought to be contributing to the symptoms or where spinal nerve root irritation, compression or tension are involved. The major concern is whether the symptoms to be treated have a local cause or are referred, or, as occasionally happens, there is a dual origin. While the medical diagnosis frequently localizes the source of the symptoms, it does not always, and much time and effort is often wasted if the physiotherapist fails to follow up the medical diagnosis with specific localising tests, e.g. 'inversion sprain of right ankle' does not include the fact that such an injury frequently involves the calcaneocuboid joint. If the physiotherapist does not realize this and test for it, but treats the lateral ligament only, then part of the patient's symptoms are likely to persist, even when he has regained good inversion and ankle stability. Likewise, a patient with 'backache and sciatica' may be found to require treatment principally directed to the mobility of the pain-sensitive structures in the spinal and intervertebral canal, as opposed to the vertebral joint structures themselves.

   The diagnosis, as stated before, will not necessarily direct the physiotherapist to the most suitable and effective treatment in such a case, but aspects of their own examination will.

2. **Is the pain (area by area) severe or not severe?** Severity may be assessed by marking a linear scale (see Chapter 2, p. 6) or by assessing the degree to which activities are curtailed by the pain (e.g. the patient must stop walking because of the pain, cannot concentrate when it is bad, wakes up at night with the pain and then has difficulty sleeping because of it etc.).

3. **Is the condition, and are the symptoms, irritable?** Since mechanically based pain and that associated with inflammation can be aggravated by certain movements, activities or postures depending on how much is undertaken

(including time), an assessment can be made of the way the symptoms have reacted to a given amount (vigour and time) of those provoking actions or postures. Irritable symptoms are those which can be easily provoked (i.e. a small amount of the provoking activity), have a high intensity or severity and do not settle immediately after the activity is stopped but continue for a time. This assessment of irritability is most commonly used with regard to musculoskeletal symptoms (Maitland. 1986), but is well worth trying to apply in other situations as a further degree of insight into the patient's problems may be gained.

4. **What is the nature of the problem?** Some insight is needed into the mechanisms which are giving rise to the patient's symptoms. One example, already discussed, is the degree to which mechanical, inflammatory or other factors are responsible for the pain. While the underlying causes of some symptoms are not always easily determined with certainty, some hypothesis should be made which seems to explain a group of findings. The hypothesis will be supported if the patient reacts in the predicted way to a certain line of management and treatment.

Another example in terms of the nature of a patient's pain is that met when treating brachial plexus lesions (see Chapter 14). Clearly, the physiotherapist will not be in the strongest position to select the most appropriate measures unless he or she has a good understanding of how and why the pathological process involved is manifesting itself in the particularly intense pain so characteristically complained of in these cases.

The effort taken to decide the degree of severity and irritability of the patient's condition as well as the attempt to fathom the nature of the patient's problem is well rewarded by the rational guidelines which can then be drawn to indicate how the physical examination should be carried out, i.e. will it need to be searching, extended and even vigorous or kept to a minimum, and carried out with a few selected tests and palpation?

The physical examination

In a book such as this, which deals with a variety of types of pain arising from different causes, it is not appropriate to recommend a detailed specific format for the physical examination. Commonly, but by no means exclusively, where pain is a prime concern, it is a part of the musculoskeletal system which is at fault and requires a detailed physical examination. Aspects of this examination are discussed in Chapter 17.

Whatever form the physical examination takes, it must always start with a detailed **observation** of the patient. In particular, with regard to pain, protective or antalgic postures, willingness to move, facial expressions and the position in which the patient prefers to be in an attempt to gain relief must all be carefully noted. Next, a comprehensive and systematic **testing** of appropriate movements and structures should seek to identify abnormalities, particularly with regard to the precise behaviour of the symptoms complained of in relation to particular active and passive movements or actions. The most succinct graphical recording and discussion of these relationships is that of the so-called 'movement diagrams' (Maitland, 1986). These movement diagrams demonstrate, by a clear and simple method, the way in which the three factors being explored – pain (local and referred), muscle spasm and inert tissue resistance – are interrelated in any given movement examined passively.

The final section of the physical examination, **palpation**, seeks to identify various tissue abnormalities, such as undue tissue tenderness, soft tissue thickening, bony abnormalities and generalized or discrete muscle spasm, as well as attempting to reproduce the patient's symptoms. In this last instance, the reproduction of the patient's pain or other symptoms is only attempted **if the severity, irritability and nature** allows. In most instances it does and the information gathered from skilful palpation is invaluable, forming, in many cases, the most informative part of the whole examination.

Where the examination of a painful joint condition is being carried out, an assessment of the characteristics of the various accessory movements of that joint forms a very significant part of the palpation section.

Response to treatment

During a course of treatment for a painful condition it is firstly more relevant to ask the patient 'How have you been?' than to inquire 'How are you?' The response of the patient's symptoms to the treatment and alterations in their signs shown on testing are the factors by which progress is assessed and upon which the next treatment is planned. While there is frequently a degree of immediate response, and this may be great or small, it is the behaviour of the symptoms between treatments which is the main factor we seek to influence. The physiotherapist needs to ask the patient three things at the start of reassessment:

'How were you in the few hours following treatment?'
'How have your symptoms been since the treatment and up to now?'
'How are your symptoms now?'

Treatment may result in the patient being:

'Better'.
'The same'.
'Worse'.

It is essential, of course, before further procedures are carried out that this is clarified for all the patient's symptoms. In other words, if the response to the question 'How have you been?' is 'Better', then what precisely has been better – all the symptoms or just some of them? Better than when or what?

In what way are the symptoms better? Are they:

Less severe?
Less irritable (i.e. taking more to provoke, and settling more quickly)?
Less widespread?
Less disturbing at night?
Starting later in the day?
Lasting a shorter period?
Enabling the patient to do more?
Requiring fewer analgesics?
Occurring less often over a period of 1 week (e.g. headache)?

In addition, the patient's **attitude** to his pain may change for the better. For example, he may be no longer terrified that the pain referred from his thoracic spine into his chest is from his heart (assuming that the patient was sent for a referred chest pain, which has mimicked a visceral problem, the latter having been excluded by his doctor).

If the patient reports that his symptoms are the **same**, then the main aspects of his subjective complaints must be repeated to refresh the memory and determine that his symptoms really *are* un-changed. Often small aspects of the patient's condition change (for better or worse) without them really being aware of it and with careful, though not laborious, questioning they will realize that something has in fact altered. If unchanged, then time should not be wasted repeating ineffectual treatment, but clearly the dosage and particular technique of administering a certain modality must be explored before it is changed entirely for something else.

A report by the patient that the symptoms have been **worse** since the last treatment must be explored carefully; they may be worse for a number of reasons. Assuming that the treatment chosen and the way it was carried out were suitable, two possibilities need to be considered:

1. The patient felt much better and so did something he should not have done and aggravated his condition.
2. The condition happens to be worse because its nature is such that there are good days and bad days and this happens to be a bad day (hence one reason to carefully clarify the behaviour of the symptoms over 24 h immediately after treatment).

The reason, whatever it is, can only be ascertained by careful questioning. It is in clarifying with the patient what aggravates and what eases his pain, and in explaining why that *prophylaxis* begins.

During the ongoing process of careful questioning, and response to the patient's questions, a subtle process of education is under way in which the patient comes to understand his symptoms more clearly. He responds by observing the behaviour of his symptoms and in doing so he is able to be more objective about them. This in turn is used by the physiotherapist who is all the while attempting to make the patient's observations of his symptoms more objective.

If the patient reports that the symptoms are worse since last time, then the current treatment session will aim to bring the symptoms and signs back to the situation existing at the start of the last treatment session. If the treatment itself seems to have aggravated the symptoms in some way, the situation can usually be rectified by altering the 'dosage' of treatment or modifying or changing the technique.

It is easy to see from the whole process briefly described here how the important role of the physiotherapist in education and prevention flows logically from their skills as communicators.

References

Davies, P.M. (1985) *Steps to Follow*, section 12.2 the painful shoulder. Springer-Verlag, Berlin

Grieve, G.P. (1975). Manipulation. *Physiotherapy*, 61(1), 11–18

Maitland, G.D. (1986) *Vertebral Manipulation*, Butterworths, London

4 The psychology and sociology of pain

SALLY FRENCH

Pain is subjective, individual and modified by degrees of attention, emotional state and the conditioning influences of past experience.

Livingstone (1943)

The intensity of the pain we experience and the way we respond to it are not merely a function of the degree of physical damage incurred. Weinman (1981) believes that 'Whatever the biological parameters of the symptoms they alone may be insufficient to explain the patient's response', and Burdette and Gale (1988) believe that pain complaint is not satisfactorily understood by reference to physical factors alone. There are individual differences in our perception of pain and the way we respond to it. Engel (1950) refers to this distinction as 'private pain' and 'public pain', and Helman (1984) describes our response to pain as 'pain behaviour'. Philips (1988) points out that the association between pain experience and pain behaviour is weak; it is possible to be in considerable pain but to hide this from others, or conversely to complain a great deal even though pain is minimal. The intensity of pain is not necessarily strongly associated with the degree of suffering either; people with minimal pain who do not know the cause of it may suffer more than those in severe pain who understand its meaning.

It would obviously be very helpful if physiotherapists could distinguish pain intensity from pain complaint in their patients, but in practice this is difficult if not impossible to achieve with any degree of accuracy. Pain is a personal and subjective experience and our knowledge of another's suffering is inevitably based on the ways in which that person responds and our own perception of this, which in turn will be influenced by the social situation. McCaffrey (1983) believes that pain is, 'whatever the patient says it is and exists wherever he says it does'.

Psychological and sociological aspects of pain are often regarded as fringe factors, merely influencing and modifying the 'real' physiological pain. The psychological and social aspects are, however, central to the experience of pain and the behaviour associated with it, as recognized by Melzack and Wall (1988) in their formulation of the pain gate theory. Edwards (1984) distinguishes 'bodily' pain from 'spiritual' pain believing that the latter has been seriously neglected in medical practice.

Factors influencing pain perception and pain behaviour

Personality

Research regarding the association between personality traits and pain experience and behaviour is inconsistent in both laboratory and natural settings. It has frequently been found, however, that extroverts express pain more freely than introverts even though they appear to be less sensitive to painful stimuli. Griffiths (1980) suggests that this may be because of their greater readiness to accept the social disapproval that is likely to be met in British society when emotions are openly displayed. Petrie (1967) found pain tolerance to increase with extroversion, and Eysenck (1961) found that during labour and childbirth introverts felt pain sooner and more intensely than extroverts, yet complained less. They also tended to remember the pain more vividly afterwards. Barsky and Klerman (1983) found considerable individual differences in the degree of attention people pay to normal bodily sensations which may have implications regarding the experience of pain.

The Social Context

The social context in which the injury occurs or in which the pain is felt can greatly influence the individual's experience of it and response to it. During the Second World War Beecher (1959) observed the behaviour of soldiers severely injured in battle. The majority said they were in no pain or very little pain with only one in three complaining enough to warrant the administration of morphine. However, they complained as much as anyone else over routine medical procedures. Beecher (1959) also observed civilians with similar injuries; the majority complained of severe pain, with most wanting morphine. He explained this in terms of the social context; the soldiers were thankful or even euphoric at still being alive whereas for the civilians the injury was a very depressing and disruptive event. It is also likely that the military role demands greater stoicism than the civilian role.

In a similar way, the pain resulting from injuries sustained in a road traffic accident may well be more severe than the pain following elective surgery, even if the physical injury resulting from the accident is less. In the case of elective surgery the patient will have had the opportunity to prepare himself for the event, he can look forward to an improved state of health and will probably be thankful that the operation is over; whereas the victim of the road traffic accident has experienced a sudden, very disturbing and negative event.

If a person's attention is fully occupied she may not feel any pain despite considerable injury, as Weinman (1981) explains, 'attention in one sensory source can reduce or abolish awareness of another source'. This can occur in the case of sportsmen and sportswomen who continue to play despite considerable injury. Similarly, Rachman and Philips (1978) note that a standard injection which is given following childbirth to aid the expulsion of the placenta is rarely felt. Masochists, on the other hand, tend to label as enjoyable what others would regard as painful, though this too is dependent on the social setting. Another example of how the social context affects pain perception and response is the tolerance people demonstrate towards injuries inflicted as part of various rituals and ceremonies – Melzack and Wall (1988), Helman (1984), Mathews and Steptoe (1988). Huxley (1952) notes that some people who were burned at the stake appeared to experience ecstasy rather than pain.

Many practitioners, for example Peck (1982), encourage people with chronic symptoms to practise focusing their attention away from the pain and to participate in enjoyable activities, as a way of relieving it. Wynn Parry (1980) reports that people suffering pain following brachial plexus injuries find the most effective way of reducing it is to absorb themselves in their work.

Culture

People seem to have a uniform sensory threshold. Sternbach and Tursky (1965) measured sensory threshold, using electric shock as the stimulus, in American women from four ethnic groups; Italian, Jewish, Irish and Old American. There was no difference in when they first reported feeling the sensation. According to Zborowski (1969), however, cultural background does have an effect on pain perception, that is, when people first report feeling pain. Hardy et al. (1952) found that radiant heat, described by Jewish and Italian people as painful, was described as merely warm by Northern Europeans. Zborowski (1952) found that Old Americans had an accepting, stoical attitude towards pain, tending to withdraw when it became intense and preferring to be alone. Conversely Jewish and Italian people were inclined to complain openly and seek support. The underlying attitudes of the latter two groups were, however, different. The Jewish people were most concerned about the cause and the meaning of the pain, whereas the Italian people were concerned about receiving immediate relief. Zola (1966) found attitudinal differences towards symptoms; Italian people were most concerned if the symptoms interfered with their social lives whereas Irish and Anglo-Saxon people were most concerned if they interfered with work.

Interesting though these findings are, care must be taken when interpreting them and acting upon them as there is a danger of unfairly stereotyping people according to their cultural or ethnic origins. It should be remembered that there is more variability within cultural groups than between them. Zborowski (1952) points out that any differences there are tend to disappear over time in cosmopolitan societies and that other factors, such as educational background and occupation, may have an affect on pain behaviour. Pilowski and Spence (1977) suggest that any differences which exist among cultural groups, in regard to their experience and expression of pain, may be due to their immigrant status and the difficulties they experience in adapting to the majority culture which may be hostile to their needs. Thus the immediate social situation may influence cultural patterns. In addition, Wolff and Langley (1977) warn of the poor research design of many of these studies.

Attitudes and behaviour of health professionals

Health practitioners, including physiotherapists, will have their own notions of appropriate pain behaviour, based on personal and occupational factors. In an American study Rosengren and DeVault (1976) describe how, in an obstetric hospital, the only place where pain was legitimated, sanctioned and defined as such, was in the delivery room. The expression of pain was deemed inappropriate in any other area, including the labour room. Thus professionals have considerable power to define and manage pain according to their own attitudes and beliefs, although considerable negotiation between patients and professionals occurs. Grieve (1987) warns us not to impose our own stereotypes on patients. It is all too easy to dismiss or become impatient with those who do not fit the stoical British ideal. Helman (1984) states:

> People will receive maximum attention and sympathy if their pain behaviour matches the society's view of how people should draw attention to their suffering – whether by an extravagant display of emotion or a quiet change of behaviour.

Hough (1987) believes that, 'western culture has a tendency to view the open expression of emotion with some distaste' and is of the opinion that this has resulted in the overuse of drugs in hospitals. Davitz and Davitz (1981) found that nurses from various cultural groups viewed their patients' pain differently and were also influenced by such factors as the patient's social class, how responsible he was judged to be for his condition and the ease or difficulty of diagnosis. Fagerhaugh and Strauss (1977) found that physiotherapists and nurses tend to assess the severity of patients' low back pain by interpreting their behaviour rather than believing what they say. Saxey (1986) warns that we should not judge how much pain someone is in by her behaviour alone as many people learn to adapt to pain and live relatively normal lives even though it is quite severe. Price (1990) believes that the monitoring of pain should be given as much importance as the monitoring of physiological measures.

Graffam (1979) is of the opinion that patients suffer postoperative pain unnecessarily and that this is partly because nurses are unjustifiably anxious about the possibility of drug addiction. Williams (1987) found the same tendency among paediatric nurses and believes that this results in children experiencing unnecessary pain after surgery. Price (1990) makes the point that children tend to be given less analgesia than adults following similar surgical procedures and believes that the whole issue of children's pain is a neglected area. Walsh and Ford (1989) are of the opinion that nurses do not believe that complete pain control is possible after surgery and Saxey (1986) asks, 'Are we guilty of thinking that the patient has to somehow "earn" the injection by suffering pain?'

Baer et al. (1970), Lenburg et al. (1970) and Johnston et al. (1987) found considerable differences in the judgements of various professional groups regarding the degree of pain experienced by real and hypothetical patients. Nurses tend to rate patients' pain higher than either physiotherapists or doctors. Pitts and Healy (1989) found that physiotherapists infer less pain in hypothetical patients than nurses but more pain than doctors. Their ratings were, however, nearer to those of the doctors. These results could not be explained in terms of gender although female doctors did infer more pain than male doctors.

It is all too easy for patients to become negatively stereotyped, making it all the more difficult for them to convince others of the pain they are experiencing. Peck (1982) points out that patients may end up being blamed for their pain both by medical staff and their families and are 'left with the burden of having to prove their innocence'. Hasler (1985) and Hargreaves (1987) emphasize the importance of good communication skills, both verbal and non-verbal, in clinical practice. It should be appreciated, however, that the organization of medical practice – lack of time, lack of autonomy, work schedules and so on – pose considerable restraints on medical personnel, including physiotherapists, making it difficult for them to respond adequately to patients whose symptoms or behaviour are atypical.

Past experience

As well as the influence of wider cultural factors on pain perception and response, Griffiths (1980) points out that the individual's unique past history is also of considerable importance. Some families focus great attention on very minor injuries whereas others tend to minimize or ignore quite serious ones. We thus learn how to interpret pain and respond to it by observing others. There are also differences in the degree and manner to which children are encouraged or discouraged from openly responding to pain. These early experiences may influence our sensitivity to potentially painful stimuli and our pain behaviour throughout life. As with other areas of social life we are guided in our interpretations and influenced in our behaviour by the interpretations and behaviour of others. Festinger (1954) described this process as one of 'social comparison'; Oster (1972) and Violon and Gilurgea (1984) found that family members respond to pain similarly. Past experience of medical encounters is also important. It is likely that a person who has had a painful experience on one occasion, at the dentist for example, will feel pessimistic and anxious when he returns for further treatment, if indeed he ever does. Unsuccessful treatments can lead to lack of trust in the clinician and a loss of confidence that a new treatment will help. Kent (1985) found that highly anxious dental patients remembered pain as more severe than the actual experience of it.

Understanding how personality, the social context, professional attitudes and cultural and family background affect pain perception and behaviour, may help to foster empathy and tolerance and improve communication between physiotherapists and their patients. Kotarba (1983) believes that a disease orientated model is not a suitable perspective for the management of chronic pain.

State of Mind

People who are anxious are more sensitive to pain than calm people. Kent (1986) found that anxious patients complain more of pain than others and Hill et al. (1952a, 1952b), demonstrated that the intensity of pain decreases if anxiety is reduced by giving subjects control over the situation. They also found that morphine only reduces pain if anxiety is high. The anticipation of pain, and uncertainty regarding its cause, tend to raise anxiety which in turn increases its perceived intensity. Thus a vicious circle may operate. Bond (1984) states that 'pain will be greater for patients who have a tendency to become anxious because pain causes anxiety and, in its turn, anxiety heightens pain'.

Reynolds (1978) reports that patients like to be given information about their conditions. Egbert et al. (1964) gave an experimental group of patients information regarding postoperative pain. When compared with the control group they required significantly less analgesia after the surgery, were judged to be in a better physical and psychological state and, on average, were discharged nearly 3 days earlier. Janis (1971) reported a reduction in postoperative pain if patients were given information before their surgery. Langer et al. (1975) and Melzack and Wall (1988) point out, however, that knowledge alone may increase anxiety because of the expectation of pain it creates. They suggest that patients must be provided with skills to cope both with their anxiety and with their pain.

If the person understands what is causing her pain, for example that chest pain is the result of indigestion rather than heart disease, she is less likely to be anxious about it. Similarly pain is better tolerated, and probably perceived as less intense, if the person believes it is temporary or 'normal'. Examples of 'normal' pain is that caused by exercise, childbirth or menstruation. What is and what is not regarded as a 'normal' symptom, however, varies considerably among different individuals and groups (Calnan, 1987).

Hall and Stride (1954) found that the appearance of the word 'pain' in a list of instructions increased the subjects perception of pain, possibly by raising their level of anxiety. The subjects reported a sensation as painful which was not regarded as such when the word was absent from the instructions. This gives rise to a contradiction of significance to physiotherapists; on the one hand it seems that focusing attention on pain – giving information about it preoperatively, informing people that they are in control of how much pain they receive and so on – decreases their anxiety and perception of pain but, on the other hand, it seems that focusing attention on pain may raise levels of anxiety and pain perception.

Anxiety may be relieved and pain reduced by giving patients control, for example allowing them to terminate a procedure at any time if it becomes uncomfortable. Wright (1987) and Flint (1988) point out that familiarity reduces anxiety, so it is important, if at all possible, that the patient be treated by the same physiotherapist on each visit. Williams (1987) believes that children should be made familiar with the hospital they are to attend beforehand and that familiarity with hospitals should be part of their general education. She is also in favour of unlimited visiting of hospitalized children. Others, for example Ainsworth (1989) and McKee (1989), believe that allowing animals in the ward, including patients' own pets, can reduce their anxieties and promote recovery.

Anxiety can be reduced by giving patients information, for example explaining the nature of their illness or giving details of the treatment. Many studies indicate that patients are dissatisfied with the degree of information they receive (McGhee, 1961; Cartwright, 1964; Kincey *et al.*, 1975; Hart, 1985; Ley, 1988) and that giving information is beneficial. Hayward (1975) found that informed patients needed less analgesia and Johnson et al. (1978) found that exercise instruction given preoperatively reduced postoperative pain. The benefit of giving information to individual patients, however, is difficult to ascertain as a sizable minority prefer not to know and people differ regarding the depth of information they want. Weinman (1981) believes that some patients' pain tolerance may well be lowered if information is forced upon them or if they are not helped to cope with it. In addition, great sensitivity and skill are required when imparting sad or unpleasant news.

Every effort should be made to keep unpleasant procedures to a minimum. Creagh (1986) found that children may deny pain if analgesia is to be given by injection. Sparshott (1989) believes that pain in newborn babies should be taken very seriously so as to prevent psychologial harm. She advocates minimal medical procedures, low noise and lighting levels, making the baby feel secure by ensuring that he is fully supported and by playing tape recordings of familiar voices which he may have heard when in the womb. Williams (1987) emphasizes the importance of play for acting out children's anxieties and for explaining and preparing them for coming events.

Sensitivity to pain is also increased if the person is depressed. This is due to the unpleasant nature of pain, the tendency for it to impose inactivity on the individual, thus reducing enjoyment and leading to a focusing of attention upon it, and the feeling of loss of control. Peck (1982) points out that guilt, despondency and self-criticism frequently accompany depression, only serving to intensify it. In such a situation the person in pain will tend to perceive it as more intense that she would do otherwise, thus a vicious circle may develop.

Mathews and Steptoe (1988) explain that pain can be secondary to depression and can be relieved by anti-depressant drugs. They state that emotion and pain 'appear to be inextricably entangled'. Davison and Neale (1978) point out that depression and anxiety are frequently linked. There is a great danger, however, in assuming that pain is secondary to depression and anxiety. Melzack and Wall (1988) warn that:

'The patients with the thick hospital charts are all too often prey to the physician's innuendoes that they are neurotic and that their neuroses are the cause of the pain . . . All too often the diagnosis of neurosis as the cause of pain hides our ignorance of many aspects of pain mechanisms.'

Depression may be relieved and pain reduced both by empathizing with the patient and involving him in the treatment. People commonly feel in better spirits after engaging in physical activity. Although the mechanism behind this altered mood is not fully understood, exercise is thought to be a way of releasing tension as well as improving self-esteem. The trip in the ambulance and the visit to the physiotherapy department may, in themselves, be sufficient to reduce pain by redirecting the patient's attention and improving his morale by providing enjoyable companionship. Although physiotherapists may despair of patients who attend 'for social reasons', in reality all patient/therapist encounters are social events and as such have the potential to be highly therapeutic.

There is a danger, however, that repeated contact with health professionals and the constant search for a medical cure may be detrimental to the person with chronic pain. Although many people expect health professionals to cure or alleviate their symptoms, repeated contact with them may actually increase pain by focusing the person's attention upon it, as well as encouraging the idea that a medical cure is possible when this may not be so. Furthermore, Peck (1982) believes that it may sap the person's energy, which could be better used to develop realistic coping strategies.

Avoidance behaviour and cognitive processes

The avoidance of physical activity is perfectly rational while pain is acute and while tissues are healing, but this pattern of behaviour sometimes persists and intensifies in those with chronic pain. Philips (1987) believes that this decreases patients' sense of control over the pain and increases their expectations that exposure to activity will create more pain. Over time, the avoidance behaviour intensifies.

Avoidance does not merely concern physical activities but also involves social interaction, hobbies and work. Philips and Jahanshahi (1986) studied people suffering from headaches and found that avoidance was the most common behaviour reported, in particular social withdrawal. There is little evidence that avoidance behaviour reduces chronic pain; over time, avoidance behaviour may become worse even though the symptoms remain static or improve. Philips (1987) believes that this behaviour is a consequence of the patient's beliefs and memories, which are often distorted, rather than a consequence of the pain itself and that these beliefs and memories are in turn reinforced by the avoidance behaviour.

Philips (1987) believes that this behavioural response is of great significance to the therapist and the patient. The patient believes she is controlling her pain by the avoidance behaviour and that the behaviour is a consequence of her pain. The therapist, on the other hand, may view the behaviour as an index of disability and an indication that the patient has developed inadequate and inappropriate coping strategies. Conversely the therapist, for fear that the patient's conditions might recur, may encourage avoidance behaviour by emphasizing the need to avoid certain activities and to take care.

Psychological treatment strategies

Physiotherapists are in a position to incorporate psychological measures into their treatment programmes. Various ways in which this can be achieved have already been discussed, for example, reducing anxiety and depression by giving the patient information and control. It is a mistake to think that the psychological treatment of pain is only indicated if the patient is coping inadequately or if the cause of the pain cannot be found. Pain is as much a psychological as a physiological phenomenon and, therefore, psychological strategies are likely to help the patient control and cope with her pain in many instances.

Physiotherapists may use psychological strategies to help their patients, either as the sole treatment technique, or by incorporating them into a programme of physical treatment. The physiotherapist must recognize when the patient needs to be

referred to a psychiatrist or clinical psychologist; he may well work alongside these professionals in some settings, for example in pain clinics. There is considerable overlap between the techniques of various health professionals and alternative practitioners in the management of pain. Some of these techniques will now be discussed.

The placebo effect

Spiro (1986) defines the placebo as, 'a substance or a procedure that is administered with suggestions that it will modify a symptom or sensation, but which, unknown to the recipient, has no specific pharmacological impact on the reaction in question'.

All treatments given by physiotherapists and others can be assumed to contain some placebo element. Weinman (1981) claims that even with pain associated with serious disease, more than one-third of patients report relief following treatment with a placebo. Melzack and Wall (1988) point out that the type of pain is important, for example they claim that 52% of headache sufferers are helped by placebos. Physiological changes such as slowing of the pulse rate are frequently observed (Griffiths, 1980). Beecher (1959) found that severe postoperative pain could be relieved in 35% of patients by the administration of a placebo whereas morphine relieved pain in about 75% of cases.

The placebo response varies greatly from one individual to the next and in the same individual from time to time and according to circumstances. Most people are susceptible to some degree. As belief in the treatment or the person administering it is central to the placebo response, the effectiveness of specific placebos will be culturally and temporally limited. Thus in our culture at the present time, taking placebos in the guise of drugs is likely to be effective.

It is likely that the placebo effect is enhanced or even produced by the degree of understanding, empathy and enthusiasm of the clinician prescribing or dispensing it, as well as his own belief in it. Balint (1964) believes that the clinician can be a more powerful therapeutic agent than the treatment he administers and Morgan (1982) states that it is the social relationship between doctor and patient that engenders this powerful therapeutic effect. Benson and McCallie (1979) report a 70–90% success rate in trials conducted by enthusiasts which reduced to 30–40%, the average placebo response, when conducted by sceptics. Novel treatments tend to be more effective than established ones, probably because of the enhanced enthusiasm of clinicians, thus new treatments have the power to render old ones less effective. Despite the therapeutic power that clinicians possess, Shapiro (1960) believes that they prefer to view their success as due to less personal factors. Spiro (1986) states:

> The idea that the physician brings little benefit to his patients and his patient's disease except as he brings him pills and procedures has been growing since modern medicine began to become scientific and focus on disease rather than on the patient.

The setting in which the treatment is given also has an effect. Uniforms, stethoscopes, the smell of disinfection and impressive-looking equipment may all act as powerful symbols of healing which can foster belief, according to the culture and expectations of the patient. Investigations of treatment carried out in the laboratory can show very different results from those conducted in the clinical setting. Frank (1975) emphasizes how operating theatres foster belief in the efficacy of surgery. He explains that 'These rooms contain spectacular machines that bleep and gurgle and flash lights, or emit immensely powerful but invisible rays, thereby impressively evoking the healing powers of science.' Brody (1980) refers to the setting as the 'healing context'. Many of the machines used by physiotherapists, for example the interferential machine, look impressive and mysterious and one wonders how important this is in producing their therapeutic effects.

Helman (1984) refers to the 'total drug effect' as being dependent on the following four factors:

1. The attributes of the drug itself.
2. The attributes of the person dispensing the drug.
3. The attributes of the person receiving the drug.
4. The setting in which the drug is administered.

These four factors apply equally to the success of many other types of treatment.

The placebo has proved itself to be an extremely powerful tool in the treatment of patients with a very wide range of conditions, leading Kaunitz (1985) to believe that:

> It is his [the clinician's] responsibility to influence to the best of his ability the patient's psychological mechanisms and external environment so that nature's forces can bring to the fore the individual's underlying strength.

Relaxation

Relaxation may be used to reduce stress, anxiety and depression. Melzack and Wall (1988) state that relaxation reduces activity in the sympathetic and motor nervous systems. The mechanisms of pain reduction may be physiological, for example when the patient succeeds in relaxing tense muscles, or cognitive, for example when the patient manages to direct his attention away from the pain. There is considerable evidence that relaxation training brings about pain reduction (Flaberty and Fitzpatrick, 1978; Blanchard et al., 1987; Hellsing and Linton, 1989). Relaxation techniques have been traditionally used by physiotherapists, particularly in relation to ante-natal education and respiratory disease. A similar approach is likely to be helpful in the management of pain.

Biofeedback

This technique is used if it is thought that the patient's pain is the result of physiological processes such as tense muscles. By giving the patient feedback concerning his physiological state he may learn to control it. Roberts (1974) found that 80% of patients with low back pain improved with biofeedback. Melzack and Perry (1975), however, found no evidence that biofeedback is any more effective than the placebo for the relief of pain. Chapman (1986) reviewed the literature and found no advantage for biofeedback combined with relaxation than relaxation alone. Smith (1987), however, found that the two techniques in combination were more successful than either technique in isolation for reducing headache.

Hypnosis

Hypnotic suggestion has been used for pain relief in many branches of medicine including dentistry, terminal care and obstetrics (Hilgard and Hilgard, 1975). Physiotherapists with some additional training may use hypnosis to reduce pain. The patient is put in a trance-like state where she is highly suggestible and deeply relaxed. In this state, various ideas can be given to her regarding her pain, for example that it is not severe or that it will no longer concern her. Melzack and Wall (1988) point out that a small proportion of people can undergo surgery while under hypnosis and with many others pain relieving measures, such as drugs, can be reduced when hypnosis is part of the treatment. Melzack and Perry (1980) found that 22% of people who had chronic pain improved with hypnotic treatment compared with 14% who received a placebo. They found that when hypnosis was combined with biofeedback the improvement was considerably greater than when hypnosis alone was given.

Counselling

There are many counselling courses available to physiotherapists and a large variety of counselling techniques which can be learned.

In non-directive counselling the therapist creates a warm and empathic relationship and environment whereby the patient can talk and work through his own problems and difficulties with encouragement but little interruption or direction from the therapist. In this way the person in pain may come to the conclusion that the best way to cope is to try to ignore it, or that his pain is being maintained by important secondary gains.

In cognitive counselling the therapist takes a more active role, concentrating on the patient's thoughts and feelings in relation to her pain and attempting to change them. For example, the patient may be continually telling herself that she cannot cope because of the pain or that she is unattractive to others because of it. These negative messages may be causing anxiety and depression, making the pain worse. It is the task of the therapist to help the patient realize that she is responsible for her own thoughts and feelings and to help her develop a more positive outlook by devising a suitable treatment programme for her to work through.

Behaviour modification

This technique is focused on changing pain behaviour rather than pain perception. It is assumed that the person's pain brings about various rewards which he wants to maintain, albeit subconsciously. Whether the patient feels less pain following this treatment is open to question. Behaviour modification is a technique whereby behaviour which is approved of is rewarded while behaviour which is disapproved of is ignored. In this way behaviour is 'shaped'. It may be the case, for example, that the patient has become very isolated because he talks of nothing but his pain, so to reduce this behaviour he will be rewarded when talking about other matters and ignored when his pain is mentioned. The patient may be fully aware of the aims and objectives of the behaviour modification programme and may even have helped to structure it, conversely it may be covert. Crabbe (1989) claims a 90% success rate and cites evidence from abroad that maintenance of improvement is of the order of 50%. How it compares with other methods or the placebo, however, is still uncertain.

There are important ethical issues of which the physiotherapist should be aware when considering the use of behaviour modification programmes or participating in them, especially if they are covert.

Group therapy

According to the patient's temperament, group therapy may have a very positive psychological effect, with the result that pain is reduced or managed more effectively. Human beings are social animals and may be greatly encouraged by working with other people who are experiencing similar difficulties. By seeing others, a person's own suffering may be put into perspective and other group members may act as models for him to follow. Some people are motivated by competition which the group experience may provide, or may simply feel less anxious and depressed by virtue of enjoyable companionship. Thus the dynamics of the group, for example in back schools or group hydrotherapy, may have important effects in reducing the person's pain or helping him cope with it.

A combined behaviour modification and group therapy programme has been developed by Williams (1989) for patients with chronic pain who are defined as displaying abnormal pain behaviour and who have not been helped by traditional medical or physiotherapy treatments. Patients take part in a fitness programme in a busy physiotherapy gymnasium. All exercises are directed away from their area of pain. Activity, cheerfulness and effort are praised whereas any demonstration of pain behaviour believed to be abnormal is ignored. Williams claims that most of these carefully selected patients show marked improvement within 3 weeks. She believes that concentrating on physical activity is particularly helpful as most patients strongly resent the suggestion that their pain is 'all in the mind'. No psychotherapy or counselling is given and professionals such as clinical psychologists are not involved. Thus the patient's view of the physiotherapist as someone who is concerned with his physical condition seems to help the programme work. This raises an important ethical issue, for clearly the patients are not fully aware of the purpose behind the treatment.

Williams (1989) believes that patients awaiting compensation claims are particularly likely to display abnormal pain behaviour. However, Mendelson (1984) and Melzack et al. (1985) found that patients waiting for compensation did not differ psychologically from other patients and Melzack and Wall (1988) point out that pain tends to persist after compensation claims are settled. They warn of the danger of giving people inappropriate labels.

Group dynamics can work in a negative as well as a positive direction. For example, members may feel obliged to conform to the group norm or some members may succeed in gaining the attention of the physiotherapist while others are ignored. Not everyone feels happy or confident in a group, or enjoys being treated with other people. Their wishes should be respected, any attempt to force them into a group situation is likely to be counterproductive.

Music

Music brings about physiological and psychological effects and may serve to direct the patient's attention away from his pain. Rozzano and Locsin (1981) found that music of the patient's own choosing aided recovery following surgery and Melzack and Wall (1988) make the point that music and rhythmic drumming often accompany healing ceremonies and probably have a hypnotic effect. Physiotherapists do use music, mostly to stimulate people when exercising in groups, but perhaps the use of music could be extended to help bring about pain relief.

Improving confidence and morale

It is sometimes the case that people reduce their activities, not so much because of the physical limitations of their illness, but because of fear and lack of confidence in their abilities. The person who has recovered from a myocardial infarction, for example, may be afraid to resume even mild physical activity for fear that his chest pain will return. Similarly the person with osteoarthritis may be suffering more from the fear of pain than the pain itself.

Physiotherapists often devise programmes for such people designed to increase their exercise tolerance and reduce their pain by means of carefully graded exercises, along with health education and other treatments when appropriate. Although the programme is usually devised to bring about physiological improvement it is likely that in many cases the improvements seen are equally or more concerned with psychological change. The person who has had a myocardial infarction, for example, will realize that the physiotherapist is not alarmed at the prospect of him walking several miles a day, going back to work or riding his bicycle. Thus over a period of time patients undergoing programmes such as these may become confident in their ability to cope with their condition and may eventually define themselves as well rather than ill.

Other techniques

There are many other psychological methods which can be used to help the person in pain. These are not traditionally part of the physiotherapist's work but with the blurring of role boundaries and the growing availability of training, some physiotherapists may become involved. These techniques include psychoanalysis, family therapy, assertiveness training, visual imagery, acupuncture, aromatherapy, homoeopathy, reflexology, meditation, various types of massage, diets and faith healing. The precise ways in which each of these therapies work and whether they are purely placebic is a matter of dispute. Much the same can be said, of course, of many of the more orthodox treatments which have been discussed. Many researchers, including Melzack and Wall (1988), have found that combining several methods for the relief of pain leads to greater success than relying on just one. This has important implications for the work of physiotherapists; it is probably unwise to become too devoted to any one technique.

Conclusion

There is no doubt that social and psychological strategies can be used either to reduce the patient's pain or to help him or her cope with it. Such strategies can be combined with each other or with the more familiar physical approaches of physiotherapy practice. To separate psychological from physical treatment is artificial; all of our treatments affect the patient psychologically, however technical they may seem. It is therefore vitally important that physiotherapists understand the nature of pain in all its complexity and treat the patient with this in mind. As Wall (1982) reminds us, 'the simplest of pains is not simple'.

References

Ainsworth, H. (1989) And the guinea-pig came too. *Nursing Times*, **85** (39), 54–6

Baer, E., Davitz, L.S. and Lieb, R. (1970) Inferences of pain and psychological distress in relation to verbal and non-verbal communication. *Nursing Res.*, **19**, 388–92

Balint, M. (1964) *The Doctor, His Patient and the Illness*, Pitman, London

Barsky, A.J. and Klerman, J.L. (1983) Overview: hypocondriasis, bodily complaints and somatic style. *Am. J. Psychiat.*, **140** (3), 273–83

Beecher, H.K. (1959) *Measurement of Subjective Responses*, Oxford University Press, Oxford

Benson, H. and McCallie, D.P. (1979) Angina pectoris and the placebo effect. *N. Eng. J. Med.*, **300**, 424–29.

Blanchard, E.B., Applebaum, K.A., Guarnieri, P. *et al.* (1987) Five year prospective follow-up on the treatment of chronic headache with biofeedback and/or relaxation. *Headache*, **27** (10), 580–3

Bond, M.R. (1984) *Pain: Its Nature, Analysis and Treatment*, 2nd edn, Churchill Livingstone, London

Brody, H. (1980) *Placebos and the Philosophy of Medicine*, University of Chicago Press, London

Burdette, B.H. and Gale, E.N. (1988) Pain as a learned response: a review of behavioral factors in chronic pain. *J. Am. Dent. Assoc.*, **116** (7), 881–5

Cartwright, A. (1964) *Human Relationships in Hospital Care*, Routledge and Kegan Paul, London

Calnan, M. (1987) *Health and Illness: the Lay Perspective*, Tavistock Publications, London

Chapman, S.L (1986) A review and clinical perspective on the use of EMG and thermal biofeedback for chronic headaches. *Pain*, **27**, 1–43

Crabbe, G. (1989) Crossing the pain threshold. *Nursing Times*, **85** (47), 16–17

Creagh, T. (1986) Just a little jab. *Nursing Times*, **82** 49–50

Davison, G.C. and Neale, J.M. (1978) *Abnormal Psychology*, John Wiley and Sons, New York

Davitz, L.J. and Davitz, J.R. (1981) *Nurses' Response to Patients' Suffering*, Springer, New York

Edwards, R.B. (1984) Pain and the ethics of pain management. *Soc. Sci. Med*, **18**, 515–23

Egbert, L., Battit, G., Welch, C. and Bartlett, M. (1964) Reduction of post-operative pain by encouragement and instruction of patients. N. Engl. J. Med., **270**, 825–7

Engel, G.L. (1950) 'Psychogenic' pain and the pain-prone patient. *Am. J. Med.*, **26**, 899–909

Eysenck, S.G.B. (1961) Cited in Rachman, S.L. and Philips, C. (1978) *Psychology and Medicine*, Penguin Books, Harmondsworth

Fagerhaugh, S.Y. and Stauss, A. (1977) *Politics of Pain Management: Staff–Patient Interaction*, Addison-Wesley, Wokingham

Festinger, L.A. (1954) Theory of social comparison processes, *Human Relations*, **7**, 117–40

Flaberty, G. and Fitzpatrick, J. (1978) Relaxation techniques to increase comfort levels of post-operative patients. *Nursing Res*, **27**, 352–5

Flint, C. (1988) Know your midwife. *Nursing Times*, **84** (38), 28–32

Frank, J.D. (1975) The faith that heals. *Johns Hopkins Med. J.*, **137**, 27–31

Graffam, S. (1979) Nurse response to patients in pain. *Nursing Leadership*, **2**, 23–5

Grieve, G.P. (1987) Psychological aspects of benign spinal pain. *Physiotherapy*, **73**(9), 499–501

Griffiths, D. (1980) *Psychology and Medicine*, Macmillan Press, London

Hall, K.R.L. and Stride, E. (1954) The varying response to pain in Psychiatric disorders: a study in abnormal psychology. *Br. J. Med. Psychol.*, **27**, 48–60

Hardy, J.D., Wolff, H.G. and Goodell, H. (1952) *Pain Sensations and Reactions*, Williams and Wilkins, New York

Hargreaves, S. (1987) The relevance of non-verbal skills in physiotherapy. *Physiotherapy*, **73** (12), 85–8

Hart, N. (1985) *The Sociology of Health and Medicine*, Causeway Press, Ormskirk

Hasler, J.C. (1985) Communication and relationships in general practice. *Physiotherapy*, **71** (10), 35–6

Hayward, J. (1975) *Information – A Prescription Against Pain*, Royal College of Nursing, London

Helman, C. (1984) *Culture, Health and Illness*, John Wright, Bristol

Hellsing, A. and Linton, S. (1989) Chronic headache treatment in an occupational setting: a pilot study. *Physiotherapy Practice*, **5** (1), 3–8

Hilgard, E.L. and Hilgard, J.R. (1975) *Hypnosis in the Relief of Pain*, Kaufmann, Los Altos, Ca

Hill, H.E., Kornetsky, C.H., Flanary, H.G. and Wikler, A. (1952a) Effects of anxiety and morphine on discrimination of intensities of painful stimuli. *J. Clin. Invest.*, **31**, 473–9

Hill, H.E., Kornetsky, C.H., Flanary, H.G. and Wikler, A. (1952b) Studies of anxiety associated with anticipation of pain. *Arch. Neurol. Psychiat.*, **67**, 612–7

Hough, A. (1987) Communication in health care. *Physiotherapy*, **73** (2), 56–9

Huxley, A. (1952) *The Devils of London*, Harper, London

Janis, I. (1971) *Stress and Frustration*, Harcourt Brace, New York

Johnson, J.E., Rice, V.H., Fuller, S.S. and Endress, P.M. (1978) Sensory information: instruction in a coping strategy and recovery from surgery. *Res. Nursing Hlth*, **1** (1), 4–17

Johnston, M., Bromley, I., Boothroyd-Brooks, M. *et al.* (1987) Behavioural assessment of physically disabled patients: agreement between rehabilitation therapists and nurses. *Int. J. Rehabil. Res.*, **10**(5), 205–13

Kaunitz, P. (1985) The favourable prognosis. *Conn. Med. J.*, **49**, 453

Kent, G. (1985) Memory of dental pain. *Pain*, **21**, 187–94

Kent, G. (1986) Effect of pre-appointment inquiries on dental patients post-appointment ratings of pain. *Br. J. Med. Psychol.*, **59**, 97–100

Kincey, J., Bradshaw, P. and Ley, P. (1975) Patients' satisfaction and reported acceptance of advice in general practice. *J. R. Coll. Gen. Pract.*, **25**, 558–62

Kotarba, J.A. (1983) *Chronic Pain: Its Social Dimensions*, Sage, Beverley Hills, Ca

Langer, E., Janis, I.L. and Wolfer, J.A. (1975) Reduction of psychological distress in surgical patients. *J. Exp. Soc. Psychol.*, **11**, 155–65

Lenburg, C.B., Glass, H.P. and Davitz, L.J. (1970) Inferences of pain and psychological distress in relation to the stage of illness and occupation of the perceiver. *Nursing Res.*, **19**, 392–8

Ley, P. (1988) *Communicating with Patients*, Croom Helm, London

Livingstone, W.K. (1943) *Pain Mechanism*, Macmillan, London

Mathews, A. and Steptoe, A. (1988) *Essential Psychology for Medical Practice*, Churchill Livingstone, London

McCaffrey, M. (1983) *Nursing the Patient in Pain*, 2nd edn, Harper and Row, London

McGhee, A. (1961) *The Patient's Attitude to Nursing Care*, E. and S. Livingstone, Edinburgh

McKee, E. (1989) Till death do us part. *Nursing Times*, **85** (39), 57–9

Melzack, R. and Perry, C. (1975) Self-regulation of pain: the use of alpha-feedback and hypnotic training on the control of chronic pain. *Exp. Neurol.*, **46**, 452–69

Melzack, R. and Perry, C. (1980) Psychological control

of pain, cited in Melzack, R. and Wall, P. (1988) *The Challenge of Pain*, Penguin Books, Harmondsworth

Melzack, R. and Wall, P. (1988) *The Challenge of Pain*, Penguin Books, Harmondsworth

Melzack, R., Katz, J. and Jeans, M.E. (1985) The role of compensation in chronic pain: analysis using a new method of scoring the McGill Pain Questionnaire. *Pain*, **23**, 101–12

Mendelson, G. (1984) Compensation pain complaints and psychological disturbance. *Pain*, **20**, 169–77

Morgan, M. (1982) The doctor–patient relationship. In *Sociology as Applied to Medicine* (eds D.H. Patrick, and G. Scambler), Bailliere Tindall, London

Oster, J. (1972) Recurrent abdominal pain, headache and limb pains in children and adolescents. *Pediatrics*, **50** (3), 429–36

Peck, C. (1982) *Controlling Chronic Pain*, Fontana, London

Petrie, A.A. (1967) *Individuality in Pain and Suffering*, University of Chicago Press, Chicago

Philips, H.C. (1987) Avoidance behaviour and its role in sustaining chronic pain. *Behav. Res. Ther.*, **25**, (4), 273–9

Philips, H.C. (1988) Changing chronic pain experience. *Pain*, **32**, 165–72

Philips, H.C. and Jahanshahi, M. (1986) The components of pain behaviour report. *Behav. Res. Ther.*, **24**, 9117–25

Pilowski, I. and Spence, N. (1977) Ethnicity and illness behaviour. *Psychol. Med.*, **7**, 447–52

Pitts, M. and Healy, S. (1989) Factors influencing the inferences of pain made by three health professions. *Physiother. Pract.*, **5** (2), 65–9

Price, S. (1990) Pain: its experience, assessment and management in children. *Nursing Times*, **86** (9), 942–5

Rachman, S.J. and Philips, C. (1978) *Psychology and Medicine*, Penguin Books, Harmondsworth

Reynolds, M. (1978) No news is bad news: patients' views about communication in hospital. *Br. Med. J.*, **1**, 1673–6

Roberts, A.H. (1974) Biofeedback techniques: their potential for the control of pain. *Minn. Med.*, **57**, 167–71

Rosengren, W.R. and DeVault, S. (1976) The sociology of time and space in an obstetrical hospital. In *Basic Readings in Medical Sociology* (eds D. Tuckett and J.M. Kaufert), Tavistock Publications, London

Rozzano, G.R.A.C. and Locsin, A.C. (1981) The effect of music on the pain of selected post-operative patients. *J. Adv. Nurs.*, **6**, 19–25

Saxey, S. (1986) Nursers' response to post-op pain. *Nursing Times*, **3**, 377–81

Smith, W.B. (1987) Biofeedback and relaxation training: the effect on headache and associated symptoms. *Headache*, **27** (9), 511–14

Sparshott, M. (1989) Minimising discomfort of sick newborns. *Nursing Times*, **85** (42), 39–42

Spiro, H.M. (1986) *Doctors, Patients and Placebos*, Vale University Press, London

Sternbach, R.A. and Tursky, B. (1965) Ethnic differences among housewives in psychophysical and skin potential responses to electric shock. *Psychophysiology*, **1**, 241–6

Violon, A. and Gilurgea, D. (1984) Familial models for chronic pain. *Pain*, **18**, 199–203

Wall, P. (1982) Introduction. In Peck C., *Controlling Chronic Pain*, Fontana, London

Walsh, M. and Ford, P. (1989) It can't hurt that much. *Nursing Times*, **85** (42), 35–8

Weinman, J. (1981) *An Outline of Psychology as Applied to Medicine*, John Wright, Bristol

Williams, J. (1987) Managing paediatric pain. *Nursing Times*, **83** (36), 36–9

Williams, J. (1989) Illness behaviour to wellness behaviour. *Physiotherapy*, **75** (1), 2–7

Wolff, B.B. and Langley, S. (1977) Cultural factors and the response to pain. In *Culture, Disease and Healing: Studies in Medical Anthropology* (ed. D. Landy), Macmillan, New York

Woods, M. (1989) Pain control and hypnosis. *Nursing Times*, **85** (7), 38–40

Wright, S. (1987) Patient-centred practice. *Nursing Times*, **83** (38), 24–7

Wynn Parry, C.B. (1980) Pain in avulsion lesions of the brachial plexus. *Pain*, **9**, 41–53

Zborowski, M. (1952) Cultural components in responses to pain. *J. Soc. Iss.*, **8**, 16–30

Zborowski, M. (1969) *People in Pain*, Jossey Bass, San Francisco

Zola, I.K. (1966) Culture and symptoms: an analysis of patients' presenting complaints. *Am. Soc. Rev.*, **31**, 615–38

5 Ergonomics and the management of pain

JEFFREY D. BOYLING

Introduction

The management of pain has been traditionally thought of in clinical terms. In the case of acute pain, the tissue or tissues responsible is identified and treatment appropriate for the condition undertaken. Chronic pain management has required a broader approach in view of secondary tissue changes and behavioural changes. However, the prevention of pain has not really received adequate attention. In particular, proper attention has not been given to pain which is work-related. With increasing levels of spinal dysfunction and upper limb disorders in the workplace the management of pain should not be considered an afterthought. The prevention of work-related pain should be a priority.

Pain in the Workplace

Pain in the workplace is not a new phenomenon. Descriptions of disorders in crafts and tradesmen, scribes and notaries can be found in the work of the Italian physician Ramazzini (1713). Over 250 years later pain in the workplace was still being documented. Ferguson (1967) reported on the musculoskeletal discomfort experienced by telegraphists. In the office Maeda and others (1980) described the localized fatigue reported by accounting machine operators. More recently, spinal pain has been reported in groups as diverse as sheep shearers (Gmeinder, 1986) and staff of a district health authority (Turnbull *et al.*, 1992). Isernhagen (1988) has written on the management and prevention of work injury. Buckle (1987), as well as Hagberg and Kilbom (1992), have published material from conferences devoted to the problem of musculoskeletal disorders at work.

The extent of pain in the workplace (i.e. prevalence) and its significance needs to be studied if prevention is to be undertaken. Pheasant (1991) has suggested that the prevalence of work-related aches and pains may be in the range of 70–90%. This does not necessarily mean all those individuals will progress to having a clinical condition. However, a progression from occasional discomfort through frequent and daily discomfort to moderate or severe pathology with decreasing levels of prevalence could be expected to occur. One problem in establishing this data is to distinguish point prevalence from period prevalence and lifetime prevalence. The former deals with the percentage of workers suffering pain at the time of the survey while the latter deals with pain suffered at some time or another during the worker's life. Period prevalence refers to those workers suffering pain over a specified period of time.

The above indicates that the clinician dealing with pain in the workplace needs to have a basic knowledge of epidemiology and how to undertake research, in which case reference to the work of Alderson (1983) and Partridge and Barnitt (1986) respectively will help the physical therapist. However, the prevention of work-related pain needs to draw upon skills not always available to the clinician. There needs to be an awareness of the role of ergonomics. But, this raises two questions. Can the application of ergonomics prevent pain? Can the application of ergonomics decrease pain when it is present? To answer these questions an understanding of ergonomics is a prerequisite.

Ergonomics

Ergonomics is derived from the Greek words '*ergo*' meaning work and '*nomos*', according to natural laws. Other definitions have also been suggested for ergonomics. Murrell (1965) described ergonomics as the 'scientific relationship between the person and the working environment'.

ANATOMY

Anthropometry   The dimensions of the human body

Biomechanics   The application of forces

PHYSIOLOGY

Work physiology   The expenditure of energy

Environmental physiology   The effects of the physical environment

PSYCHOLOGY

Skill psychology   Information processing and decision making

Occupational psychology   Training, effort and individual difference

Fig. 5.1   Components of ergonomics.

Grandjean (1982) in his book entitled *Fitting the Task to the Man* stated that ergonomics was the study of man's behaviour in relation to his work. Pheasant (1991) has defined ergonomics as the science of matching the job to the worker and the product to the user. To fulfil these definitions knowledge of several disciplines is required.

Singleton (1972) has indicated that ergonomics is a broad profession which draws upon the disciplines of anatomy, physiology and psychology. Within these three categories there are subcategories and these are shown in Figure 5.1. Knowledge of other subjects such as systems, statistics and instrumentation is also required. Related fields include work study and time and motion study. The main point to note, however, is the relationship between the person and the working environment. There must be an appreciation of the physical as well as the mental aspects of this relationship, i.e. the man–machine interface. Figure 5.2 illustrates this.

The application of ergonomics to the problem of pain in the workplace is increasing and there are cost benefits to be achieved. Organizations as well as individuals can reduce costs (see Figure 5.3) and improve productivity by looking at the problem of work-related pain. A case study showing

the benefits of ergonomics in reducing musculoskeletal pain at work has been published by Spilling *et al.* (1986). The United Kingdom Health and Safety Executive (1993) has published data on the potential savings.

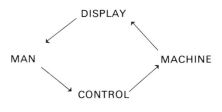

Fig. 5.2   The man–machine interface.

Work-related Pain

The regions of pain commonly reported by workers are the spine and the upper limbs. The aetiology of back pain and upper limb disorders is complex and

	Direct Cost	Indirect Cost
Insured	employer's liability public liability damage to plant damage to vehicles treatment costs	product liability business interruption
Uninsured	sick pay product losses treatment costs	overmanning replacement staff staff training loss of goodwill

Fig. 5.3 Costs of work-related musculoskeletal disorders.

Table 5.1 Anatomical region of injuries due to manual handling

Anatomical region	Percentage of injuries
Back	45
Finger/thumb	16
Arm	13
Lower limb	9
Rest of torso	8
Hand	6
Other	3
Total	100

Source: Health and Safety Executive, 1992a.

multifactorial. Not all the factors responsible for the onset, progression and resolution of these problems will be work-related. However, the likelihood of onset, rate of progression and speed of recovery can be influenced by the application of ergonomics in the workplace as well as elsewhere.

Spinal Pain

Until recently the approach to spinal pain in the context of manual handling has been to focus on the weight. This is not applying ergonomics, for the reason it is considering a single factor in isolation. Fraser (1989) has reported other approaches, including the epidemiological approach, the biomechanical approach, the physiological approach and the psychophysical approach. In isolation these approaches only consider limited aspects of the problem of pain due to manual handling.

The ergonomic approach to the reduction of pain due to manual handling considers a wide range of factors. It also acknowledges the fact that not all manual handling injuries result in spinal pain. Data published by the United Kingdom Health and Safety Executive (1992a) from the period 1990/91 for over 3-day injuries show that only 45% involved the back. Table 5.1 shows the distribution of injuries according to anatomical region. Consequently, the application of an ergonomic approach will have benefits in terms of reducing spinal pain in addition to pain sustained in other anatomical regions.

The ergonomic approach to the reduction of pain due to manual handling considers a number of aspects and these are the task, the load, the working environment, individual capability and other factors. These factors have been incorporated into the latest manual handling legislation in the United Kingdom (Department of Employment,

1992). Australia, New Zealand, the United States and other countries are also placing greater emphasis on ergonomics in an attempt to reduce manual handling injuries.

The Task

Analysis of the task can lead to a reduction in the risk of injury. In particular reducing the distance the load is held or manipulated at relative to the trunk can lead to a decreased injury risk. Another factor to consider is the importance of posture. Twisting, stooping, reaching upwards or a combination of these postures needs to be reduced so as to lower the risk of injury. Distances that the load is moved through, be it vertical or horizontal, can increase the dynamic and static load applied to the spine. Reducing the distance by automation, mechanization or improved workplace design can help. Pushing and pulling can increase the potential for slipping and tripping type incidents. These can be minimized by attention to the interface between the floor and the foot as well as ensuring that the hand grip is below shoulder height but above hip height. Small loads handled frequently can result in a high cumulative load being applied to the spine as well as other parts of the body. The potential for fatigue and hence injury is higher. The nature of the work may impose a rate which is beyond the physical capacity of the worker. Work undertaken while seated or in a team is not without risk. Seated work precludes the use of the powerful leg muscles or involves twisting reaching activities to handle the load. Team lifting can lead to injury if there is a mismatch in the physical capabilities of the lifters or a breakdown in communication.

The Load

Loads can be heavy, bulky, unwieldy, difficult to grasp, unstable or potentially damaging. The lifting of heavy loads should be avoided. Loads can be light but bulky. Consequently, they may be difficult to hold close to the body in which case the risk of injury is increased. Alternative means of manual handling should be adopted. Human loads are not supplied with handles nor are a range of inanimate loads. The lack of grips can lead to injuries of the upper limbs. Alternatively, poor grips can lead to the load being dropped with damage to the feet being the likely outcome. Spinal strain trying to hold a load is another possible outcome. Loads lacking rigidity can move without warning as can patients. Both increase the risk of injury and hence pain.

The Working Environment

Lack of space can force the person to adopt unsatisfactory postures or move awkwardly. The underfoot surface may be slippery, uneven or unstable and all can lead to slips, trips and falls. Variations in the thermal environment may mean the individual's capacity to work is reduced. Alternatively, cold or sweaty hands may have trouble gripping the load leading to an increased injury risk. Gusts of wind can suddenly shift the load leading to potential pain producing injury. Poor lighting can limit the visibility and increase the risk of tripping accidents.

Individual capability

Individuals vary in terms of their physical dimensions as well as their strength. Matching the task to the individual is of importance if the risk of pain is to be reduced. Similarly, acknowledging the variations due to ill health or pregnancy is necessary if the risks of injury are to be minimized. Knowledge or training are of importance if systems of work or special pieces of equipment are to be used.

Other Factors

Personal protective equipment and the clothing worn can influence manual handling. The avoidance of equipment which restricts free movement is important. The wearing of equipment to protect the person from the load may result in a better grip being adopted, with the load held closer to the body.

Spinal Pain: Summary

The potential to reduce the risk of pain due to injury, be it acute or the result of cumulative loading, exists. The application of ergonomics can convert this potential to reality. Ergonomics can prevent pain by matching the task to the worker with respect to the physical and mental capabilities of the worker. At the same time ergonomics can reduce spinal loading and this in itself can decrease pain by reducing the stress on injured tissues.

Upper Limb Disorders

In 1990 the Health and Safety Executive of the United Kingdom decided to adopt the term 'upper limb disorder' (ULD) to cover a range of different conditions where pain and other symptoms are reported in the soft tissues of the hand, wrist, arm and shoulder (Health and Safety Executive, 1990). Unlike spinal pain, which causes no problem with regard to terminology, upper limb disorders do. Therefore, an understanding of the terminology used to describe these conditions is necessary before any consideration is given to the application of ergonomics.

What is an 'Upper Limb Disorder'?

To answer this question it is necessary to look at the terminology used. Table 5.2 shows numerous descriptive terms which are used and which apply to the same thing. The problem with these terms is that they do not give any clear indication as to the structure(s) causing the problem. Furthermore, in terms of the mechanisms suggested, they may be misleading. They are umbrella terms to cover what can be an ill-defined symptom complex. Frequently, upper limb disorders are considered to be in the hand and forearm and other terms such as those listed below are used:

Carpal tunnel syndrome	Compression neuropathy
Tendinitis	Tenosynovitis
Lateral epicondylitis	Medial Epicondylitis
Bursitis	De Quervain's

These terms are diagnostic labels for clearly defined clinical conditions. Each one of the descriptive

Table 5.2 Descriptive terms for upper limb disorders

Description	Abbr.	Country
Repetitive strain injury	RSI	Australia
Repetition strain injury	RSI	Australia
Repetitive motion injury	RMI	Canada
Cumulative trauma disorder	CTD	United States
Occupational cervicobrachial disorder	OCD	Sweden, Japan
Occupational overuse disorder	OOD	Australia

and diagnostic terms will have a set of symptoms and signs. In each case these will vary from patient to patient and in each patient the symptoms and signs may change from day to day.

Various symptoms have been reported for ULDs, including discomfort, aching, pains, paraesthesia, anaesthesia, heaviness, swelling/fullness and burning. These symptoms can be reported in the conditions already mentioned above as well as in other conditions which are not listed. This leads to an important point in the management of upper limb disorders. People with the above symptoms should not be labelled as having an upper limb disorder (ULD) until a thorough medical examination has been conducted. This is important because one of the problems with ULDs is the unnecessary anxiety that can be created by inappropriate use of terms. This same anxiety is not associated with spinal pain. Therefore, a key element in the overall management is a thorough examination of any individual with symptoms so as to establish an accurate diagnosis. This is where physical therapists need continually to update their skills to keep abreast of the latest knowledge (see Sahrmann, 1987; Butler, 1991).

In summary, ULD is a collective term for those conditions characterized by discomfort or persistent pain in muscles, tendons and other soft tissues. This means an 'upper limb disorder' can be a clearly defined clinical condition or an ill-defined symptom complex. However, in the interests of the patient, only use the term upper limb disorder if a clinical diagnosis cannot be applied. Fortunately, the application of ergonomics to prevent the pain of ULDs should not be affected by terminology.

Principles of Management

The management of ULDs involves prevention of the problem and rehabilitation of those individuals with symptoms. In the case of the former, prevention in the workplace means the application of ergonomics. It should also be noted that the workplace is not restricted to certain activities. The titles of some books (Huskisson, 1992) would suggest that an upper limb disorder is a keyboard disease. This is not the case. A wide range of occupations ranging from those undertaken in the office to the factory as well as leisure pursuits can be involved.

Prevention

The seriousness of upper limb disorders has been recognized in a number of countries and steps taken to minimize the problem. In Australia a code of practice was established by Worksafe in 1986. In New Zealand guidance has also been on what was called Occupational Overuse Syndrome (Department of Labour, 1991). With regard to the office and the use of display screen equipment, i.e. computers, the United Kingdom introduced legislation in 1992 (Health and Safety Executive, 1992b), and similar legislation was enacted across the European Community.

The main principle of management is prevention and this is where ergonomics can help. Unfortunately, many physical therapists do not really understand what ergonomics is. In the office attention is frequently directed at the chair and desk with no thought given to other factors which may have a bearing on the development of an upper limb disorder. This occurs to a lesser extent in the factory. Therefore, prevention of upper limb disorders requires a detailed assessment of the workplace to identify physical, environmental and organizational factors that could result in musculoskeletal disorders. Prevention revolves around one key question: does the workplace fit the worker in all aspects?

It is worth while to distinguish the office from the factory because different activities are undertaken. Unfortunately, changes in both areas are sometimes made only after symptoms such as pain have developed in the workers. In this situation, prevention and rehabilitation are needed.

Upper Limb Disorders in the Office

In the office, upper limb disorders are usually, although not exclusively, associated with the use of computers. Due to the increasing use of computer keyboards, there has been an increase in the number of people reporting symptoms. This is regrettable in view of the fact that upper limb disorders are preventable. The prevention of the pain and associated symptoms of upper limb disorders demand the application of ergonomics. Standards to assist people in the introduction of visual display terminals to the office have been published (AS3590, 1990; BS7179, 1990). Unfortunately, standards are usually provided for guidance and do not have any legal implication. Members of the European Community have now been issued with a directive which has to be incorporated into legislation within the individual countries. In the UK this has resulted in the Health and Safety (Display Screen Equipment) Regulations 1992 (HSE, 1992b).

The application of ergonomics in the office and in particular with regard to display screen equipment needs to focus on a number of areas. These areas are the equipment, the environment and the interface between the computer and user.

Equipment

The quality and location of the display screen can cause users to develop upper limb disorders. The pain and associated symptoms can be avoided by ensuring that the screen is of a high quality which means the characters are easy to see and there is no perceptible flicker. It is also important that the screen is adjustable in terms of height, tilt and swivel, so that it can be positioned in a location which is comfortable for the user. It is also important that the screen is free of reflections and that the user is not subjected to glare whilst operating the screen. Both reflection and glare can cause the operator to adopt an awkward or constrained posture and hence develop symptoms.

The keyboard should be separate from the computer and capable of tilting. This is to allow the user to adopt a comfortable posture and this is enhanced by allowing for space in front of the keyboard. The keyboard should not be of an excessive thickness otherwise that will result in unbalanced joint positions at the wrists and static postures being adopted by the forearms. The keyboard should have a matt finish and this should also apply to the work surface.

The work desk or surface should be of sufficient size to allow the user to undertake all the tasks required. Frequently, new technology is placed on existing desks which were designed for paper-based operations and are unsuitable for display screen equipment operations. The resulting congestion forces operators to maintain awkward constrained postures and this leads to the onset of symptoms. The key is to ensure that the operator can adopt a comfortable posture. This may mean the addition of a document holder so that items referred to are well positioned. Chairs need to be adjustable so that the operators can position themselves in a suitable location with regards to the keyboard and screen. It must be recognized that individuals come in different shapes and sizes and, therefore, the chair chosen should have adequate flexibility to accommodate this range. For some users a footrest may be necessary. Otherwise the user may adopt a posture which is not conducive to the work they are undertaking, resulting in the development of symptoms. Workstation adjustment and an efficient working posture are shown in Figure 5.4.

Environment

Factors such as space, lighting, reflections and glare, noise, heat, radiation and humidity need to be considered. A thermal environment which is comfortable for the user is important. The provision of adequate lighting will also assist the user in being able to see what is on the screen as well as hard copy that they may be referring to. Noise can be distracting and consequently stress producing. This can lead to increased muscular tension and the onset of symptoms.

Computer–user interface

In the office attention is frequently directed at the chair and the desk but no thought given to other factors which may have a bearing on the development of an upper limb disorder. In particular, physical therapists do not appreciate the breadth of ergonomics and therefore ignore such factors as the interface between the computer and the user. Software can be poorly designed and this can result in unnecessary mental stress as well as physical stress to operate the system. Both can lead to the development of symptoms, manifesting in an upper limb disorder. The application of ergonomics to the design of the software is therefore very important. In particular the software must be suitable for the task, it must be easy to use and adaptable to the level of knowledge or experience of the user. Feedback to the user in a form which is understandable is also important.

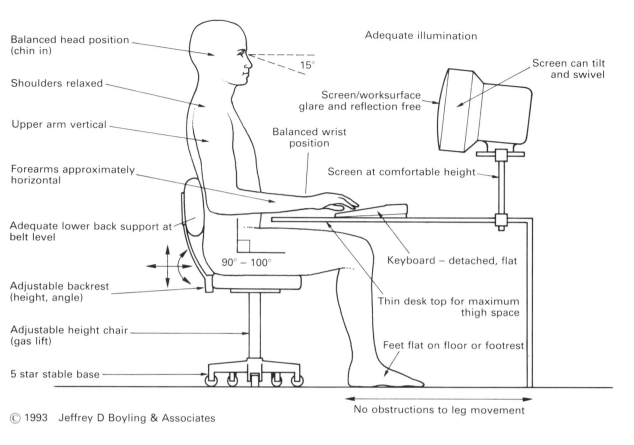

Balanced head position
(chin in)

Adequate illumination

15°

Screen can tilt
and swivel

Shoulders relaxed

Screen/worksurface
glare and reflection free

Upper arm vertical

Balanced wrist
position

Forearms approximately
horizontal

Screen at comfortable height

Adequate lower back support at
belt level

90° – 100°

Keyboard – detached, flat

Adjustable backrest
(height, angle)

Thin desk top for maximum
thigh space

Adjustable height chair
(gas lift)

Feet flat on floor or footrest

5 star stable base

No obstructions to leg movement

© 1993   Jeffrey D Boyling & Associates

Fig. 5.4   Workstation adjustment and efficient working posture.

Upper Limb Disorders in The Factory

Putz-Anderson (1988) and the Health and Safety Executive (1990) have both given guidance on prevention of upper limb disorders, especially those encountered in the factory. Greater emphasis on ergonomics is found in the latter publication and predisposing work conditions are listed. The factors associated with an increased risk of upper limb disorder (Health and Safety Executive, 1990) can be grouped into three general categories.

1. Force – the application of undesirable manual force.
2. Frequency and duration of movement – including unsuitable rates of working or repetition of a single element.
3. Awkward posture of the hand, wrist, arm or shoulder.

These risk factors can occur in isolation but usually they are found to occur in combination. McAtamney and Corlett (1992) have produced a guide and methods to reduce the pain of work-related upper limb disorders.

Force

Poor design of tools, the work place or the task itself can lead to excessive force being exerted either via the tools or the hands. Attention needs to be given to the characteristic of the material being worked upon (i.e. pliability) as well as the tools being used. With regard to the latter, the sharpness of the tools needs to be maintained so as to reduce forces required to cut the material. Excessive force is sometimes required by virtue of the fact that the operator has to hold the tool while operating the control switch. This can be overcome by the use of suspension devices and jigs.

Frequency and duration

Highly repetitive motions, machine pacing and bonus payment systems are all risk factors for the development of painful upper limb disorders. Highly repetitive motions with short cycle times usually require a high speed and therefore less tension can be developed by the muscle. Consequently greater effort is required but there is a lack of sufficient recovery time. Machine pacing assumes that all workers are capable of matching the pace of the machine. Self-pacing reduces the risk. Payment systems and flexible time working can also produce the problem of pain in the workplace by virtue of the fact that the operator is trying to reach a certain level to achieve a payment and this may be beyond the physical capability of the person. Alternatively, a worker may not be taking rest breaks so as to accumulate the working time and hence leave work early.

Posture

Fixed postures or constrained postures overload the muscles and tendons and can also lead to compression of nerve tissue. Joints have to work in an uneven or asymmetrical manner and the nature of the muscle contraction is static rather than dynamic. The avoidance of these practices by applying ergonomic principles will lead to less pain in the workplace.

Other work-related factors

There are numerous other factors which can contribute to the development of an upper limb disorder. Some of these are vibration, cold environments, poor training, lack of training. Attention to all factors is part of the ergonomic approach.

Preventative measures

Those jobs suspected of causing upper limb disorders need to be assessed so that risks can be identified and remedial action taken. The application of ergonomics is of great benefit and in particular it needs to be incorporated into part of the corporate structure. Attention to work design and organizational arrangements is very important.

Work design

Attention should be focused on the reduction of force levels, reduction of highly repetitive movements and postural changes. The strategies to achieve this will vary depending on the task, but basic principles can be applied.

Organizational arrangements

Effective training and instruction are essential for people to perform tasks in a safe and healthy way consistent with the need to achieve quality and production standards. Training needs to be structured. However, training alone cannot compensate for job and equipment design. Therefore, thought should be given to the training requirements and this should include the teaching of ergonomic principles. It is worth noting some key anatomical principles:

1. Adopt balanced joint positions.
2. Avoid static muscle work.
3. Do not compress the nerves.
4. Reverse the posture regularly.

New employees need to be introduced to the workplace at a pace that will allow them to condition themselves to the work undertaken. This should also apply to any individual returning to work after a period away. This could cover people returning from holidays, ill health or special leave.

Job rotation is often suggested to alleviate some of the problems found on the factory floor. It does have benefits in terms of altering the work undertaken in mental terms. However, it does not always mean that there will be a change in physical activity. If job rotation is to be undertaken careful thought needs to be given to the physical demands placed upon the individual in each job and it needs to be organized in such a way that there is a variation in the physical demands.

Upper Limb Disorder: Summary

The potential to reduce the risk of pain due to the cumulative loading, be it in the factory or in the office, exists and it can be achieved with the application of ergonomics. Ergonomics can minimize the mismatch between the person and the task. It is important that tools, workstations and jobs are assessed. The guiding principle as set out by Putz-Anderson (1988) is to make the job fit the person, not to make the person fit the job.

Treatment of Work-related Pain

The need for treatment can be reduced by the application of ergonomics. However, it will not solve all problems. Consideration of age-related changes, less than ideal workers in terms of physical construction and injuries sustained outside the workplace is still required. Approaches to treatment of spinal pain have been documented by Grieve (1988) as well as Boyling and Palastanga (1994). The treatment of upper limb disorders has also been documented (Elvey *et al.*, 1986; Butler, 1991).

Treatment of spinal pain as well as upper limb disorders needs to be based on an accurate examination of the patient. Without this any treatment method is doomed to failure or, worse, the prolonging of the patient's problem. This is particularly important for a subset of ULDs, i.e. the ill-defined symptom complex. These have been described by Elvey *et al.* (1986) and this work highlighted the role of nerve tissue in symptom production. More advanced information on the role of the nervous system is found in Butler (1991). Physiotherapists should note that Butler's work assumes a thorough understanding of musculoskeletal examination. It is very easy to exacerbate the patient's problem with inappropriate handling and/or treatment.

There are a number of problems seen in the treatment of this condition. Frequently, patients have been treated with a variety of modalities (especially electrotherapy) directed at the site of the symptoms. Electrotherapy is a valuable tool when used properly. Treating the site of the symptoms and not the source of the symptoms can delay recovery.

Another problem seen is the patient whose symptoms have subsided but then return when the patient attempts to do anything. The reason for this relates to the structure at fault. A lot of patients (particularly the chronic cases) have lost the mobility of the nerve tissue. When the nerve tissue is moved/stretched it produces the symptoms at the time or the resulting inflammation produces them later. The flare-up! Failure to treat the tissues at fault delays recovery and hence return to the workplace.

The inability of the therapist to acknowledge that a patient's condition is beyond their professional skills is another problem. Professionalism is the ability to seek the assistance of a more experienced colleague and not say that no more can be done for the patient.

Some patients may be able to continue working while receiving treatment. In other cases the severity and irritability of the condition may require the person to have time off. It is essential that contact between the person and the workplace is maintained during this phase.

Treatment should then include the question of return to work. Careful consideration needs to be given to any return to work situation. Questions that arise include when will the person be fit to return, what will the person be capable of doing when at work. This is where rehabilitation experts and not ergonomists can assist in the rehabilitation process. Essential elements include ensuring that a return to work as soon as possible is a normal expectation, provision of suitable duties/employment where practicable for an injured worker as an integral part of the rehabilitation process and consultation with management, workers and any representative of the workers.

Ergonomics can go a long way to preventing pain which is work-related but in terms of reducing pain when it is present, that is much harder. It is dependent upon the severity and irritability of the condition. It is also dependent on other factors, such as the attitude of the employee to the workplace as well as the attitude of the management to the problem. Therefore, applying ergonomics may not necessarily resolve the problem of pain.

Conclusion

Spinal pain and upper limb disorders are preventable and treatable. Prevention demands a full understanding of ergonomics. Rehabilitation depends on early identification/referral, accurate diagnosis of structures involved, accurate management of those structures, patient education, accurate identification of any causative factors, early return to the workplace and cooperation of all parties involved. Physical therapists have a major role to play in the prevention and rehabilitation of upper limb disorders. The application of ergonomics by physical therapists is the foundation for prevention and reduces the need for rehabilitation of painful work-related conditions.

References

Alderson, M. (1983) *An Introduction to Epidemiology*, 2nd edn, Macmillan, London

AS3590 (1990) *Screen Based Workstations*. Standards Australia, Sydney

Boyling, J.D. and Palastanga, N. (eds) (1994) *Grieve's Modern Manual Therapy*, 2nd edn, Churchill Livingstone, Edinburgh

BS7179 (1990) *Ergonomics of Design and Use of Visual Display Terminals (vdts in offices)*. British Standards Institution, Milton Keynes

Buckle, P. (ed.) (1987) *Musculoskeletal Disorders at Work* (Proceedings of a conference held at the University of Surrey, Guildford), Taylor and Francis, London

Butler, D.S. (1991) *Mobilisation of the Nervous System*, Churchill Livingstone, Melbourne

Department of Employment (1992) *The Manual Handling Operations Regulations, 1992*. HMSO, London

Department of Labour (1991) Occupational Overuse Syndrome. Occupational Safety & Health, Wellington, NZ

Elvey, R.L. Quintner, J.L. and Thomas, A.N. (1986) A clinical study of RSI. *Aust. Family Phys.*, **15** (10), 1314–15, 1319 and 1322

Ferguson, D.A. (1967) *Report on Health Survey of Telegraph Officers*. School of Public Health and Tropical Medicine, University of Sydney

Fraser, T.M. (1989) *The Worker at Work*, Taylor and Francis, London

Gmeinder, G.E. (1986) Back complaints among shearers in Western Australia. *Aust. J. Physiother.*, **32**(3), 139–44

Grandjean, E. (1982) *Fitting the Task to the Man: an Ergonomic Approach*, Taylor and Francis, London

Grieve, G.P. (1988) *Common Vertebral Joint Problems*, 2nd edn, Churchill Livingstone, Edinburgh

Hagberg, M. and Kilbom, A. (ed.) (1992) International Scientific Conference on the Prevention of Work-related Musculoskeletal Disorders. PREMUS, Sweden, Arbets Miljo Institutet

Health and Safety Executive (1990) *Work Related Upper Limb Disorders: A Guide to Prevention*, HMSO, London

Health and Safety Executive (1992a) *Manual Handling: Guidance on Regulations*, HMSO, London

Health and Safety Executive (1992b) *Display Screen Equipment Regulations*, HMSO, London

Health and Safety Executive (1993) *The Costs of Accidents at Work*, HMSO, London

Huskisson, E. (1992) *Repetitive Strain Injury: the Keyboard Disease*, Charterhouse Conference and Communications Limited, London

Isernhagen, S.J. (1988) *Work Injury: Management and Prevention*, Aspen Publishers, Rockville, Md

Maeda, K., Hunting, W. and Grandjean, E. (1980) Localized fatigue in accounting machine operators. *J. Occup. Med.*, **22**, 810–16

McAtamney, L. and Corlett, E.N. (1992) *Reducing the Risks of Work Related Upper Limb Disorders: a Guide and Methods*. The Institute for Occupational Ergonomics, University of Nottingham, Nottingham

Murrell, K.F.H. (1965) *Ergonomics: Man in his Working Environment*, Chapman and Hall, London

Partridge, C.J. and Barnitt, R.E. (1986) *Research Guidelines: A handbook for Therapists*, Heinemann Physiotherapy, London

Pheasant, S.T. (1991) *Ergonomics: Work and Health*, Macmillan, London

Ramazzini, B. (1713, 1940) *De Morbis Artificum* (Diseases of Workers), trans. W.C. Wright, University of Chicago Press

Sahrmann, S.A. (1987) Posture and muscle imbalance. *Postgraduate Advances in Physical Therapy*, APTA I–VIII

Singleton, W.T. (1972) *Introduction to Ergonomics*, WHO, Geneva

Spilling, S. Eiterheim, J. and Aaras, A. (1986) Cost benefit analysis of work environment investment at STK's telephone plant at Kongsvinger. In *The Ergonomics of Working Postures* (eds, E.N. Corlett, J. Wilson and I. Manencia), Taylor and Francis, London, pp. 380–97

Turnbull, N., Dornan, J., Fletcher, B. and Wilson, S. (1992) Prevalence of spinal pain among the staff of a district health authority, *Occup. Med.*, **42**, 143–8

Worksafe Australia (1986) *Repetition Strain Injury: A Report and Model Code of Practice*, Australian Government Publishing Service, Canberra

6 *Acute and chronic pain and assessment*

DAVID BOWSHER

Introduction

Touch, hearing and sight are **sensations** because we have sense organs specifically activated by mechanical, sound and light energy respectively. Pain is also a specific sensation brought about by damage or threat of damage), although, of course, there is no outside form of energy called 'pain'. Other forms of energy, such as (harmless) magnetism or (harmful) ionizing radiation do not produce any sensations because we have no sense organs specifically activated by them. There are nerve endings in muscle (muscle spindles) which are activated by lengthening, and yet we are not consciously aware of their excitation, because the central connections of the spindles in the spinal cord and brain do not bring their activity to consciousness.

These self-evident considerations immediately illustrate two things about *all* sensations: (1) there must be a form of energy which specifically activates a sense organ (receptor); and (2) the connections within the spinal cord and brain which convey the impulses coming from the receptor must be so arranged that their activity becomes conscious.

A receptor may in general terms be defined as a structure, usually a nerve ending, which converts some specific form of energy into nervous impulses. Specific receptors for pain will be described in Chapter 7.

A third factor, **modulation**, should also be considered. Modulation means that information from a receptor can be changed, enhanced, diminished, or even suppressed, either in the periphery or in the brain. For example, we cease to be aware of the contact of our clothes, although they excite touch receptors, because the receptors themselves cease to respond; this is a form of peripheral modulation called **adaptation**. When concentrating on a television programme, our auditory receptors may fail to inform us that the telephone is ringing; this is a form of central modulation whereby auditory information is suppressed within the brain so that we can concentrate on the audiovisual content of the programme which occupies our attention.

Acute and chronic pain

Pain has been defined by the International Association for the Study of Pain (IASP) as 'an unpleasant sensory and emotional experience associated with actual or potential tissue damage, or described in terms of such damage'. A damaging stimulus is a **noxious** (*noxa* = harm, damage) stimulus, and may produce pain in a normal conscious subject; but an anaesthetized patient, for example, does not feel pain inflicted by the surgeon's knife, though the stimulus remains noxious. Only the highest (conscious) centres of the nervous system have been functionally inactivated by the anaesthetic, so the functionally intact peripheral nerves are still carrying messages engendered by noxious stimulation – these are **nociceptive** (i.e. damage-signalling) messages – even though pain is not consciously felt. Because pain is a private and subjective experience, we can only know that animals other than man have **nociceptors**, i.e. receptors responding specifically to noxious stimuli; but we may deduce from their behaviour that they probably feel pain as well.

Like all other sensations, pain has a threshold; that is to say, noxious stimulation must reach a certain intensity before pain is felt. This is the **pain perception threshold**, strictly defined as the **least** intensity of noxious stimulation at which a subject consciously perceives pain. Large numbers of psychophysical experiments carried out on normal healthy subjects with artificial (but measurable) stimuli, such as electric shock, radiant heat, or mechanical pressure show that the pain perception threshold, like other sensory thresholds, is fairly constant from person to person. Using radiant heat applied to the skin, for example, pain is perceived at about 45°C.

We cannot be certain that experimentally inflicted pain in normal subjects can be equated with pathological pain in ill patients; but so far as the pain perception threshold is concerned, it is probably so. One very obvious reason why this is uncertain is because people do not seek therapeutic help at the very moment of feeling the first mild twinge of pain.

From the clinical point of view, a far more important threshold is the **pain tolerance level**, defined as the **greatest** intensity of noxious stimulation an individual can bear; it might have been better to have called it the pain **intolerance** level. This varies widely from person to person, and in the same person under different conditions. Factors, such as cultural background, motivation and emotional significance of pain can alter tolerance level. For instance, someone may experience little or no pain while rescuing a child from a burning house, while the same individual might understandably regard having a lighted match applied to the skin for no reason whatsoever as intolerably painful. The important fact to bear in mind from the clinical point of view is that patients do not seek help until their pain has gone *beyond* tolerance level.

Patients describe pain in very different terms if left to their own devices. This makes interpretation very difficult at times. It must, however, be regarded as axiomatic in clinical practice that any pain feels as bad to the sufferer as he or she says it does. The practical problem posed by such considerations is how to assess a patient's pain as objectively as possible.

Pain assessment

Of the many methods devised, three are in fairly widespread use, and are described below.

The McGill Pain Questionnaire

In order to overcome the differing values attributable to different patients' own descriptions, Melzack (1975) devised a list of words arranged in 20 groups (Figure 6.1). The patient is asked to underline or circle not more than one word in any group (or every group, if he wishes) which applies to or describes his pain. This is believed to be more objective because the patient is forced to use words defined or at least chosen by the physiotherapist, not by the patient. Groups 1 to 10 are **somatic** words defining the physiological characteristics of the pain; groups 11 to 15 are **affective** words defining its subjective characteristics; group 16 is **evaluative** describing intensity; and groups 17 to 20 are miscellaneous.

Scoring is relatively simple, and is done both for all 20 word groups taken together, and separately for the groups in each of the four categories described above. The first parameter is the **total number of words chosen** (maximum 20). An **intensity score** is calculated by assigning the value 1 to the first word in any group, 2 to the second, and so on; the intensity score is the sum of all these values. It only takes a patient about 10 minutes to fill in the McGill pain questionnaire. Many workers find that it is a useful diagnostic aid if administered at a patient's first visit. Whether the progress of therapy can be satisfactorily assessed by subsequently administering the questionnaire at regular intervals is a matter of debate; some physiotherapists are enthusiastic, others sceptical.

The Submaximal Effort Tourniquet Test

This is a remarkable way of 'matching' a patient's pain (Smith *et al.*, 1966). A sphygmomanometer cuff is inflated on the patient's elevated arm to above systolic arterial pressure. The patient then clenches and unclenches the fist rhythmically. In order to standardize this procedure, a grip dynamometer must be used to ensure constant force, and a metronome to ensure constant rate. As the muscles contract in the ischaemic arm, a cramp-like pain develops. The patient is instructed to stop when this is judged to be of the same intensity as the pathological pain complained of. The time from start to finish measures the intensity of the pain at that moment. The remarkable feature of this test, according to its proponents, is that virtually all patients, even though their pathological pain may not be in the least cramp-like, can nevertheless 'match' it. Again, the test can be repeated at every session in order to evaluate progress. However, the method is extremely time-consuming, and is rarely used outside the experimental laboratory.

Look carefully at the twenty groups of words. If any word in any group applies to *your* pain, please circle that word — but do not circle more than *one word in any one group* — so you must choose the *most suitable word* in that group.

In groups that do not apply to your pain, there is no need to circle *any* word — just leave them as they are.

Group 1	Group 2	Group 3	Group 4	Group 5
Flickering	Jumping	Pricking	Sharp	Pinching
Quivering	Flashing	Boring	Gritting	Pressing
Pulsing	Shooting	Drilling	Lacerating	Gnawing
Throbbing		Stabbing		Cramping
Beating		Lancinating		Crushing
Pounding				

Group 6	Group 7	Group 8	Group 9	Group 10
Tugging	Hot	Tingling	Dull	Tender
Pulling	Burning	Itching	Sore	Taut
Wrenching	Scalding	Smarting	Hurting	Rasping
	Searing	Stinging	Aching	Splitting
			Heavy	

Group 11	Group 12	Group 13	Group 14	Group 15
Tiring	Sickening	Fearful	Punishing	Wretched
Exhausting	Suffocating	Frightful	Gruelling	Blinding
		Terrifying	Cruel	
			Vicious	
			Killing	

Group 16	Group 17	Group 18	Group 19	Group 20
Annoying	Spreading	Tight	Cool	Nagging
Troublesome	Radiating	Numb	Cold	Nauseating
Miserable	Penetrating	Drawing	Freezing	Agonising
Intense	Piercing	Squeezing		Dreadful
Unbearable		Tearing		Torturing

Fig. 6.1   The McGill pain questionnaire. Patients are asked to underline not more than one word from any or all of the 20 groups which best describe their pain. The simplest scoring methods involve: (1) total number of words underlined; (2) intensity, measured by allotting score 1 to the first word in any group, 2 to the second, and so on. The first 10 groups of words are somatic (describing what the pain feels like), 11–15 are affective, 16 is evaluative, and 17–20 miscellaneous.

The Visual Analogue Scale (VAS)

Because of the ease and simplicity of its administration, this is by now the most widely used method of measuring pain (Bond and Pilowsky, 1966). The patient is presented with a strip of paper on which is a line 10 cm long (Figure 6.2). At one end is written 'no pain' and at the other 'the worst pain I ever felt', and the patient is asked to mark the line at the point corresponding to the intensity of pain at that very moment. Plastic VAS scales with a slider which the patient moves, and with a ruler on the reverse side where the therapist can read it, are now available. The remarkable thing about the visual analogue scale is its constancy; even though a patient only sees the scale for as long as it takes to mark it, if the pain intensity is the same, it will be marked in exactly the same

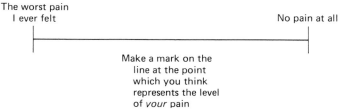

The worst pain
I ever felt   No pain at all

Make a mark on the
line at the point
which you think
represents the level
of *your* pain

Fig. 6.2   The visual analogue scale used to determine the severity of the pain experienced by the patient. This is all there is to it! Simple, but very useful.

Table 6.1   The Characteristics of First and Second Pain

Function	First, rapid (or ?acute) pain	Second, slow (or ?chronic) pain
Adequate stimulus	Pinprick, heat	Tissue damage
Nerve fibres	A-delta (small myelinated)	C (unmyelinated)
Conduction velocity	5–15 m/s (11·0–33·5 mph)	0·5–2·0 m/s (1·0–4·5 mph)
Distribution	Body surface (including mouth and anus)	All tissues except brain and spinal cord
Reflex response	Withdrawal (flexion), phasic muscle contraction	Spasm, rigidity, tonic muscle contraction [a]
Biological value	Causes organism to avoid possible tissue damage	Brings about enforced rest of damaged part, so promoting natural healing
Effect of morphine	Very little	Suppression of pain sensation, abolition of spasm

[a] Note that this reflex reaction involves both agonists and antagonists, which is part of the definition of spasm or rigidity; it is a pathological rather than a physiological reaction.

place the next day. The VAS is thus an extremely useful, and of course very rapid, method of evaluating the effects of treatment. Its disadvantage is that it cannot be used for comparing one patient with another, since two individuals with apparently the same intensity of pain will mark the line in different places. However, its value in tracing the progress of a single patient is immense.

Types Of Pain

In 1894 Goldscheider noted that when a painful stimulus is applied to a hand or foot, most (but not all) people experience a double pain sensation – at first, sharp, well-localized pain which ceases as soon as the transient stimulus (e.g. a pin or heat spot) is removed, followed by a dull, poorly localized ache which continues for some time after withdrawal of the stimulus. These phenomena have been called **first** or **rapid** and **second** or **slow** pain respectively. Like other sensory modalities, they can be dissociated by ischaemia. If an arm is made ischaemic by a sphygmomanometer cuff inflated to above systolic pressure, sensation disappears in inverse proportion to the size (and therefore the oxygen/metabolic requirement) of the afferent nerve fibres concerned. Thus, low-threshold mechanical sensations (touch, vibration, joint position sense etc.) carried by large A-beta nerve fibres are the first to disappear; pricking or first pain sensations disappear a little later when small myelinated or A-delta nerve fibres are inactivated; tissue-damage or second pain, associated with unmyelinated or C peripheral afferent nerve fibres, is the last to disappear. It may be noted that when ischaemia is reversed (e.g. by removal of an intervertebral disc which has been pressing on a

nerve root), sensations return in the reverse order. More recently, direct proof of these correlations has been provided by the technique of **microneurography**, whereby needle electrodes are inserted through the skin directly into peripheral nerve bundles, and are able to record from single nerve fibres in response to appropriate distal stimulation. In 1972, two pairs of workers (van Hees and Gybels, 1972; Torebjörk and Hallin, 1972) succeeded in recording human A-delta and C fibres; their work has been confirmed and extended many times since, and more recently they have been able to stimulate single nociceptive fibres in man (see p. 44).

The critical, and unanswered, question is: to what extent can experimental or induced first and second pain be equated with acute and chronic clinical pain? Acute clinical pain is accompanied by a number of phenomena, such as increased heart rate, raised blood pressure and pupillary constriction – all signs of sympathetic activity – while chronic pain does not have such an accompaniment. Experimental first and second pain, perhaps because they are too evanescent, are unaccompanied by autonomic activity, except when the subject is apprehensive. However, apart from this, first and second pain have features which are not only very similar to acute and chronic pain, but of considerable significance for the understanding of their characteristics (Bowsher, 1982). These are shown in Table 6.1.

Whether or not first and second pain can be equated with acute and chronic pain, it is certainly the case that all these types of sensation are produced by the activation of receptors (nociceptors) which generate nervous impulses in their associated nerve fibres; receptor and fibre together constitute a sensory unit. The same sensory units are certainly concerned in the production of experimental and clinical pains, though it is possible that in the latter case additional sensory units may also be involved.

Clinically, there is a third type of pain which is completely different from all others. This is **neurogenic pain**, which is not caused by activation of peripheral receptors, but by damage to the peripheral or central nervous system (excluding acute compression, such as may occur in prolapsed intervertebral disc). Neurogenic pain is usually of a burning and/or shooting nature; it is virtually unresponsive to opioid (narcotic) analgesics; it is accompanied in most cases by autonomic disturbances, and despite its severity does not usually interfere seriously with sleep (Bowsher, 1991). Examples of neurogenic pain are post-herpetic neuralgia, causalgia, trigeminal neuralgia, and thalamic syndrome. There is no muscle spasm in neurogenic pain.

References

Bond, M.R. and Pilowsky, I. (1966) The subjective assessment of pain and its relationship to the administration of analgesics in patients with advanced cancer. *J. Psychosomat. Res*, **10**, 203

Bowsher, D. (1982) A note on the distinction between first and second pain. In *Anatomical, Physiological, and Pharmacological Aspects of Trigeminal Pain* (eds B. Matthews and R.G. Hill), Excerpta Medica, Amsterdam, pp. 3–6

Bowsher, D. (1991), Neurogenic pain syndromes and their management. *Brit. Med. Bull.*, **47**, 644–66

Melzack, R. (1975) The McGill pain questionnaire: major properties and scoring methods. *Pain*, **1**, 277–99

Smith, G.M., Egbert, L.D., Markowitz, R.A. *et al.*, (1966) An experimental pain method sensitive to morphine in man: the submaximum effort tourniquet technique. *Pharmacol. Exp. Therap.*, **154**, 324–32

Torebjörk, H.E. and Hallin, R.G. (1972) Activity in C fibres correlated to perception in man. In *Cervical Pain* (eds C. Hirsch and Y. Zotterman), Pergamon Press, Oxford, pp. 171–8

van Hees, J. and Gybels, J.M. (1972) Pain related to single afferent C fibers from human skin. *Brain Res.*, **48**, 397–400

7 Nociceptors and peripheral nerve fibres

DAVID BOWSHER

Introduction

It has already been stated that pain receptors (nociceptors) are associated with small myelinated and unmyelinated nerve fibres in the periphery. It is of some importance to consider more closely the mechanisms and connections of these sensory units.

A-delta nociceptors

A-delta nociceptors are mostly distributed fairly superficially on the body surface (skin), including its infoldings into the mouth and anus at either end of the alimentary canal; but they have also been described in small numbers in joints and muscle. Organized non-neural receptors associated with A-delta nerve terminals have been described in the skin of experimental animals (Kruger and Rodin, 1983). These receptors, which transduce high-intensity stimuli into nerve impulses, are distributed as a series of sensitive spots within the receptive field separated by insensitive areas. The majority of these nociceptors are sensitive only to high-intensity mechanical stimuli; a small number are also sensitive to noxious temperature changes (above 45°C). A-delta fibres carry these messages to the spinal cord or brainstem at an average speed of 15 m/s (just under 35 mph or 55 km/h). It is not yet known with certainty what the transmitter substance in these sensory units is.

C Polymodal nociceptors

Nociceptors with unmyelinated fibres have been very intensively investigated both in man and experimental animals. They are found in the deeper part of the skin and in virtually every other tissue except the nervous system itself. These nociceptors, which account for over 90% of primary afferent C fibres in primates, have fairly small but homogenous receptive fields. They are frequently sensitive to mechanical, thermal and chemical noxious stimuli, and so have come to be called **polymodal nociceptors**. They are not really separately sensitive to different forms of energy, but to a factor common to damaged tissue, however the damage is caused. The nature of the actual chemical substance which excites the nerve endings is unknown, but prostaglandins are involved and pain-producing chemicals such as bradykinin are active in extraordinarily low concentrations.

C polymodal nociceptors are the well-known 'free nerve endings' in which the nerve terminals themselves are the receptors. The sensory units are commonly silent unless activated by noxious stimulation. The unmyelinated nerve fibres conduct the nociceptive messages towards the central nervous system at an average velocity of about 1 m/s (2.25 mph = 3.5 km/h).

Nociceptors and pain sensation

Torebjörk and Ochoa (1980) have been able to stimulate single A-delta and C nociceptors in cutaneous nerves in the human arm. When A-delta fibres are activated, sharp pricking or stinging sensations are referred to small punctiform areas of skin, while C fibre stimulation produces dull aching pain in larger skin patches 5–10 mm in diameter. The production of burning pain requires the coactivation of C polymodal nociceptors and heat receptors, which form another group of sensory units with unmyelinated fibres.

When polymodal nociceptors are stimulated repeatedly, or the tissue which they innervate is damaged, they show sensitization; that is to say, they either respond at lower intensities of stimulation and/or respond at higher rates than before to

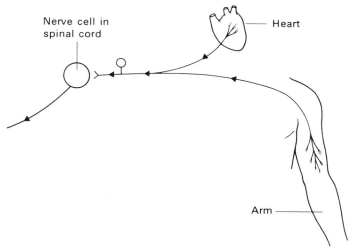

Fig. 7.1   Referred pain due to branched sensory neurons. The primary afferent shown has branches supplying both heart and arm.

a given stimulus. A-delta nociceptors also some-times show sensitization, but to a lesser degree. These phenomena may partly explain the hypersen-sitivity of injured tissue. However, it is believed that chemical substances travelling along afferent nerve fibres coming from damaged/inflamed tissues may also sensitize wide dynamic range central cells in the spinal cord (see Chapter 8, p. 49) so that they respond to almost any peripheral stimu-lus with a 'pain-type' discharge pattern. This must not be confused with peripheral (denervation) supersensitivity, when partly or relatively dener-vated muscle becomes hyperexcitable due to pathol-ogy of the efferent (motor) neurons. But there is also frequently concomitant disorder of the afferent (sensory) fibres, so that afferent sensitization may be added to effector (i.e. muscle) supersensitivity, producing a very marked motor and sensory effect when trigger spots are stimulated.

Both A-delta and C nociceptors have their cell bodies, of course, in the spinal dorsal root or trigemi-nal nerve ganglia. The proximal parts of all the A-delta axons and 70% of the C polymodal axons enter the central nervous system through the dorsal (or sensory trigeminal) roots, as classically de-scribed. But 30% of C polymodal proximal axons double back to the mixed nerve and enter the spinal cord or brainstem through the ventral (motor) root (Coggeshall *et al.*, 1975). This may provide at least part of the explanation for the failure of dorsal rhizotomy (cutting of dorsal root) to abolish pain,

though, of course, all other sensory fibres are cut. The C fibres which have entered through the ventral root ascend within the substance of the spinal cord or brainstem and terminate in the same manner as those fibres which have entered through the dorsal (sensory) root. Details of spinal cord circuitry will be described in Chapter 8 (Figure 8.2a, p. 48); but here it is necessary to describe those features which are responsible for referred pain in the periphery.

Referred Pain

Two mechanisms are known which may account for the phenomenon of referred pain, whereby tissue damage in one location is felt as pain in another. The simpler, but more recently discovered basis is the existence of **bifurcated axons** in periph-eral sensory nerves (Taylor *et al.*, 1984). They and other workers have demonstrated, both anatomi-cally and physiologically, sensory units which have one branch supplying skin and another branch coming from muscle or some other subcutaneous structure. Such branched sensory units have a single cell body in a dorsal root ganglion and a single proximal axon travelling to the spinal cord from the ganglion cell (Figure 7.1).

The second mechanism consists of the **conver-gence** of separate peripheral sensory units onto the same cell in the spinal cord (Figure 7.2). This phenomenon has recently been extensively

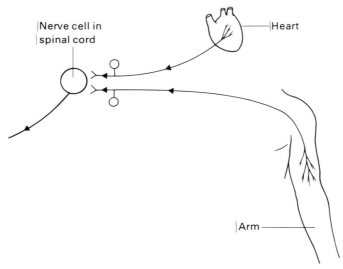

Fig. 7.2 Referred pain due to convergence. The nerve cell in the spinal cord receives input from two different peripheral neurons, one supplying the arm, the other the heart. Since the central cell is more 'used' to getting input from the arm, input from the heart may be interpreted as coming from the arm.

reinvestigated and found to be very widespread. Thus, nociceptors coming from viscera and travelling to the spinal cord in sympathetic or splanchnic nerves contact the same dorsal horn cells as do nociceptors coming from skin and travelling in somatic nerves. Many of the classical referred pains, such as heart to left upper limb and gallbladder to shoulder have been shown to be due to somatovisceral convergence.

References

Coggeshall, R.E., Applebaum, M.L., Fazan, M. *et al.* (1975) Unmyelinated axons in human ventral roots; a possible explanation of the failure of dorsal rhizotomy to relieve pain. *Brain*, **981**, 157–66

Kruger L. and Rodin B.E. (1983) Peripheral mechanisms involved in pain. In *Animal Pain* (eds R.L. Kitchell and H.E. Erickson), American Physiological Society, Maryland, USA, pp. 1–26

Taylor, D.C.M., Pierau, Fr-K. and Mizutani, M. (1984) Possible bases for referred pain. In *The Neurobiology of Pain* (eds A.V. Holden and W. Winlow), Manchester University Press, Manchester, pp. 143–56

Torebjörk, H.E. and Ochoa, J.L. (1980) Specific sensations evoked by activity in single identified sensory units in man. *Acta Physiol. Scand*, **110**, 445–7

8 Central pain mechanisms

DAVID BOWSHER

Introduction: pain pathways

The main pathways responsible for relaying information about noxious stimulation to higher centres have been known for some time, though contemporary research continues to refine the details. Most recent experimental investigations have been concentrated on trying to understand what goes on at the immediate point of entry of nociceptive afferents into the spinal cord or brainstem.

The Dorsal Horn of the Spinal Cord

The grey matter of the spinal cord can be seen, particularly in thick stained sections, to be divided into nine **laminae** or layers: or ten counting the grey matter surrounding the central canal (Figure 8.1). In addition to the connections to be described, two general principles of spinal lamination should be borne in mind:

1. Each lamina contains several, or indeed in some cases many, morphologically and functionally different types of cell; so that the input–output characteristics of any given lamina are not homogeneous. When, below, it is stated that 'neurons' in lamina . . . receive afferents from . . . and send their axons to . . .', this does not mean *all* neurons in the lamina behave in this way, but merely that there is a group which does.

2. Wherever else they send axons (and most axons are branched, sometimes very extensively), cells of each lamina send axon branches to laminae deeper in the grey matter.

Cells bordering the tip of the dorsal horn constitute the narrow **marginal zone**, or lamina I; deep to it is the **substantia gelatinosa** (SG) or lamina II. The rest of the dorsal horn is made up of laminae III, IV, V and VI, which collectively used to be known as the **nucleus proprius** of the dorsal horn. All six laminae of the dorsal horn receive primary afferent fibres from the periphery, whereas the **intermediate grey matter** made up of laminae VII and VIII

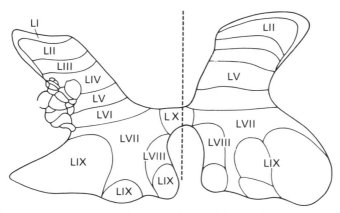

Fig. 8.1 Laminae (LI–X) in the grey matter of the dorsal horn of the adult human spinal cord – in the cervical region on the left and in the lumbar region on the right.

consists of interneurons which neither receive from nor project to structures outside the central nervous system; their input comes from more superficial laminae or from axons descending from higher brain centres. The **ventral (anterior) horn** contains the motor neurons of lamina IX, whose axons, of course, leave the spinal cord to innervate muscles in the periphery.

Unmyelinated (C) peripheral afferent axons, and therefore polymodal nociceptors, end in lamina II (Figure 8.2a). Indeed, it is the lack of myelin in lamina II which gives it its gelatinous appearance and hence the name of substantia gelatinosa. Small myelinated (A-delta) high-threshold mechanical or mechanothermal nociceptors terminate in lamina I (as do a minority of unmyelinated polymodal nociceptors) and in the lateral part of lamina V, in the 'neck' of the dorsal horn. Other, non-nociceptive, myelinated primary afferents end in lamina V as well as in other dorsal horn laminae (except laminae I and II).

Because cells in lamina I mostly receive their

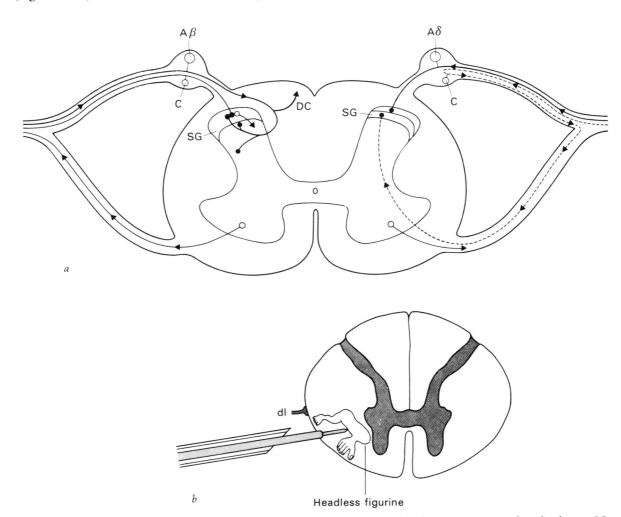

Fig. 8.2   *a* and *b*, A diagrammatic representation of the human spinal cord is shown in *a*. DC = dorsal column; SG = Substantia gelatinosa. *b* represents the 'pain pathway' in the second cervical segment (after Lahuerta, 1985, personal communication); it can be compared to a headless figurine, and shows how the body below the head is represented in the anterolateral funiculus of the white matter. The surgeon, guided by the dentate ligament (dl), can insert an electrode as shown, and coagulate (i.e. destroy) the 'pain fibres' of the mixed spinothalamic and spinoreticulodiencephalic pathways (see text).

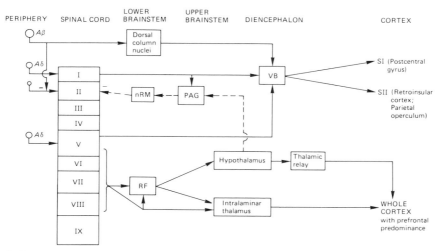

Fig. 8.3 Block diagram to show connections responsible for pain sensation (input from A-delta and C peripheral nociceptors), and also low-threshold mechanoreceptive pathway (peripheral A-beta fibres); other innocuous pathways are not shown. RF, reticular formation; nRM, nucleus Raphe magnus; PAG, periaqueductal grey matter; VB, ventrobasal nuclear complex of thalamus; SI and SII are the first and second somatosensory areas of the cerebral cortex, the locations of which are shown in brackets on the diagram. Dashed lines represent descending pathways, the ultimate effect of which is inhibitory in lamina II of the spinal cord, as indicated by the minus sign next to the arrow head. Collaterals from primary A-beta fibres also inhibit C fibre terminals; this is also shown by a minus sign.

input only from nociceptors, they respond only to noxious stimuli and so are said to be **nocispecific**. Many cells in lamina V and deeper, on the other hand, show convergence of (often indirect) input from both nociceptive and non-nociceptive primary afferents. They respond therefore to both noxious and non-noxious input, though with a different pattern of impulses; they are known as **wide dynamic range** (WDR) cells. A third category of spinal neurons is made up of those cells which respond only to non-noxious (or **innocuous**) peripheral stimuli; but these are not dealt with here.

Ascending Pathways (see Figure 8.4)

For pain to become conscious, the nervous activity engendered in the spinal grey matter by nociceptive afferent excitation must travel up to the brain. Since it has been known for three-quarters of a century that surgical section of the anterolateral quadrant of the spinal white matter (Figure 8.2*b*) abolishes pain on the opposite side of the body below the level of operation (Spiller and Martin, 1912), a practical way to explore pain pathways is to consider the origins and destinations of ascending fibres in the anterolateral funiculus (bundle of

white matter). This whole subject has recently been reviewed by Vierck *et al.* (1985).

Terminations in the Brain

Destinations were investigated earlier than origins using the various methods available at different times for tracing fibres which degenerate following anterolateral cordotomy (see, e.g., Bowsher, 1957; Boivie, 1979), or the forward (anterograde) transport of tracer substances from the level of section (see, e.g., Mantyh, 1983). Essentially fibres in the anterolateral funiculus terminate in three main supraspinal destinations (Figure 8.3):

1. The **medial reticular formation** of the lower brainstem.
2. Some of the **intralaminar nuclei** of the thalamus.
3. The **ventrobasal nuclear complex** of the thalamus.

To these should be added a fourth minor, but important, target:

4. The **periaqueductal grey matter** (PAG) of the upper brainstem.

Since these terminal areas are all below the cortex, further relays (which will be discussed later in this chapter) must carry noxiously generated impulses to the cerebral cortex, and thus to consciousness. Before considering this aspect, however, it seems reasonable first to look at the origins of the four pathways contained in the spinal anterolateral funiculus. This has become possible because of the fairly recent discovery that the enzyme horseradish peroxidase, when injected into the region of axon terminals, is transported back along the fibres to the cells of origin, where it can be rendered visible by a histochemical process. Of course this technique cannot be employed in man, but Willis and his colleagues have employed it extensively in the monkey – in which the pathways, together with their origins and terminations, are believed to be identical to those in man.

The results of such experiments have been reviewed by Willis (1985). To take them in the same order as the destinations which have been summarized above, cells marked by horseradish peroxidase injected into:

1. The medial brainstem reticular formation are mainly in laminae VII and VIII of the spinal grey matter, and to a lesser extent in lamina V.
2. The intralaminar thalamic nuclei are also chiefly in laminae VII and VIII, with small quantities in laminae V and I.
3. The ventrobasal nuclear complex of the thalamus are mostly in laminae I and V.
4. The periaqueductal grey matter are principally in lamina I, and to a slighter extent in lamina V.

It will be noted that cells in lamina V project to all destinations. They are not necessarily the same cells, since human lamina V contains at least eight different neuron types (Abdel-Maguid and Bowsher, 1985). However, physiological experiments in various animal species have shown that some axons branch to the intralaminar and ventrobasal thalamus, and others to the reticular formation and intralaminar thalamus, and yet others to the periaqueductal grey matter and ventrobasal thalamus. The input–output relationships of the spinal grey matter are illustrated diagrammatically in Figure 8.3 which also shows some other important connections:

1. The brainstem reticular formation projects on to the intralaminar thalamus, and also the hypothalamus, which has also recently been shown to receive direct projections from the spinal cord.
2. The ventrobasal thalamus actually receives its major input from low-threshold non-nociceptive mechanical receptors in the periphery (A-beta fibres), which relay through the dorsal column (gracile and cuneate) nuclei in the lower brainstem.

Therefore, when we see that the ventrobasal thalamus projects mainly to the principal somatosensory area (SI) in the postcentral gyrus, it is perhaps not surprising to learn that lesions in this part of the brain abolish almost every kind of somatic sensation *except* tissue damage pain (but including pinprick sensation).

Mechanisms of Pain Sensation

Nociceptors activated by tissue damage send their impulses mainly through the reticular formation and intralaminar thalamus to the whole cerebral cortex (Figure 8.4), though predominantly to prefrontal regions. This is too big an area for a natural or surgical lesion to abolish pain. Note also that a parallel projection from the reticular formation to the hypothalamus also reaches the prefrontal cortex. This may explain why there are autonomic concomitants to acute tissue damage type pain.

Lastly, it should be noted that although peripheral C fibre input is principally to spinal grey lamina II, output to the tissue–damage–pain pathway is chiefly from WDR cells in laminae VII and VIII. This means that convergent intraspinal circuitry must exist between input and output, and several synapses are known to be involved. This may help to explain why pain elicited by activation of C polymodal nociceptors is less well localized than pinprick sensation (which excites A-delta nociceptors).

The mechanisms so far described may be adequate to explain how messages from externally applied noxious stimuli are processed, but they certainly do not explain chronic pain. For instance, inflamed joints or broken bones are exquisitely painful if they are simply handled in a gentle manner, activating only low-threshold mechanoreceptors which certainly do not normally give rise to painful sensations.

Guilbaud and her collaborators have examined virtually all fibres, pathways and relays concerned with pain in the peripheral and central nervous

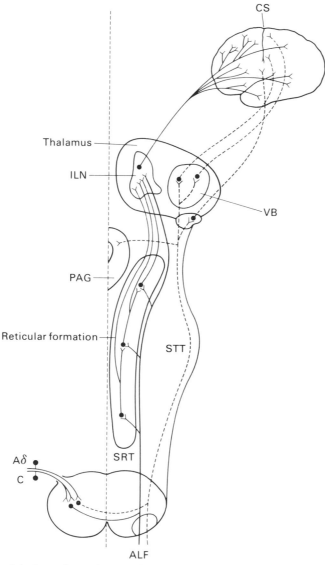

Fig. 8.4 Diagram of central 'pain pathways'. Input from both A-delta and C nociceptors is relayed to the opposite anterolateral funiculus (ALF) of the spinal white matter. The mainly A-delta-driven spinothalamic pathway (STT) is shown as a broken line, giving off collateral branches to the periaqueductal grey matter (PAG) on its way to the ventrobasal thalamus (VB), whence it relays to the postcentral gyrus behind the central sulcus (CS). The spinoreticulodiencephalic pathway is shown as a solid line (SRT) projecting to the reticular formation and thence to the intralaminar nuclei (ILN) of the thalamus. These relay to virtually the whole cortex, but with prefrontal predominance. Note how the two pathways, inextricably mixed in the spinal cord, 'come apart' above it – which is why destructive operations for pain relief cannot be satisfactorily performed above spinal cord level.

system of rats with allergic polyarthritis. In the periphery they found that primary afferent nociceptors, normally silent except when stimulated, are continuously active, and that low-threshold (non-nociceptive) mechanoreceptors from joints discharge at very high rates (Guilbaud *et al.*, 1985). More significantly perhaps, WDR cells in the dorsal horn discharge with a 'nociceptive pattern' when activated via these non-noxious peripheral afferents (Iggo *et al.*, 1984).

Why do WDR cells change their firing pattern? Circumstantial evidence has led Morley (1985) to speculate that primary nociceptive afferents in damaged areas may be chemically altered, and that some chemical modulator substance (perhaps present normally, but now in higher concentration) released from central terminals within the spinal cord or brainstem is able, directly or indirectly, to 'sensitize' WDR cells in the cord so that they respond abnormally to input from normally innocuous primary afferent messages. Such a mechanism may be implicit in the demonstration by Mense (1982) that aspirin raises the peripheral threshold of primary nociceptive afferents.

Neurogenic Pain

The foregoing refers to pain elicited by the stimulation of nociceptors – which in their turn are excited as a result of tissue damage. Some pains, however, are caused *not* by tissue damage but by malfunction of the nervous system itself. Examples of such pains are causalgia, reflex sympathetic dystrophy, partial avulsion of nerve roots (usually the brachial plexus, as a result of RTAs with motor cycles), postherpetic neuralgia, painful diabetic neuropathy, and trigeminal neuralgia, all apparently in the periphery; and cerebral infarction following stroke or subarachnoid haemorrhage more obviously involving the central nervous system (Bowsher, 1991).

These pains, which are referred to as **neurogenic** (= arising from the nervous system), have a certain number of common features. We should, however, begin by pointing out the obvious – since there is no nociceptor activation, these pains do not follow the classical 'pain pathways' described above, and so do not pass by its opioid-sensitive synapses; they are therefore *not* alleviated by conventional analgesics, including the strongest narcotics.

Neurogenic pain is frequently (but not always) described as burning and/or shooting by sufferers. There is autonomic instability, evidenced by the fact that the pain is exacerbated by physical (e.g. cold) or mental (e.g. anxiety) stress and alleviated by relaxation – these patients can nearly always drop off to sleep, though they may wake in agony.

Except in the case of trigeminal neuralgia, there is always a sensory deficit in cases of neurogenic pain. The deficit *always* involves either or both of the 'small-fibre' modalities of pinprick and temperature (warm and cold) sensations – though pain produced by very hot objects is not usually changed to any significant degree. There may or may not be a deficit for 'large-fibre' modalities such as touch – but this is irrelevant for neurogenic pain; touch deficits can exist without there being any neurogenic pain.

Many patients with neurogenic pain suffer from **allodynia** – pain produced by a non-painful stimulus, such as light touch or contact with a cool object. Although not all cases demonstrate it, it *only* occurs in neurogenic pain; so that when observed, it is pathognomonic of the condition.

Medically, the best treatment for neurogenic pains (except trigeminal neuralgia) are the first-generation tricyclic drugs amitriptyline or desipramine. The sooner they are administered, the more effective they are – so valuable time should not be wasted trying, unsuccessfully, to alleviate these pains with analgesics. Trigeminal neuralgia is of course treated with the anticonvulsant carbamazepine.

Transcutaneous nerve stimulation and high-frequency vibration (Lundeberg, 1983) are often effective in neurogenic pain, as are some forms of manual physiotherapy (see Chapter 14). Acupuncture, on the other hand, which activates opioidergic mechanisms, is not.

Some conditions, notably malignant disease, but sometimes also such conditions as brachial plexus avulsion, may produce a mixture of tissue damage and neurogenic pain. In such conditions, a burning element may be noticed when the tissue damage element has been wholly or partly relieved. This is a sign *not* to persist with the treatment that has relieved the tissue damage pain, but to undertake specific therapy for the neurogenic element.

References

Abdel-Maguid, T.E., and Bowsher, D. (1985) The grey matter of the dorsal horn of the adult human spinal cord, including comparisons with general somatic and visceral afferent cranial nerve nuclei. *J. Anat.*, **142**, 33–58

Boivie, J. (1979) An anatomical reinvestigation of the termination of the spinothalamic tract in the monkey. *J. Comp. Neurol.*, **186**, 343–69

Bowsher, D. (1957) Termination of the central pain pathway in man: the conscious appreciation of pain. *Brain*, **80**, 606–22

Bowsher, D. (1991) Neurogenic pain syndromes and their management. *Brit. Med. Bull.*, **47**, 644–66

Guilbaud, G., Iggo, A. and Tegner, R. (1985) Sensory receptors in ankle joint capsules of normal and arthritic rats. *Exp. Brain Res.*, **58**, 29–40

Iggo, A., Guilbaud, G. and Tegner, R. (1984) Sensory mechanisms in arthritic rat joints. In *Advances in Pain Research and Therapy*, vol. 6 (eds L. Kruger and J. Kiebeskind, J.), Raven Press, New York, pp. 83–93

Lundeberg, T.C.M. (1983) Vibratory stimulation for the alleviation of chronic pain. *Acta Physiol. Scand.*, Suppl. 523, 1–51

Mantyh, P.W. (1983) The spinothalamic tract in the primate: a re-examination using wheatgerm agglutinin conjugated to horseradish peroxidase. *Neuroscience*, **9**, 847–62

Mense, S. (1982) Reduction of the bradykinin-induced activation of feline group III and IV muscle receptors by acetylsalicylic acid. *J. Physiol.*, **326**., 269–84

Morley, J.S. (1985) Peptides in nociceptive pathways. In *Persistent Pain: Modern Methods of Treatment*, vol. 5 (eds S. Lipton and J.B. miles), Academic Press, London, pp. 65–91

Spiller W.G. and Martin E. (1912) The treatment of persistent pain of organic origin in the lower part of the body by division of the anterolateral column of the spinal cord. *J. Am. Med. Assoc.* **58**, 1489–90

Vierck, C.J., Greenspan, J.D., Ritz, L.A., and Yeomans, D.C. (1985) The spinal pathway contributing to the ascending conduction and the descending modulation of pain sensations and reactions. In *Spinal Afferent Processing* (ed. T.L. Yaksh), Plenum Press, New York, pp. 275–330

Willis, W.D. (1985) Nociceptive pathways: anatomy and physiology of nociceptive ascending pathways. *Phil. Trans. R. Soc. Lond.*, **B308**, 253–86

9 Modulation of nociceptive input

DAVID BOWSHER

Introduction

The phenomenon cited at the end of the preceding chapter, namely that aspirin raises the threshold of peripheral nociceptors, is an example of **peripheral modulation** (see Chapter 8 p. 51) It is now known that morphine can also act at the peripheral (receptor) end of primary afferent neurons – and has been exploited by the intra-articular injection of morphine in painful arthritis. Most other forms of pain modulation take place within the central nervous system (CNS).

Pain modulation

The gate control theory

This theory of pain modulation was put forward by Melzack and Wall in 1965. Although the details are still much disputed by research workers, the theory has proved enormously fruitful not only in our understanding of pain mechanisms and their modulation, but also in enabling us to devise methods of controlling pain on a rational basis. At its simplest, the theory postulates that within the spinal cord there are mechanisms which may 'open the gate' to impulses generated by noxious stimulation, so that we become abnormally aware of them (e.g. banging an inflamed joint), and others which tend to 'close the gate' so that we are less aware of noxious input (Figure 9.1).

A simple, obvious and well-known example of the latter is the everyday phenomenon of 'rubbing a pain better'. This obviously works (to a greater or lesser extent), otherwise the whole human race would not do it instinctively! It appears that low-threshold cutaneous mechanoreceptors (A-beta fibres), the main central axons of which pass up the dorsal columns without synapse until they reach the gracile and cuneate nuclei, give off segmental collaterals on entering the spinal cord (Figure 9.2). These axon collaterals terminate *on* the terminals of A-delta and C nociceptor fibres in the outer laminae of the spinal grey matter. When low-threshold mechanoreceptors are activated by rubbing, their collateral endings partially excite the nociceptor terminals, so that when impulses come along the nociceptor fibres, they find the terminals in a refractory state, i.e. in a state of reduced excitability, so that the quantity of transmitter substance released from the nociceptor terminals in response to impulses coming along their own fibres is reduced or even abolished. This way of 'closing the gate' is an example of the physiological mechanism of **presynaptic inhibition**.

Transcutaneous Electrical Nerve Stimulation (TENS)

It will be seen immediately that this mechanism is the basis of pain relief by transcutaneous electrical nerve stimulation, and indeed TENS was the first (and very successful) deliberate application of the gate control theory (Wall and Sweet, 1967). TENS is **high-frequency low-intensity** stimulation – low intensity because it only activates the largest low-threshold cutaneous nerve fibres; and high-frequency because not only are these large fibres capable of carrying impulses at higher rates than smaller fibres, but because TENS is in fact most effective at relatively high stimulation rates. The anatomical arrangement of these A-beta fibres (see Figure 9.2) means that the segmental collaterals can also be activated by excitation travelling backwards (*antidromically*) down the dorsal column fibres; so that *dorsal column stimulation* (DCS) also works, at least in part, by the same mechanism.

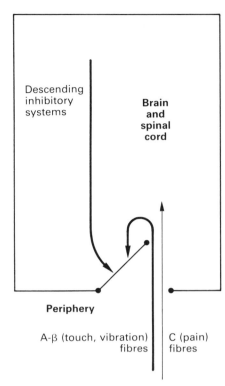

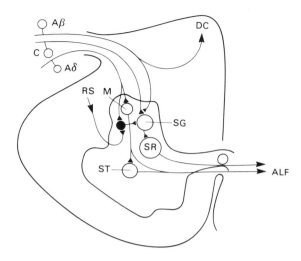

Fig. 9.2 Spinal cord circuitry. C polymodal nociceptors excite cells in the substantia gelatinosa (SG), which converges on to spinoreticular cells (SR) in deeper layers. Acting on the C terminals are terminals of collateral axons of A-beta fibres, whose main fibres pass up the dorsal columns (DC). Thus TENS stimulation applied to peripheral A-beta fibres or antidromic stimulation of DC fibres in the spinal cord will presynaptically inhibit C terminals. A-delta fibres end on marginal layer (M) cells in lamina I, as well as on deeper (lamina V) spinothalamic (ST) cells; but they also have collaterals reaching inhibitory enkephalinergic interneurons (solid black) in the substantia gelatinosa, which inhibit relay cells (SG) in the substantia gelatinosa. Since the inhibitory interneurons are driven by A-delta primary afferents, the effective stimulus will be pinprick (i.e. acupuncture); fibres descending from the brainstem (RS) also reach these inhibitory interneurons; since they are enkephalinergic, their action is reversible by naloxone. ALF, anterolateral funiculus.

Fig. 9.1 Gate control theory. Impulses in small C fibres in the periphery, generated by potentially painful stimuli, push open the gate into the central nervous system and can thus enter into consciousness; the more impulses, the harder they push, and the more intense the resultant sensation. There are two mechanisms which can act to close the gate, partially or completely. The first is 'pulling it to' from the outside; this is done by impulses in large ('touch') fibres, and can be activated by 'rubbing it better', vibration and TENS, as well as indirectly by dorsal column stimulation (DCS). The second mechanism, equivalent to closing the gate from the inside, is carried out by inhibitory mechanisms within the central nervous system. These can be activated by endorphins which are released by procedures such as acupuncture, and so-called psychological mechanisms such as the failure to feel pain in moments of great excitement; endorphins are also imitated by drugs such as morphine and many other analgesics.

Lundeberg (1983) with particular reference to pain, and found to be a very useful alternative to TENS.

It is now realized that there are several different 'gate mechanisms' within the spinal cord, and indeed at higher levels of the nervous system as well. The following paragraphs will examine some of them.

Vibration

Electricity is not the only way of exciting peripheral A-beta fibres; they can be selectively activated by vibration. Vibration has long been used in physiotherapy, but has recently been reinvestigated by

Pharmacological Pain Modulation (Opioids)

Looking at pain modulation from another aspect, it has been known for centuries that morphine abolishes tissue damage type pain – but not pin-prick sensation or neurogenic pain. In the early 1970s, several research groups discovered that certain neurons have morphine *receptors* or *binding sites*. These pharmacological receptors must not be confused with physiological peripheral receptors, which transduce external energy into nerve impulses. Pharmacological receptors are in fact sites on the membrane of the nerve cell or its processes (dendrites) at which a particular substance (in this case morphine) acts either to excite or to inhibit the neuron. In this sense, all transmitter substances in presynaptic nerve terminals act at specific receptors, which are in fact postsynaptic sites on target neurons. Morphine, of course, is not a naturally occurring transmitter substance; but it imitates naturally occurring transmitters, the first of which, the *enkephalins*, were discovered in 1975. Other subsequently discovered natural *opioid* substances include beta-endorphin and dynorphin.

Morphine binding sites are not only found in *some* (but not all) neurons in pain pathways, but also in some neurons in the respiratory and vomiting centres, which is why respiration is depressed and nausea elicited by morphine. This is a useful example of the general, and important, axiom that no transmitter and no type of receptor or binding site is specific to a single functional system, such as the 'pain system'.

Based on the facts given in earlier chapters, it is easy to predict that morphine binding sites will be found on neurons in the spinoreticulodiencephalic pathway chiefly responsible for the perception of tissue damage type pain, but *not* to any great extent in the direct spinothalamic pathway mainly responsible for the perception of sharp pricking pain.

In fact, a heavy concentration of opiate receptors is found in the substantia gelatinosa (lamina II) near the tip of the dorsal horn of the spinal grey matter. Since this is close to the surface of the spinal cord, opiates introduced into the spinal subarachnoid space by intrathecal (or even epidural) injection or infusion easily seep into the substantia gelatinosa and produce analgesia, hopefully without producing less desirable effects by action at higher levels of the CNS.

It is, of course, implicit that the naturally occurring transmitters imitated by morphine, and therefore morphine itself (and other narcotic analgesics) **inhibit** the neurons upon which they act. It is now known that within the substantia gelatinosa there are short-axoned **enkephalinergic interneurons**, the terminals of which make contact with other neurons in laminae I and II which they thus inhibit. It is therefore of interest to enquire how these inhibitory enkephalinergic interneurons are activated.

Acupuncture

It transpires that A-delta primary afferent nociceptors make synaptic contact with the interneurons; such contacts may be collateral branches of axons terminating in laminae I and/or V. Peripherally, A-delta nociceptors are activated by pinprick stimuli; within the spinal cord, their synaptic action is most effective at a stimulation rate of 2 or 3/s (2–3 Hz). Pinprick stimulation at 2 or 3 Hz is commonly known as acupuncture; it is more accurate and helpful to consider it (in contrast to TENS) as **high-intensity low-frequency** stimulation. Acupuncture points appear to be where small bundles of A-delta afferents (accompanied by sympathetic efferents) pierce the deep fascia. They can of course be stimulated electrically; unfortunately this is sometimes called 'acupuncture-like TENS', which is confusing as TENS and acupuncture are almost opposites. Since acupuncture is enkephalinergic, its effects can be reversed by the opioid antagonist drug naloxone (Sjölund and Eriksson, 1979).

This explanation, however, is only true for acupuncture applied within the same segment as the pain (segmental acupuncture); the mechanism of remote acupuncture must be different (Figure 9.3).

The other known input to enkephalinergic interneurons in the substantia gelatinosa is from fibres descending from the brainstem. One group of such fibres uses 5-hydroxytryptamine (serotonin) as its transmitter. These brainstem serotoninergic neurons appear to be driven from the periaqueductal grey matter (PAG) in the midbrain. It will be recalled that the PAG obtains an input, probably a collateral input, from the direct spinothalamic pathway – particularly that part arising from cells in lamina I of the dorsal horn, in which A-delta primary afferent nociceptors terminate. Thus a pinprick-stimulus-generated loop from the marginal layer (lamina 1) to the PAG and back again, relaying through the lower brainstem to the substantia gelatinosa (lamina II) may explain remote (non-segmental) acupuncture (see also Chapter 8).

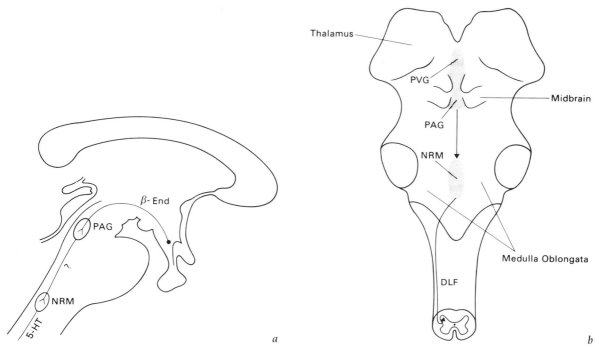

Fig. 9.3   *a*, Descending inhibitory pathways. Beta-endorphinergic (*β*-End) cells in the hypothalamus project to the periaqueductal grey matter (PAG); thence fibres with an unknown transmitter (?) pass to the lower brainstem (NRM), from which a final serotoninergic relay (5-HT) passes down the dorsolateral white funiculus of the spinal cord to excite the enkephalinergic interneurons shown in Figure 9.2. *b*, Dorsal view of descending inhibitory pathways from periventricular (PVG) and periaqueductal (PAG) grey matter to relay (NRM) in the medulla oblongata, whence serotoninergic fibres pass in the dorsolateral funiculus (DLF) down the spinal cord to enkephalinergic interneurons in the substantia gelatinosa (see Figure 9.2).

Neurochemical Pain Modulation

It may be mentioned that a group of fibres descending from neurons in the brainstem to the dorsal horn are noradrenergic, i.e. their transmitter is noradrenaline. They too have an analgesic action, but it is by direct inhibition of dorsal horn nociceptive neurons, not via an enkephalinergic interneuron. Some tricyclic drugs also reduce noradrenaline removal, so they promote this kind of non-opioid analgesia as well. Perhaps this is why these tricyclics are one of the few drugs which are useful in neurogenic pain, which is resistant to narcotic (opioid) analgesics.

When considering the lamina I → PAG → brainstem → lamina II circuit (figure 9.3), an interesting neurochemical feature is that a microinjection of morphine into the PAG produces a very profound analgesia (Tsou and Jang, 1964). It is now known that there is a pathway from the hypothalamus (to

which the prefrontal cortex projects) to the PAG; and that the transmitter substance in this pathway is beta-endorphin. Since opioids, including beta-endorphin, are universally inhibitory, it has been supposed that inhibitory PAG interneurons are inhibited by the hypothalamus, thus disinhibiting (i.e. exciting) the projection neurons from the PAG to the lower brainstem. Neurosurgeons have succeeded in suppressing pain by implanting stimulating electrodes in the PAG.

In this chapter, a number of ways in which pain can be modulated have been briefly reviewed. We have seen that nociceptive circuitry can be interfered with by several manoeuvres – by high-frequency low-intensity stimulation (vibration or TENS), low-frequency high-intensity stimulation (mechanical or electrical acupuncture), or by chemical manipulation. All of these change pain tolerance level, not the pain perception threshold;

the latter is modulated only by aspirin and morphine acting peripherally at the receptor (physiological transducer).

It must not be imagined that these methods must all be used independently of one another. For instance, electrical stimulators are often used at variable parameters so as to attempt to produce analgesia almost simultaneously by TENS and by electroacupuncture.

The time factor remains to be mentioned. If all the modulatory mechanisms worked only in the ways described in this chapter, their duration of analgesic action should only exceed the duration of the eliciting stimulus by quite a short time. Yet, in fact, analgesia often lasts a remarkably long time after stimulation has ceased. This can only be explained by a mechanism akin to that described in Chapter 8 (p. 52), but this time probably within the CNS. Just as neuromodulatory chemicals, probably peptides, may be responsible for long-lasting pain, so long-term chemical changes within the neurons must presumably be responsible for long-lasting pain relief, by changing the responsiveness of the neurons themselves. The nervous system does not live by electricity alone!

References

Bowsher, D. (1991) Neurogenic pain syndromes and their management. *Br. Med. Bull.*, **47**, 644–66

Lundeberg, T.C.M. (1983) Vibratory stimulation for the alleviation of chronic pain. *Acta Physiol. Scand.*, Suppl. 523; 1–51

Melzack R. Wall, P.D. (1965) Pain mechanisms: a new theory. *Science*, **150**, 971–9

Sjölund, B.H. and Eriksson, M.B.E. (1979) The influence of naloxone on analgesia produced by peripheral conditioning stimulation. *Brain Res*, **173**, 295–302

Tsou K. and Jang C.S. (1964) Studies on the site of analgesic action of morphine by intracerebral microinjection. *Sci. Sinica.*, **131**, 1099–109

Wall, P.D. Sweet, W.H. (1967) Temporary abolition of pain in man. *Science*, **155**, 108–9

10 Neuropharmacology of the pain pathway

JOHN W. THOMPSON

Introduction

The two major components of the nociceptive pathway are (i) the nociceptors and their associated peripheral nerve fibres and (ii) the central nociceptive (pain) pathways, which include ascending nociceptive pathways extending to the thalamus, hypothalamus, limbic system and sensory cortex; and the descending pain inhibitory pathways running from the midbrain via the brainstem and medulla to the dorsal horn at all levels of the spinal cord (see Chapters 7, 8 and 9). Communication between these neural pathways takes place by means of chemical transmitters, commonly called neurotransmitters. The main purpose of this chapter is to discuss the nature, distribution and mechanism of action of these neurotransmitters together with the ways in which their functions can be modified by external factors in order to achieve pain control. It is important for the reader to realize that at the present time the subject of the neuropharmacology of pain is under intensive study and is therefore in a state of flux. The overall picture contains many gaps which need to be filled; as a consequence, this account is unavoidably incomplete and, in places, necessarily conjectural. The neuropharmacology of the pain pathway will be discussed on a neuroanatomical basis under four headings: the nociceptors; the primary afferent neuron; the neurons of the dorsal horn; and the neurons of the descending pathways.

Neuropharmacology of nociceptors

The microscopic structure and molecular mechanisms of both the A-delta and C nociceptors are as yet unknown. By contrast, much is known about the physiological characteristics of the nociceptive neurons to which the nociceptors are connected and which represent the primary afferent neuron transmitting nociceptive information to the dorsal horn of the spinal cord. It is well established that there are major differences between the pharmacological properties of the two groups of nociceptors. Thus, A-delta nociceptors, also known as A-mechano-heat nociceptors (AMH), respond mainly, as their name implies, to mechanical and thermal stimulation although they will also respond to some pharmacological agents (e.g. bradykinin). The other, and numerically larger group, is the C-polymodal nociceptors which respond to all three types of noxious stimuli namely chemical, thermal and mechanical. The non-myelinated sensory fibres at whose distal end the C-polymodal nociceptors reside, are rich in neuropeptides and these are released during activity. In addition, this group of nociceptors become sensitized with repeated exposure to heat, a property that may explain in part the well-known phenomenon of hyperalgesia (an increased response to a normally painful stimulus, IASP 1986) which follows tissue injury, for example, sunburn.

Chemical stimulants of the nociceptors

Although the C-polymodal nociceptors are sensitive to chemical, thermal and mechanical stimuli, it seems probable that, with the exception of the most transient mechanical stimulus, these nociceptors are mainly stimulated by chemical agents released as a result of local tissue damage. Thus mechanical or thermal damage trigger inflammatory responses as a result of which various potent pharmacological agents are released which stimulate the C-polymodal nociceptors.

The principal substances that stimulate or sensitize nociceptors are:

1. Protons (H^+)
2. Certain neurotransmitters – 5-hydroxytryptamine (serotonin)
   histamine
   acetylcholine

3. Polypeptides – bradykinin
                    kallidin
4. Eicosanoids – prostaglandins (E and F)
5. Cellular metabolites – adenosine triphosphate
                    (ATP)
                    adenosine diphosphate
                    (ADP)
                    lactic acid ($\rightarrow H^+$)
                    potassium ions (K^+)
6. Spicy plants – capsaicin (red peppers)
                    capsicum (black pepper)

This list includes many of the chemical agents released during acute and chronic inflammation (Nos. 1–5). It is evident that these tissue damage transducers respond to a very wide range of different chemical classes. Some general comments about these agents will now be made; for a detailed account the reader is referred to Rang *et al.* (1991).

It is a matter of common knowledge that acidic solutions (rich in protons) readily cause pain; and experiments have shown that this is associated with brief depolarization (i.e. excitation) of the sensory nerve fibre (Krishtal and Pidoplichko, 1980). Of the more complex agents, some such as 5-hydroxytryptamine (5HT$_3$ receptor), ATP and capsaicin act directly by opening the ion channels of the nociceptive neuron whereas others, for example, 5-hydroxytryptamine (5HT$_1$ receptor), bradykinin and histamine, act by stimulating a second messenger system. Prostaglandins and leukotrienes act indirectly, the former by sensitizing the nociceptors to the polypeptide bradykinin and the latter by causing the release of other neuroactive agents from polymorphonuclear leukocytes (Levine *et al.*, 1986). ATP and other metabolites released from active cells may stimulate nociceptors directly by opening ion channels or indirectly by releasing neuroactive agents, or both; knowledge in this area is incomplete. By contrast, red peppers are well known to cause a burning taste in the mouth which is due to the active agent capsaicin (8-methyl-N-vanillyl-6-nonenamide). On local application to skin or mucous membrane this activates a specfic receptor which depolarizes the C-fibre to cause brief pain and a longer-lasting hyperalgesia. In addition, capsaicin releases the algogenic polypeptide Substance P (SP) (see below).

The primary afferent neuron

In spite of intensive research efforts, the neurotransmitters released from the central endings of the A-delta and C primary afferent neurons have not yet been identified unequivocally. The neurotransmitters acetylcholine (ACh) and noradrenaline (NAd), so familiar in other parts of the nervous system, are clearly not involved, likewise 5HT and dopamine (D). This leaves as possible candidates amino acids, peptides and ATP. However, the excitatory amino acids L-glutamate and L-aspartate are probably not involved because specific antagonists of these compounds fail to block the activation of dorsal horn neurons by C-fibres (although these antagonists have been shown to block transmission systems in which the afferents are large-diameter myelinated neurons). The most likely candidate is Substance P (SP) or one of the other larger peptides such as vasoactive intestinal peptide (VIP), cholecystokinin (probably as the C-terminal octapeptide CCK-8), or somatostatin; or possibly all three are involved. It has been suggested that SP is the neurotransmitter released at the central endings of the C-fibres which originate from somatic structures, while VIP is released at the endings of those primary afferents which originate from visceral structures. Progress is likely to be hindered until specific antagonists are developed which can be used to identify whether SP, VIP, CCK or possibly ATP are involved as neurotransmitters at this crucial link in the chain of nociceptive neurons

The neurons of the dorsal horn

The neuroanatomical basis which underlies modulation of nociceptive input within the spinal cord has been described earlier in Chapter 9 (see Gate control theory). The interactive control between the different neurons involved is achieved pharmacologically by the synaptic release of appropriate excitatory and inhibitory neurotransmitters. For example, the synaptic transmission of nociceptive information from neuron A to neuron B may be temporarily blocked as a result of the action of an inhibitory neurotransmitter released from the endings of an adjacent neuron C which prevents the release of the neurotransmitter from the endings of neuron A, a mechanism known as presynaptic inhibition. We must now consider the possible candidates involved in this process. The number of amino acids and peptides which are added to the list of putative neurotransmitters in the dorsal horn continues to grow! Table 10.1 contains a list of possible candidates which have been classified both chemically (amino acids or peptides) and pharmacologically (excitatory or inhibitory).

Table 10.1   List of some possible neurotransmitters in the dorsal horn of the spinal cord

Chemical class	Excitatory	Inhibitory
Amino acids		
Aspartate	+	
Glutamate	+	
Gamma-aminobutyric acid (GABA)		+
Glycine		+
Peptides		
Substance P (SP)	+	
Vasoactive intestinal peptide	+	
Cholecystokinin (CCK)	+	
Somatostatin	+	
Bombesin	+	
Neurotensin	+	
met/leu-enkephalin		+
Dynorphin		+

In considering this formidable list, it is important to note that at any given synapse *more than one transmitter may be involved*. Indeed, evidence suggests that several transmitters may be released simultaneously (so-called co-release), with each neurotransmitter carrying out a particular function at the synapse. It is therefore the final blend of pharmacological 'soup' that determines the quantitative and temporal behaviour of synaptic transmission, i.e. the content, duration and timing of the information transmitted. Aspartate and glutamate excite most dorsal horn cells and it is therefore unlikely that these agents are involved *exclusively* in the transmission of nociceptive information. On the other hand, there is now strong evidence that aspartate acts on specific NMDA receptors (based on the abbreviation n-methyl-d-aspartate, a chemical derivative of aspartate which is selective for, and therefore used to map out, these receptors). Furthermore, NMDA receptors in conjunction with SP (acting on tachykinin receptors) apparently mediate a phenomenon known as 'windup' in which nociceptive signals arriving in the dorsal horn undergo a cumulative increase in magnitude. This is probably an important mechanism in the expansion of painful areas that is so characteristic of clinical chronic pain states (Woolf, 1991).

GABA and glycine are two important inhibitory neurotransmitters and the evidence available suggests that GABA is involved in the modulation of nociceptive transmission. Figure 10.1 illustrates the location of GABAergic interneurons from the endings of which GABA is released and which in turn, by presynaptic inhibition, stops the release of excitatory neurotransmitter(s) from the endings of the nociceptive C-fibres. This prevents onward transmission of nociceptive information to cells in the substantia gelatinosa (SG) and therefore to the brain.

The role of each peptide found in the dorsal horn (see Table 10.1, which is not exhaustive!) has yet to be determined. As mentioned earlier, it appears that these agents are co-released from nerve endings and through their admixture subtly control synaptic transmission of nociceptive (and non-nociceptive) information. However, the greatest advances in knowledge about neurotransmitters in the dorsal horn concerns the opioid peptides which were first isolated by Kosterlitz and Hughes in 1975 (Hughes *et al.*, 1975). The subject of the opioid peptides has become a vast area of its own and only a brief summary can be given here.

Opioid peptides and the receptors upon which they act are widely distributed throughout the brain and spinal cord, as indicated in Table 10.2. There are three types of opioid receptors named mu (μ), delta (δ) and kappa (κ) to which should be added a fourth type known as sigma (σ) which does not belong to the opioid receptor family but is important because some of the side-effects produced by opioids (for example, pentazocine) are probably due to stimulation of these sigma receptors. The opioid peptides can be classified into three groups on the basis of their chemical and pharmacological properties and also on their anatomical distribution (Thompson, 1984a, 1990), as set out in Table 10.2. Each opioid peptide is formed by cleavage from a large precursor protein molecule. Thus beta-endorphin is formed from pro-opiomelanocortin (from which ACTH is also formed); both met-enkephalin and leu-enkephalin are cleaved from pro-enkephalin; and dynorphins A and B are formed from prodynorphin. At one time it was thought that each opioid peptide acted as a specific endogenous agonist at only one of the three types of opioid receptors, i.e. mu, delta or kappa, but this is now known to be incorrect. In reality, all these opioid peptides possess some degree of activity at all three types of receptor, although each peptide is relatively selective for one of the three opioid receptors. For example, as indicated in Table 10.2, beta-endorphin is the most potent peptide at mu receptors followed by, in decreasing order, dynorphin A, met-enkephalin and leu-enkephalin. Table 10.2 also shows that stimulating each type of receptor produces its own

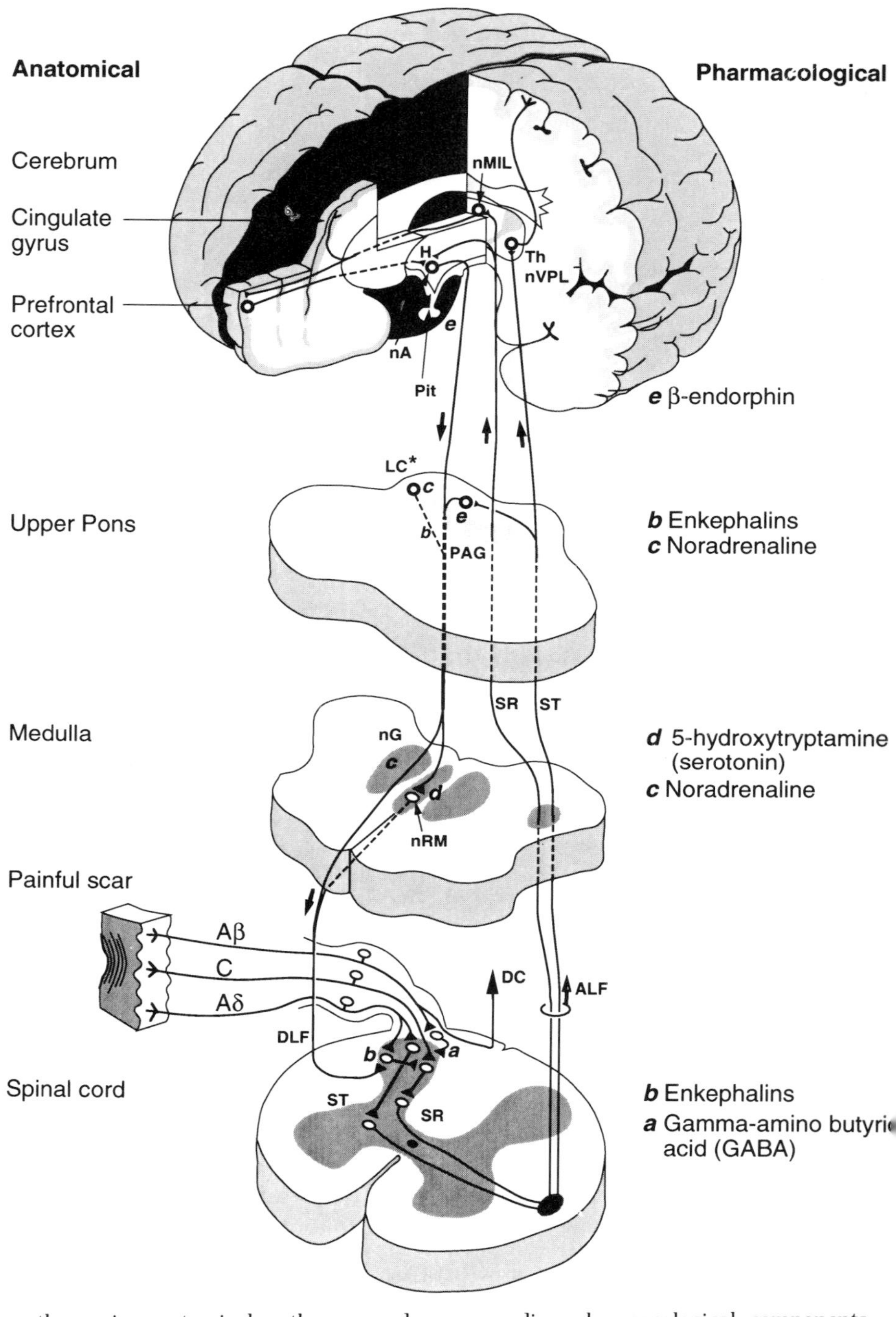

Abbreviations: $A\beta$, C and $A\delta$ represent afferent neurones conducting information from tactile receptors, polymodal nociceptors and high threshold mechanoreceptors, respectively; ALF = anterolateral funiculus; nA = arcuate nucleus of hypothalamus; DC = dorsal column (cuneate and gracile tracts); DLF = dorsolateral funiculus; H = hypothalamus; LC* = locus ceruleus; the asterisk denotes that LC is included in this section for diagrammatic convenience although in reality lies in the mid-pontine region caudal to PAG; nA = arcuate nucleus of the hypothalamus; nG = nucleus gigantocellularis; nMIL = medial intralaminar nucleus of the thalamus; Pit. = pituitary gland; nVPL = ventroposterior lateral nucleus of thalamus; PAG = periaqueductal grey; nRM = nucleus raphe magnus; SR = spinoreticular tract; ST = spinothalamic tract; Th = thalamus.

(This figure is based on the publications of: Bowsher 1985, 1987; Cousins, 1991; Fields and Basbaum, 1994; Han and Terenius, 1982; Jones et al. 1991; Le Bars et al. 1979; and Thompson and Filshie, 1993). © Audio Visual Centre, University of Newcastle Upon Tyne, UK, 1994.

Fig. 10.1 Diagram to show the main anatomical pathways and corresponding pharmacological components (neurotransmitters and neuromodulators a to e; see figure) of the nociceptive system at the levels of the spinal cord, medulla, upper pons and cerebral hemisphere. The left cerebral hemisphere has been sectioned coronally and the portion anterior to the section removed apart from a medial saggital slice which has itself been partly cut away for demonstration purposes.

The **ascending** pathways (↑) involved in transmitting nociceptive information from the skin to the higher centres (sensory cortex), prefrontal cortex and cingulate gyrus) via the dorsal horn, the anterolateral funiculus and the thalamus are shown. The **descending inhibitory** pathways (↓) from the pre-frontal cortex to the dorsal horn via the arcuate nucleus of the hypothalamus, the periaqueductal grey and dorsolateral funiculus are also shown. **Connections** between the spinothalamic tract and the descending inhibitory pathway via the periaqueductal grey are shown, as also are those between the spinoreticular tract and the hypothalamus.

Table 10.2 Classification of opioid peptides and opioid receptors

Receptors	Mu (μ)	Delta (δ)	Kappa (κ)	Sigma (σ)[a]
Putative endogenous agonists	β-endorphin (β-end)	met-enkephalin (met) leu-enkephalin (leu)	Dynorphin A1–13 (dyn A) A1–8 Dynorphin B	?
Distribution of peptidergic neurones	Anterior pituitary Hypothalamus	Striatum Preoptic hypothalamus Limbic system Raphe nuclei Spinal cord Adrenal medulla Sympathetic ganglia Myenteric ganglia	Posterior pituitary Hypothalamus Spinal cord Submucous plexus of GI tract	
Potency order of endogenous agonists	β-end > dyn A > met > leu	met = leu = β-end > dyn A	dyn A $\gg$ β-end $\gg$ leu = met	
Synthetic agonist	Morphine	DPDPE (experimental)	Pentazocine	Phencyclidine Pentazocine
Antagonist	Naloxone	Naloxone; but less potent than at mu	Naloxone; but less potent than at mu	Naloxone; but less potent than at mu
Effector pathway	cAMP$\downarrow$	cAMP$\downarrow$	?	?
Ion channel action	K$^+$ channel activator	K$^+$ channel activator	Ca^{2+} channel inhibition	?
Effects				
Analgesia	Supraspinal analgesia	Analgesia	Spinal analgesia	No analgesia
Psychotropic	Euphoria[b]	Euphoria[b]	Sedation	Dysphoria $\pm$ hallucinations
Respiration	Respiratory depression	Respiratory depression	Respiratory depression	Respiratory stimulation
GI tract	Constipation (central)	Constipation (peripheral)		
Pupil	Miosis		Miosis	Mydriasis
Motor		Motor functions		Motor stimulation
Dependence	Physical dependence		Physical dependence (nalorphine type)	

[a] Sigma receptors are not considered to belong to the family of opioid receptors. However, they are important because some of the side-effects produced by opioids are probably due to stimulation of sigma receptors.
[b] With clinical opioid analgesia the word 'euphoria' implies a sense of peaceful well-being that accompanies the relief of pain. By contrast, with opioid abuse (especially intravenous administration = 'mainlining') the word 'euphoria' implies a temporary state of ecstasy.
DPDPE = D-penicillamine D-pencillamine enkephalin.
Source: Reproduced from Thompson (1990) in *Opioids in the Treatment of Cancer Pain* (ed. D. Doyle), by kind permission of Royal Society of Medicine Services Ltd.

profile of effects but with a considerable degree of overlap. Two of the receptors (mu and delta) operate by opening potassium (K^+) channels whereas the third (kappa) acts by inhibiting calcium (Ca^{2+}) channels in the relevant neuronal membranes (the mechanism underlying the non-opioid sigma receptor is as yet unknown). The overall action of opioid peptides is to *inhibit* the nerve cell or synapse upon which they act. It remains undecided as to whether this inhibitory action is pre-or postsynaptic. Thus, a presynaptic action of the opioid peptide would block synaptic transmission by interfering with the release of the appropriate neurotransmitter(s) whereas a postsynaptic action would act by rendering the membrane of the postsynaptic neuron inexcitable by the neurotransmitter(s) normally released. Although this distinction is important academically, in practice the end result is the same, namely to produce partial or complete block of synaptic transmission in the neuronal pathway under consideration.

In the gate control theory of pain, conceptualized by Melzack and Wall in 1965, a pivotal structure is an input-driven short interneuron that releases an inhibitory neurotransmitter in the vicinity of a synapse that transmits nociceptive information (see Chapter 9, and Figure 9.2). The effect of the release of this inhibitory transmitter is to control or 'gate' the amount of nociceptive information fed to the next neuron in the chain and ultimately, therefore, to the spinal cord and to the brain. More recent work has identified the input-driven cell as an enkephalinergic interneuron (see Figures 9.3a and 10.2). The weight of evidence suggests that this interneuron synthesizes met-enkephalin which, by activating the potassium (K^+) channels of the relay cells, inhibits the onward transmission of nociceptive information within the cells of the substantia gelatinosa (SG).

The neuropharmacology of the ascending connections between the dorsal horn and the medulla, pons and cerebral cortex is not known. By contrast, much is known about the neuropharmacology of the descending pathways and this will now be discussed.

The neurons of the descending pathways

As discussed earlier, opioid peptides have been shown to play a pivotal role in the regulation of nociceptive input within the dorsal horn of the spinal cord (see above). Equally, these agents have also been demonstrated to play a vital role in the descending inhibitory control exerted by the neuronal pathways that descend from the midbrain and brainstem to the dorsal horn of the spinal cord. Thus, when opiates are injected into the cerebral ventricles this produces analgesia and so indicates the presence of supraspinal sites of action of these agents. In other experiments, morphine, met-enkephalin and the opioid antagonist naloxone were precisely placed by microinjection into various areas of the midbrain and brainstem. The results demonstrated that opiates and enkephalins produce analgesia only at highly specific sites which are located within the midbrain at the ventral part of the periaqueductal grey matter (PAG) and within the caudal brainstem at the nucleus raphe magnus (NRM) and the adjacent nucleus paragigantocellularis (NRPG).

Another important finding is that the NRM contains the majority of those neurons that synthesize 5-hydroxytryptamine (5HT) and which project to all levels of the spinal cord terminating on to the

Fig. 10.2 Diagram to illustrate how the input of nociceptive information to the brain is controlled through presynaptic inhibition of chemical transmission between the primary and secondary afferent neurones in the spinal cord. *a*, **Under background conditions**: A nociceptor generates a nerve impulse which travels to its primary afferent nerve ending where it releases the chemical transmitter Substance P (SP) from its stores. The released SP activates post-synaptic SP receptors located on the cell body of the secondary afferent neuron thereby triggering off a nerve impulse which ascends the spinal cord to the thalamus. *b*, **Under conditions of noxious stimulation**: Activation of the descending inhibitory pathway (from supraspinal centres) stimulates enkephalinergic neurons in the spinal cord to release enkephalin which then activates presynaptic opioid receptors located on the primary afferent nerve endings. This inhibits the release of SP and thus blocks chemical transmission between primary and secondary afferent neurons and so prevents the onward transmission of nociceptive information to the thalamus. At spinal level, opiates (e.g. morphine) produce analgesia by mimicking the action of enkephalin on opioid receptors. There is some evidence that enkephalin may also block nociceptive transmission through a *post*synaptic mechanism which involves hyperpolarization of the postsynaptic membrane. (Reproduced from Thompson (1984b) in *Advances in Geriatric Medicine 4* (eds J. Grimley Evans and F.I. Caird), by kind permission of Churchill Livingstone.)

(a)

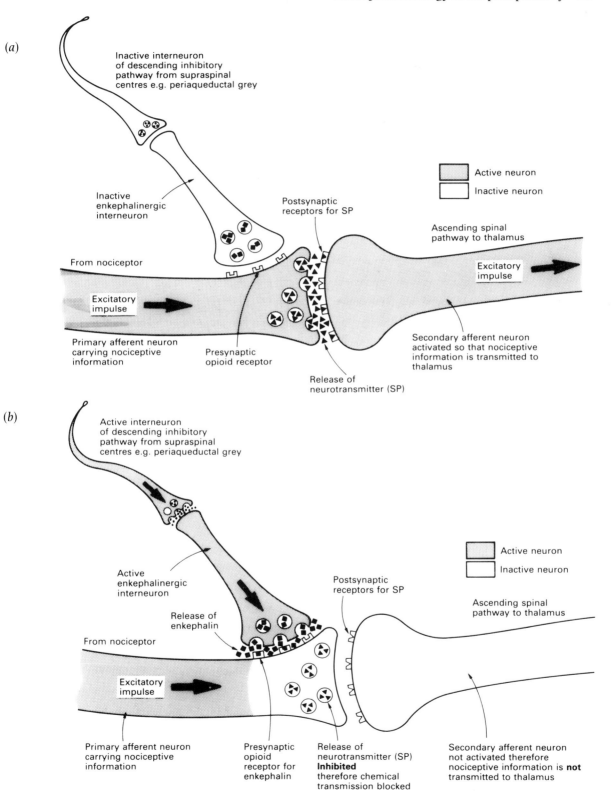

Inactive interneuron
of descending inhibitory
pathway from supraspinal
centres e.g. periaqueductal grey

Postsynaptic
receptors for SP

Active neuron

Inactive neuron

Inactive
enkephalinergic
interneuron

Ascending spinal
pathway to thalamus

Excitatory
impulse

From nociceptor

Excitatory
impulse

Primary afferent neuron
carrying nociceptive
information

Presynaptic
opioid receptor

Secondary afferent neuron
activated so that nociceptive
information is transmitted to
thalamus

Release of
neurotransmitter (SP)

(b)

Active interneuron
of descending inhibitory
pathway from supraspinal
centres e.g. periaqueductal grey

Active neuron

Inactive neuron

Active
enkephalinergic
interneuron

Postsynaptic
receptors for SP

Ascending spinal
pathway to thalamus

Release of
enkephalin

From nociceptor

Excitatory
impulse

Primary afferent neuron
carrying nociceptive
information

Presynaptic
opioid
receptor for
enkephalin

Release of
neurotransmitter (SP)
Inhibited
therefore chemical
transmission blocked

Secondary afferent neuron
not activated therefore
nociceptive information is **not**
transmitted to thalamus

neurons of the dorsal horn. This descending 5HT pathway is of fundamental importance, as shown by the fact that electrical stimulation of it inhibits the activities of convergent dorsal horn cells. Further evidence in support of the role of 5HT in pain control derives from the fact that intrathecal 5HT induces analgesia; and conversely intrathecal 5HT antagonists block analgesia induced by stimulation of the NRM. The situation seems to be that in the normal course of events, noxious stimulation activates the descending pathway which originates in the NRM and releases both 5HT and enkephalin which in turn exert an inhibitory influence on the transmission of *ascending* nociceptive information to the brain.

A controversial area is the mechanism by which the opioid and 5HT systems act together to exert their descending inhibitory control. On the basis of the results of electrical stimulation and on intuitive grounds, it has been thought for some time that exogenous opiates and endogenous opioid peptides induce analgesia by enhancing the descending inhibitory pathways. Surprisingly, the evidence available suggests that the opposite is true, namely that opioids actually *reduce* the descending 5HT-mediated activity. As Dickenson (1989) has pointed out, the solution to this paradox may depend upon the fact that a noxious input activates the descending 5HT system which in turn actually *enhances* the input of noxious signals at the expense of the non-noxious signals, i.e. to increase the noxious/non-noxious signal ratio. Under these conditions the action of morphine or enkephalin is to reduce the amount of descending inhibition which in turn reduces the noxious/non-noxious signal ratio thereby *attenuating* the amount of nociceptive information transmitted to the brain, i.e. producing analgesia.

In addition to 5HT, there are other descending control pathways, particularly noradrenergic (NAd), that project from the locus coeruleus and other brainstem noradrenergic centres. When noradrenaline is applied to nociceptive neurons in the spinal cord it inhibits their activity. It has been shown that alpha 2 (α2) adrenoceptors are involved in the presynaptic inhibitory action which noradrenaline exerts on transmission in the nerve endings of C fibres. Furthermore, procedures that interfere with noradrenergic mechanisms in the spinal cord are known to antagonize the analgesic action of morphine. From this result it may be concluded that part of morphine's action is mediated via noradrenergic mechanisms.

Implications for physiotherapy of the neuropharmacology of the pain pathway

At first sight it may seem unnecessary for the practising physiotherapist to become familiar with the extremely complex and, as yet, incomplete details of the neuropharmacology of pain. However, on reflection it soon becomes clear that there are several very important reasons why physiotherapists should try to understand the general principles involved.

1. Many of the conditions treated by physiotherapists are associated with various types of pain and understanding these is greatly assisted by a knowledge of the underlying neuroanatomy and neuropharmacology.

2. The selection of appropriate methods of treatment depends upon a knowledge of the neurophysiological and neuropharmacological mechanisms responsible for the pain. Thus nociceptive pain, such as that arising from an inflamed joint, involves the release of algogenic agents and is likely to respond to non-steroidal anti-inflammatory drugs (NSAIDs). By contrast, neurogenic or neuropathic pain (see Chapter 8) does not usually respond to either NSAIDs or morphine but will respond to certain psychotropic drugs (see Chapter 11) and to stimulation-induced analgesia such as TENS and vibration and sometimes to acupuncture (see Chapters 13 and 14).

3. Progress in understanding the neuropharmacology of pain will lead to new methods of analgesia. It is obviously important for the practising physiotherapist to keep abreast of these rational therapeutic developments and this can only be achieved with the aid of a knowledge of the fundamental mechanisms involved.

Acknowledgements

The author wishes to thank the editors and publishers who have given permission to reproduce material published elsewhere. He also wishes to express his grateful thanks to Mrs Margaret Cheek for her excellent secretarial help.

References

Bowsher, D. (1985) Sensory mechanisms. *Clinical Neuropsychology*, **45**, 227–44

Bowsher, D. (1987) The physiology of acupuncture. *Journal of the Intractable Pain Society of Great Britain and Ireland*, **5**, 15–18

Cousins, M.J. (1991) Prevention of postoperative pain. Chapter 5 in Proceedings of the Vth World Congress on Pain (eds M.R. Bond, J.E. Charlton and C.J. Woolf). *Pain Research and Clinical Management*, Vol.4. Elsevier, Amsterdam

Dickenson, A.H. (1989) Pain transmission and analgesia. In *Neurotransmitters, Drugs and Disease* (eds R.A. Webster and C.C. Jordan), Blackwell Scientific Publications, Oxford, pp. 446–64

Fields H.L. and Basbaum A.L. (1994) Central nervous system mechanisms of pain modulation. In *Textbook of Pain*, 3rd edn (eds P.D. Wall and R. Melzack). Churchill Livingstone, Edinburgh

Han, J.S. and Terenius, L. (1982) Neurochemical basis of acupuncture analgesia. *Annual Review of Pharmacology and Toxicology*, **22**, 193–220

Hughes, J., Smith, T.W., Kosterlitz, H.W., *et al.* (1975) Identification of two related pentapeptides from the brain with potent opiate agonist activity. *Nature*, **258**, 577–9

IASP (International Association for the Study of Pain) (1986) Classification of chronic pain syndromes and definitions of pain terms. *Pain*, Suppl.3, S219

Jones, A.K.P., Brown, W.D., Friston, K.T., Qi Ky, Frackowiak, R.S.J. (1991) Cortical and subcortical localisation of response to pain in man using positron emission tomography. *Proceedings of the Royal Society of London*, Series B, **244**, 29–44

Krishtal, O.A. and Pidoplichko, V.I. (1980) A receptor for proton in the nerve cell membrane. *Neuroscience*, **5**, 2325–7

Le Bars, D., Dickenson, A.H. and Besson, J.M. (1979) Diffuse noxious inhibitory controls (DNIC). II. Lack of effort on non-convergent neurons, supraspinal involvement and theoretical implications. *Pain*, **6**, 305–327

Levine, J.D., Taiwo, Y.O., Collins, S.D., and Tam, J.K. (1986) Noradrenaline hyperalgesia is mediated through interaction with sympathetic postganglionic neurone terminals rather than activation of primary afferent nociceptors. *Nature*, **323**, 158–60.

Melzack, R. and Wall, P.D. (1965) Pain mechanisms: a new theory. *Science N.Y.*, **150**, 971

Rang, H.D., Bevan S. and Dray, A. (1991) Chemical activation of nociceptive peripheral neurones. *Br. Med. Bull.*, **47**, 534–48

Thompson, J.W. (1983) Electrical stimulation: powerful relief for those chronic pains. *Pulse*, **43**, 50–1

Thompson, J.W. (1984a) Opioid peptides. *Br. Med. J.*, **288**, 259–61

Thompson, J.W. (1984b) Pain: mechanisms and principles of management. In *Advances in Geriatric Medicine 4* (eds J. Grimley Evans and F.I. Caird), Pitman, London, pp. 3–16

Thompson, J.W. (1990) Clinical pharmacology of opioid agonists and partial agonists. In *Opioids in the Treatment of Cancer Pain* (ed. D. Doyle), Royal Society of Medicine Services International Congress and Symposium Series No. 146, Royal Society of Medicine Services Ltd, London, pp. 17–38

Thompson, J.W. and Filshie, J. (1993) Transcutaneous electrical nerve stimulation (TENS) and acupuncture. *Oxford Textbook of Palliative Medicine* (eds D. Doyle, Hanks, G.W.C. and Macdonald, N.). Oxford University Press, Oxford

Woolf, C.J. (1991) Generation of acute pain: central mechanisms. *Br. Med. Bull.*, **47**, 523–33

11 *Pharmacology of pain relief*

JOHN W. THOMPSON

Introduction

Pain may be acute or chronic. Acute pain is always purposeful whereas chronic pain is sometimes purposeful but may progress to become useless and intractable. Acute pain is generally considered to become chronic when it outlasts the normal healing process; in practice this usually means within 1–2 months. Thus, by definition, acute pain is a self-limiting condition, irrespective of whether it is treated promptly and adequately, or neglected, as unfortunately so often happens. Apart from the temporal differences, acute and chronic pain differ greatly in other ways. Thus, chronic pain may be associated with secondary functional and structural changes in the nervous system such as those associated with the development of neurogenic (neuropathic) pain. This is not only responsible for the complex and particularly unpleasant characteristics of this type of chronic pain but also demands that different treatment strategies be employed.

Applying the principles of the neuroanatomy and neuropharmacology of pain described in earlier sections of this book (see Chapters 6–10), there are five methods which may be used, singly or in combination, to control pain (Thompson, 1984):

1. Remove peripheral stimulus	Surgical, e.g. ablation Cryotherapy Neurolytic, e.g. phenol, ethanol Radiotherapy, e.g. shrink neoplasm Pharmacological, e.g. NSAID, corticosteroid; antiepileptic to suppress nociceptive discharges from a neuroma

2. Interrupt nociceptive input	Pharmacological
	   non-invasive, e.g. NSAID
	   invasive, e.g. local anaesthetic
	Surgical, e.g. neurectomy

3. Stimulate nociceptive inhibitory mechanisms	Massage and spinal mobilization ⎫ TENS ⎬ touch receptors, A-β fibres Vibration ⎭ Heat, thermoreceptors, C fibres Cold, thermoreceptors, A-δ fibres Electro/acupuncture, nociceptors, A-δ fibres Counter-irritants, nociceptors, ?C fibres
4. Modulate central appreciation of pain and/or emotional concomitants	Pharmacological, e.g. opioid analgesics, psychotropic drugs, general anaesthetics Psychological, e.g. school for bravery, cognitive/behavioural, counselling, relaxation, biofeedback, hypnosis

5. Block or remove secondary factors maintaining pain	Sympathetic nerve block
	   pharmacological, e.g. adrenoceptor blockers
	   physical, e.g. chemical, surgical
	Vasodilators for pain associated with vascular spasm
	Antispastics for pain associated with spasm of skeletal muscle
	Others, e.g. pituitary ablation for widespread cancer pain

Having defined the five principal methods by which pain can be relieved, we must now consider the different agents that are available to relieve pain. These can be divided conveniently into primary and secondary analgesics, as summarized below. The chapter will then focus on discussion of each group of agents in detail.

I. PRIMARY ANALGESIC AGENTS (SYNONYM: NON-SPECIFIC ANALGESICS)

(A) Systemic
  1. Non-opioid analgesics (non-narcotics)
     (a) Non-steroidal drugs which lack anti-inflammatory properties
     (b) Non-steroidal anti-inflammatory drugs (NSAIDs)
     (c) Slow acting anti-rheumatic drugs
  2. Opioid analgesics (narcotics)
     (Opiates and opioids)
  3. General anaesthetics
(B) Local
  1. Local anaesthetics (local analgesics) including nerve blocks
  2. Stimulation induced analgesia
     (a) Massage and vibration
     (b) Heat and cold
     (c) Transcutaneous electrical nerve stimulation (TENS)
     (d) Acupuncture and electroacupuncture
     (e) Counter-irritants
  3. Ablative
     (a) Neurolytics (phenol, ethanol, cryoprobe)
     (b) Surgery and radiotherapy

II. SECONDARY ANALGESIC AGENTS (SYNONYMS: SPECIFIC ANALGESICS, CO-ANALGESICS)

(A) Pharmacological
  1. Selected psychotropic drugs
     (a) antidepressants
     (b) antiepileptics
     (c) antipsychotics
     (d) anxiolytics
  2. Antispastics
  3. Anti-inflammatory steroids
  4. Sympathetic nerve block
     (a) α and β-adrenoceptor blockers
     (b) sympathectomy (chemical, surgical)
  5. Vasodilators

(B) Psycho-social
  (a) Counselling
  (b) Cognitive/behavioural
  (c) Relaxation
  (d) Biofeedback
  (e) Hypnosis
  (f) Rehabilitation

I. *Primary Analgesic Agents* (*non-specific analgesics*)
All the agents in this group act at one or more sites on the nociceptive pathway. Each is non-specific in the sense that it can be used as an effective analgesic in the treatment of a wide variety of painful conditions of different causation. This large group of agents can be subdivided into systemic and local agents.

Systemic agents

Non-opioid analgesics (non-narcotic)

Three groups of drugs need to be considered, one without and two with anti-inflammatory properties.

Non-steroidal drugs which lack anti-inflammatory properties

Two chemically and pharmacologically unrelated drugs belong to this group.

(i) Paracetamol

Official name	Proprietary names
paracetamol	Calpol
	Disprol
	Paldesic
	Panadol
	Panaleve
	Salzone

Main uses: Paracetamol is an analgesic and antipyretic (fever reducing) drug with clinically insignificant anti-inflammatory properties. It is used to treat mild to moderate pain including headache, dysmenorrhoea and especially musculoskeletal conditions. The normal adult dose is 0.5–1 g 4–6 hourly up to a maximum total daily dose of 4 g (8 x 0.5g tablets).

Mechanism of action: The analgesic and antipyretic (but not anti-inflammatory) properties of paracetamol are similar to those of aspirin (see later). Nevertheless, neither the site nor the mode of action of the analgesic effect of paracetamol have been firmly established. The antipyretic effect is probably due to inhibition of the enzyme cyclo-oxygenese in the brain.

Adverse effects: When used in the correct therapeutic doses, paracetamol is unlikely to cause any problems. By contrast, overdose is a potentially lethal condition likely to cause liver damage (hepatotoxicity) (Prescott *et al.*, 1971).

Under normal circumstances, paracetamol is metabolized in the liver to harmless compounds that are excreted in the urine. However, following an overdose, the metabolic pathways are liable to become overloaded. As a consequence, a toxic metabolite (probably N-acetyl-p-benzoquinone) which is normally rendered inert by glutathione (an amino acid), accumulates and damages the liver cells which may be so severe as to precipitate liver failure. Acute liver damage is characterized by jaundice and disorders of blood coagulation and may lead to coma and death. It can result from a single dose of 10–15 g (20–30 tablets).

A treacherous feature of paracetamol poisoning is the delay of 24 hours or more between the ingestion of the drug and the onset of symptoms. Thus the patient and others who are fully aware that an overdose has been taken, may not realize the potential seriousness of the situation and fail to seek medical help. Early treatment is vital and includes gastric lavage and the administration of N-acetylcysteine which enables the liver to detoxify the dangerous metabolite but only if the patient receives it within 12 hours of taking the overdose.

Implications for physiotherapy

Paracetamol is a commonly used and effective analgesic for mild or moderate pain. It can be purchased over the counter in pharmacies, supermarkets and many other shops so that many patients with painful conditions, for which physiotherapy has been prescribed, are likely to be taking paracetamol. Self-medication with correct doses of this analgesic is not likely to pose any problem for physiotherapy. However, it is conceivable that the physiotherapist might be the first person to become aware of the excessive and potentially dangerous self-overdosing with paracetamol by a patient when appropriate action would need to be taken.

(ii) Nefopam

Official name	Proprietary name
nefopam	Acupan

Main uses: This analgesic is reported to be effective against moderately severe, acute and chronic pain but has neither antipyretic nor anti-inflammatory properties. It is used for postoperative pain, musculoskeletal pain and also for pain due to acute trauma and cancer. Unlike NSAIDs and opioids, it does not cause metabolic disturbances nor respiratory depression, respectively. The recommended dose of 1–3 tablets (30–90 mg) once to thrice daily should be reduced to 1 tablet three times daily in the elderly because of the risk of adverse effects (see later); it can also be administered by injection.

Complete details of its mode of action are not yet known, although it has been clearly established that nefopam is neither an NSAID nor an opioid. Some studies suggest that it activates the descending pain inhibitory pathways in the spinal cord.

Adverse effects: Nefopam is related chemically and pharmacologically to drugs used for the treatment of Parkinson's disease and therefore shares some of their pharmacological actions. Some patients tolerate nefopam well but others may develop one or more of the following adverse effects: nausea, nervousness, dry mouth, light-headedness and urinary retention; or less frequently, vomiting, blurred vision, drowsiness, sweating, insomnia, headache and tachycardia.

Implications for physiotherapy

Any patient who has achieved effective analgesia with nefopam should have no problems with physiotherapy. On the other hand, a patient who exhibits adverse effects to this drug, especially nausea, vomiting, nervousness, light-headedness, blurred vision or drowsiness is obviously liable to run into difficulties when undertaking physiotherapy. Indeed, it might prove necessary to discuss with the physician in charge of the patient the desirability of reducing or stopping medication with nefopam in order to permit the continuation of physiotherapy.

Non-steroidal anti-inflammatory drugs (NSAIDs)

NSAIDs, of which aspirin and ibuprofen are examples, comprise one of the largest groups of drugs used in therapeutics.

Official name	Proprietary names(s)
aspirin	
azapropazone	Rheumox

Official name	Proprietary names(s)
diclofenac	Rhumalgan
	Voltarol
diflunisal	Dolobid
etodolac	Lodine
fenbufen	Lederfen
fenoprofen	Fenopron, Progesic
flurbiprofen	Frobin
ibuprofen	Apsifen, Brufen, Fenbid,
	Ibular, Lidifen
	Motrin, Paxofen
indomethacin	Indocid
mefenamic acid	Ponstan
nabumetone	Rolifex
naproxen	Naprosyn, Synflex
piroxicam	Feldene
sulindac	Clinoril
tenoxicam	Mobiflex
tiaprofenic acid	Surgam
tolmetin	Tolectin

Main uses: The NSAIDs form a large group of chemical compounds of different chemical classes. Each member is characterized by possessing three major pharmacological actions:

1. analgesic effect (relieves nociceptive but not usually neurogenic pain).
2. Anti-inflammatory effect (modify inflammatory response).
3. Antipyretic effect (lower a raised body temperature).

As a consequence of these actions, the NSAIDs are particularly suited for use in musculoskeletal conditions where they relieve pain, reduce swelling and increase mobility.

Unfortunately, nearly a quarter of the adverse drug reactions reported to the Committee on Safety of Medicines in the UK are caused by NSAIDs (see below). This is partly due to the fact that these drugs are used extensively in the older age groups who are more liable to develop adverse effects to any drug; and also to the inherent toxicity of this particular group of drugs. Some patients tolerate these drugs well while others do not.

Warning: aspirin should not be given to children below the age of 12 years because of the risk of causing Reye's syndrome in which there is damage to the liver and brain.

Mechanism of action: Although the NSAIDs belong to widely differing chemical classes, their predominant action is to inhibit the synthesis of an important group of chemical mediators, known as the eicosanoids (prostaglandins, thromboxane, prostacyclin and leukotrienes) which cause or are involved in pain, inflammation and pyrexia (see Chapter 10). Other pharmacological actions of the NSAIDs that are important include their ability to inhibit inflammatory cell migration, lysosomal enzyme release, cytokine production and also to inhibit the formation of oxygen radicals (so called superoxide) which damage tissues. It seems likely that the different activity profiles of the NSAIDs against these agents may account for the differing responses to these drugs observed within and between patients. It is important to note that while NSAIDs relieve the symptoms of musculoskeletal disease, they do not alter the course of the disease (compare with slow acting anti-rheumatics, see later).

Adverse effects: Gastrointestinal irritation represents the commonest adverse effect of NSAIDs. This is largely due to the acidic nature of most of the NSAIDs. Unfortunately all NSAIDs can cause gastrointestinal ulceration and haemorrhage and to which the elderly patient is particularly at risk. Ibuprofen is the least likely to cause ulceration (and apart from aspirin, is the only NSAID sold over the counter). The introduction of slow release preparations, pro-drugs and suppositories has only partly solved the problem.

Skin rashes and allergy occur occasionally and a patient who claims to be susceptible to this type of problem should always be taken seriously.

Depression of the bone marrow is rare but agranulocytosis can occur with phenylbutazone which is therefore reserved for use only in ankylosing spondylitis.

Fluid retention sometimes occurs and may lead to oedema, hypertension and heart failure. All NSAIDs can reduce renal *function* although rarely to a severe degree. Hyperkalaemia (raised concentration of potassium in the blood) can occur and renal *damage* has been reported with one particular group of NSAIDs (propionic acid derivatives).

Central nervous system effects including headache and dizziness may occur with certain NSAIDs, especially indomethacin.

Implication for physiotherapy

On the positive side, NSAIDs can relieve pain, reduce swelling and increase mobility of muscles or joints, thereby greatly facilitating the efficacy of physiotherapy. These two therapeutic approaches are thus able to synergize.

Table 11.1   Slow-acting disease-modifying drugs in rheumatoid arthritis

Class of drug	Official name	Proprietary name	Mechanism of action	Adverse effects
(a) Gold	sodium auro-thiomalate	Myocrisin	Inhibit phagocytosis and lysosomal enzyme activity. Suppress cell-mediated immune reactions and reduce concentrations of immuno-globulins and rheumatoid factor	Diarrhoea and abdominal pain Rashes pruritus Blood dyscrasias
	auranofin	Ridaura		
(b) Penicillamine	penicillamine	Distamine	Uncertain. May involve reduction of immunoglobulin IgM concentration	Nausea, amnesia, loss of taste, mouth ulcers, hypersensitivity, oedema, proteinuria, blood dyscrasias; rarely myasthenia, fever, lupus erythematosus
(c) Antimalarial	hydroxychloro-quine	Plaqueril	Action in rheumatoid arthritis uncertain. Stabilize lysosomes thereby inhibiting release of lysosomal enzymes which would cause inflammation. Also inhibits phospholipase A2.	Corneal opacities Retinopathy and visual loss (vision must be monitored)
(d) Immuno-suppressants	azathioprine	Azamune Berkaprine Imuran	Metabolized in body to mercaptopurine which inhibits DNA synthesis	Nausea and vomiting; bone marrow depression
	chlorambucil	Leukeran	A cytotoxic alkylating agent which acts similarly to cyclophosphamide (see below)	Bone marrow depression; inhibition of spermatogenesis
	cyclophosphamide	Endoxana	A cytotoxic alkylating agent which reduces antibody-mediated and cell-mediated immune responses	Hair loss, anorexia, nausea and vomiting; haemorrhagic cystitis (10%) leading to bladder fibrosis Renal action leading to water retention and hyponatraemia
	methotrexate	Maxtrex	Inhibits the synthesis of tetrahydro-folate (THF) from dihydrofolate (DHF), an essential step in nucleic acid synthesis	Gastrointestinal disturbances, oral ulcers, pharyngitis, gingivitis, nausea and vomiting, bone marrow depression, hepatotoxicity
	sulphasalazine	Solazpyrin	A chemical combination of a sulphonamide (sulphapyridine) with a salicylate. It acts as a pro-drug for delivery of 5-aminosalicylates to the large intestine in the treatment of inflammatory bowel disease, e.g. ulcerative colitis. Also produces remission in rheumatoid arthritis where mechanism of action is unknown	Nausea, vomiting and abdominal discomfort, hyper-sensitivity (rashes, drug fever etc.), bone marrow depression

On the negative side, the occasional patient may be found unable to cooperate fully with the physiotherapist because of adverse effects, particularly gastric irritation, dizziness, headache, or heart failure which has been precipitated by medication with NSAIDs.

Slow acting anti-rheumatic drugs (*slow acting disease-modifying drugs in rheumatoid arthritis*)

Main uses: This heterogenous group of drugs (see Table 11.1) not only relieve the symptoms of rheumatoid arthritis (like NSAIDs) but also *alter the*

course of the disease. Unlike the NSAIDs, they do not have an immediate therapeutic effect but require 4–6 months to produce a full response. A good therapeutic response includes both an improvement in the signs and symptoms of arthritis and also an improvement in the extra-articular manifestations of the disease for example, vasculitis. These drugs also reduce the raised erythrocyte sedimentation rate (ESR) associated with these conditions and may also reduce the titre of the rheumatoid factor, both of which reflect a reduction in the intensity of the inflammatory process. If a particular agent has not produced any objective improvement within 6 months it is usual for it to be discontinued.

Mechanism of action: Table 11.1 contains details about the mechanism of action of each of the four classes of drug. In general, the drugs possess inhibitory effects on inflammatory or immune mechanisms, or both, thereby suppressing the destructive pathological processes that characterize rheumatoid arthritis.

Adverse effects: As indicated in Table 11.1, this group of drugs is capable of producing major and serious adverse effects. However, this is hardly surprising since their primary action is cytotoxic and, due to lack of specificity, includes actively growing healthy cells, particularly those of the gastrointestinal tract, bone marrow and hair follicles.

Implications for physiotherapy

A physiotherapy programme designed to increase the mobility of patients with rheumatoid arthritis can be greatly assisted by the concurrent use of this group of drugs. When patients with rheumatoid arthritis respond well to medication with a drug belonging to this group, physiotherapy can obviously assist by increasing mobility and reducing the swelling of affected joints. Nevertheless, when carrying out the rehabilitation programme, the physiotherapist will need to take into account carefully any physical or psychological restrictions placed on the patient by virtue of adverse effects produced by this group of drugs.

Opioid analgesics

Opium is derived from the juice of the unripe seed capsule of the oriental poppy *Papaver somniferum* and from which is extracted the alkaloids

morphine and codeine. Many chemical derivatives have been made from naturally occurring morphine and more recently endogenous (occurring naturally within the body) peptides have been discovered, isolated and synthesized.

An opiate is a product specifically derived from the juice of the opium poppy, examples being morphine and codeine. **An opioid** (= opiate-like) is a new term that has been introduced to cover all those compounds which, whatever their chemical type, possess morphine-like activity but which are NOT derived from the juice of the opium poppy; a good example is pethidine which is produced by chemical synthesis. An essential criterion of an opioid is that its effects are antagonized competitively (in effect, molecule for molecule), by the important opioid antagonist drug naloxone. This important action applies also, of course, to morphine and other opiates which are therefore by definition, also opioids. As a consequence, naloxone is a life-saving drug in opioid overdose (e.g. heroin = diamorphine) and should always be included in the contents of a doctor's medical emergency bag.

The actions of morphine are many and divided into: central nervous system action, peripheral actions and other actions.

Actions on the Central Nervous System

These consist of a mixture of depressant and stimulant effects.

Depressant effects

1. Analgesia: due to the combined effects of a small elevation of pain **threshold** and a large increase of pain **tolerance** (see Chapter 6).
2. Sedation (which can progress to anaesthesia with large doses).
3. Depression of respiration (dose-related).
4. Depression of cough reflex (anti-tussive action).
5. Bradycardia (slowing of heart rate) with hypotension (minimal except in older patient).

Stimulant effects

1. 'Euphoria' which in the context of clinical opioid analgesia, implies *a sense of peaceful wellbeing that accompanies the relief of pain.* The occasional patient reacts in the opposite way when it is called dysphoria. By sharp and important contrast, in the context of opioid abuse

(especially intravenous self-administration = 'mainlining'), the word 'euphoria' implies a temporary state of ecstasy.

2. Nausea and vomiting.
3. Miosis (constriction of the pupil).
4. Anti-diuresis (reduced urine formation due to opioid-induced release of anti-diuretic hormone = vasopressin).
5. Sweating.
6. Central excitation (rare); hallucinations and convulsions.

Peripheral actions

1. Smooth muscle stimulation, particularly of the gastrointestinal tract (including sphincters) with reduced peristalsis resulting in constipation.
2. Biliary tract: spasm of smooth muscle including sphincter of Oddi.
3. Histamine release: itching, urticaria, hypotension (with large doses).

Other actions: tolerance and dependence

For therapeutic use, opioids (including opiates) are divided into categories of **strong** and **weak** (See Table 11.2) depending upon their so-called 'ceiling of analgesia' or, put simply, whether or not a particular opioid is capable of relieving either moderate or severe pains. Some special terms need to be defined here.

Tolerance is the need to increase the dose of a drug in order to achieve the same effect as that achieved previously with a smaller dose. When morphine is being used to treat cancer pain, the first indication of tolerance developing is when the patient reports that the analgesic effect is failing to last as long as it did previously. It is important to note that tolerance develops at a different rate for each effect of the opioid. Thus it is fastest to respiratory depression followed by (in descending order) 'euphoria', sedation, nausea and vomiting, analgesia and slowest (if at all) to constipation.

Dependence is a phenomenon separate from tolerance and is often divided (somewhat artificially) into physical and psychological types. **Physical dependence** is said to occur when withdrawal of the drug results in physical effects such as, for example, the delirium tremens or 'DTs' of alcohol withdrawal. **Psychological dependence** is said to occur when the effects of withdrawal are mainly psychological, for example, as occurs with cocaine where there is anxiety or intense craving for the drug unaccompanied by physical illness.

Physical dependence is likely to develop in the majority of patients who need to take regular opioids for longer than 3-4 weeks. However, it is very important to realize that this does not indicate that the dose cannot be reduced if, at some future time, the need for an opioid lessens or ceases. Indeed, patients who need to be treated with opioids for chronic pain are usually and understandably delighted to be weaned off their opioid in the happy event that their pain lessens or disappears.

Main uses: Morphine is the reference standard not only of opiates and opioids but also of all classes of analgesics. Morphine is used to relieve a wide variety of pains ranging from moderate to severe. Thus, it is used to relieve acute pains such as those occurring with cardiac infarction or post operatively; and it is used for certain chronic pains, particularly those due to cancer. Repeated administration may lead to tolerance and dependence but contrary to general belief, these are not serious problems and are no reason why morphine (and related drugs) should be withheld from a patient in severe pain. Morphine remains second to none amongst the strong opioids. When used for chronic pain, mostly for cancer pain, its disadvantage of a short duration of action of 4 hours has been overcome by making a slow release preparation called 'Morphine Continus' or 'MST'. A single dose of this preparation provides analgesia for 12 hours.

Mechanism of action: The actions of morphine and their mechanisms are complicated. Morphine, other opiates and opioids are good examples of drugs that produce their effects as a result of acting on specific pharmacological receptors. A drug that combines with a receptor, activates it and initiates a sequence of effects is termed **an agonist**, an example being morphine. By contrast, a drug which interferes with the action of an agonist is termed **an antagonist**. Now, a **pure** antagonist can only produce an effect when in the presence of an agonist (because it has no action of its own), an example being naloxone, the morphine antagonist. To complete the picture we must mention that some derivatives of morphine possess both agonist and antagonist actions and such a drug is termed a mixed agonist-antagonist, an example being pentazocine (see Table 11.2).

Having considered the different types of drug (agonist, antagonist, mixed agonist-antagonist) we must now consider briefly the different types of receptors upon which the drugs may act. There

Table 11.2   Opioid Analgesics

Official name	Proprietary or other name	Duration of action (h)	Half-life [T½] (h)	Analgesic potency relative to morphine = 1	Adverse effects	Comments
Weak opioids codeine	Methylmorphine	4	3	0.08 (lower analgesic ceiling)	N, V, S, Dz, C, B, R, Dp (rare). Lower analgesic ceiling due to ADRs	Weak analgesic Anti-tussive Anti-diarrhoeal A pro-drug: 10% de-methylated to morphine
dihydrocodeine	DF118	4	3	0.1 (lower analgesic ceiling)	N, V, S, *Dz*, C, R, Dp (rare). Lower analgesic ceiling due to ADRs	Weak analgesic Anti-tussive Anti-diarrhoeal
dextropropoxy-phene	Doloxene	6–8	12	0.16	N, V, S, *Dz*, C, P, A, Dp. Interacts with other CNS depressants includ-ing alcohol.	Weak analgesic commonly prescribed in combination with para-cetamol and known as co-proxamol (Cosalgesic, Distalgesic, Paxalgesic)
pentazocine	Fortral	2	2	0.6	N, V, S, *Dz, P, M,* CVS Dys, Dp. Lower analgesic ceiling due to partial Kappa (κ) antagonism (see Table 10.2)	Weak analgesic
Strong opioids morphine		4	3	1	N, V, S, C, R, Mi, Dp	A strong and effective analgesic which remains the standard of reference
diamorphine	heroin	4	Very short	1	As for morphine	A strong and effective analgesic which is rapidly converted (deacetylated) to morphine (i.e. a pro-drug) and indistinguish-able from morphine
methadone	Physeptone Amidone	6–8	15 single doses; 48–72 repeated doses	1 single dose 3 repeated doses	N, V, Sr, R, Mi, Dp	A strong analgesic for acute and especially chronic pain. Probably less euphoria but cumulation may produce sedation
pethidine	Meperidine (USA) Pamergan	2	2.5	0.125	N, V, S, ? < C, R, My, Dp. Overdose causes tremors & convulsions	A strong analgesic for acute but not chronic pain Lower analgesic ceiling than morphine
buprenorphine	Temgesic	8	3.5	25–50	N, V, R?	Strong long-acting analgesic Sublingual use

Abbreviations: A, abdominal pain; ADRs, adverse drug reactions; B, biliary colic; C, constipation; CVS, cardiovascular changes; Dp, dependence; Dys, dysphoria; Dz, dizziness; M, mood changes; Mi, Miosis; My, mydriasis; N, nausea; P, psychotomimetic effects; R, respiratory depression; S, sedation; V, vomiting.
   Use of italic denotes a high incidence.

are three kinds of opioid receptor, each identified with a letter from the Greek alphabet namely, mu (μ), kappa (κ) and delta (δ). Each of the three types of receptor has (i) its own characteristic distribution in the nervous system and (ii) its own pattern of response when activated by a specific agonist (see Chapter 10, Table 10.2). Under physiological conditions, the receptors are activated by a family of endogenous peptides known as beta-endorphin, met-enkephalin, leu-enkephalin and dynorphin. The opiates and opioids produce their effects by stimulating opioid receptors which are normally activated by these endogenous peptides. All the foregoing information has been collected together and summarized in Table 10.2.

Adverse effects: These are detailed in Table 11.2.

Implications for physiotherapy

The powerful analgesic action of morphine in a patient who would otherwise be in severe pain will obviously make possible the implementation of appropriate physiotherapy. Nevertheless there are important guidelines to be observed for the patient medicated with morphine.

1. Take care that excessive or inappropriate physiotherapy is not unwittingly expected of a patient as a consequence of the presence of the analgesia induced by morphine.
2. For acute or chronic pain, opioids need to be administered regularly 'by the clock' (e.g. for morphine, every 4 hours) and never 'on demand'. It is vitally important to realize that regular opioid medication must continue and physiotherapy arranged to permit this.
3. The physiotherapist must be aware of certain opioid-induced adverse effects such as nausea, vomiting, sedation and dizziness which may affect the choice of physiotherapy for a particular patient and the ability of that patient to undertake it to a reasonable and useful degree.
4. The physiotherapist is particularly well placed to observe and monitor the performance and progress of each patient, including to note both positive and negative effects of any analgesic drug treatment received by the patient.

General Anaesthetics

This heterogeneous group of agents includes gases, e.g. nitrous oxide, volatile liquids, e.g. halothane, and intravenous agents, e.g. thiopentone sodium, which are used to render a patient unconscious and analgesic (anaesthesia) so as to permit a surgical operation or other painful procedure to be carried out without pain. While these agents are highly important, for obvious reasons they cannot be used for the prolonged treatment of acute or more particularly, chronic pain! For this reason, the pharmacology of general anaesthetics will not be discussed further.

Implications for physiotherapy

For many years the physiotherapist has made a very important contribution to the safer and more efficient use of general anaesthesia. This has been achieved through preoperative and postoperative breathing and other exercises which have improved the respiratory exchange and pulmonary elimination of general anaesthetics thus expediting the mobilization of the patient.

Local agents

Local anaesthetics

Table 11.3 gives details of local anaesthetics that are commonly used to produce diagnostic and therapeutic nerve blocks in the treatment of acute and chronic pain, including those used for palliative medicine. Lignocaine and bupivacaine are the two local anaesthetics used most frequently. The different uses, routes of administration and preparations employed, together with information about the speed of onset and duration of action (but not doses), are included in Table 11.3.

Main uses: Local anaesthetics can be used to produce many different types of nerve block (see Table 11.4), which range from simple topical blocks (e.g. local application of a spray or ointment to relieve the pain of an ulcerated mucous membrane) to technically complicated blocks (e.g. injection of a solution of local anaesthetic to block a nerve plexus or a sympathetic ganglion). A recent and important surgical use is to produce so-called pre-emptive analgesia in which the operation site is infiltrated with local anaesthetic *prior* to operation. This procedure has been found to reduce postoperative pain significantly, most probably by protecting the CNS from the surgically evoked nociceptive barrage which triggers secondary neurophysiological mechanisms that heighten postoperative pain.

Table 11.3 Local anaesthetics commonly used for the management of acute and chronic pain

Name (and synonym)	Route: Uses	Proprietary preparation available	Local anaesthetic	Vasoconstrictor	Onset of Action (min)	Duration of Action
1. lignocaine (lidocaine Xylocaine)	Injection: brief anaesthesia with maximum local diffusion	Xylocaine 1% (plain)	lignocaine hydrochloride 1%	—	1–2	15–45 min
	Injection: anaesthesia of medium duration and minimum diffusion	Xylocaine 1% with adrenaline 1:200,000	lignocaine hydrochloride 1%	adrenaline tartrate 1:200,000 = 5 μg/ml (as adrenaline)	1–2	2–4 h
	Topical: relieve pain of ulcerated mouth or throat	Xylocaine spray	lignocaine (base) 10.378%w/w	—	0.25	25–30 min
	Topical: relief of painful lesions of skin and mucous membranes	Xylocaine ointment	lignocaine 5% (base)	—	3–5	25–30 min
2. bupivacaine (Marcain)	Injection: prolonged anaesthesia with maximum diffusion; epidural, intrathecal	Marcain Plain	bupivacaine hydrochloride 0.5%	—	4	6 h
	Injection: prolonged local pain relief. e.g. intercostal nerve block; metastasis in rib	Marcain with adrenaline	bupivacaine hydrochloride 0.5%	adrenaline tartrate 1:200,000 = 5 μg/ml (as adrenaline)	4	6 h +
3. EMLA = eutectic mixture of local anaesthetics	Topical: to prepare venepuncture site; surgical treatment of localized lesion, e.g. painful scar	EMLA cream 5%	Each gram contains lignocaine base 25 mg prilocaine base 25 mg in a eutectic mixture as an oil-water emulsion	—	1 h or longer	For duration of application. Efficacy may decline after 5 hours of application

Mechanism of action: Local anaesthetics produce a reversible block of conduction in nerve endings and nerve trunks. This action is the result of stabilization of excitable nerve cell membranes which the local anaesthetic achieves by blocking the sodium channels in the membrane. Normally, nerve cell membranes are excitable, including to electrical currents, thus enabling them to conduct nerve impulses (for further details, see Chapter 7). By this means, motor and sensory nerves conduct information, the latter including nociception which, when it reaches consciousness, is interpreted as pain. The excitability of every nerve cell membrane depends critically upon the functioning of the sodium channels through which sodium ions [Na$^+$] pass. Local anaesthetics *block* the sodium channels and thereby block nerve conduction. The susceptibility of nerve endings and nerve trunks to local anaesthetics is *inversely* proportional to the diameter of the nerve fibres of which the trunk is composed. Thus, the small C fibres which transmit slow, second or tissue damage pain are blocked before the larger A-delta fibres which transmit fast, first, or pricking pain (see Chapter 7). Correspondingly, the large A-alpha motor fibres are the most resistant to local anaesthetic and are blocked last.

When present in sufficiently high concentration, local anaesthetics will also block the sodium channels present in the cell membranes of other tissues. Important examples are (i) the smooth muscle of blood vessels and (ii) the conducting system of the heart. At these sites excessive concentrations of local anaesthetic may cause, respectively, acute hypotension through widespread relaxation of vascular smooth muscle and cardiac arrhythmias (or even arrest) through interference with the cardiac conducting system. Thus it can be seen that the fundamental mechanism of action of local anaesthetics can also be responsible for producing some of the adverse effects that may be caused by these drugs (see below).

In order to prolong the duration of action of an injection of local anaesthetic, it is common practice to mix with it a small amount of a vasoconstrictor drug, usually adrenaline (as tartrate) (see Table 11.3). The vasoconstrictor not only increases the duration of local anaesthesia but, by slowing the rate of absorption of the drug into the circulation, reduces the maximum concentration attained and so lessens the risk of adverse effects.

Adverse effects: These are due either to the local anaesthetic drug or to some other factor. Furthermore, adverse effects caused by the local anaesthetic may occur in normal individuals or in individuals who are qualitatively abnormal, for example, those who have developed an allergy to this group of drugs. Paradoxically, all local anaesthetics are potential central stimulants (probably by blocking central inhibitory mechanisms) and so may cause apprehension, confusion, excitement or frank euphoria. This initial stage may be followed by muscle twitchings and convulsions which require urgent treatment. The stimulant effects just described may be followed by another adverse reaction which is central depression resulting in hypotension, loss of consciousness and respiratory depression which will require urgent artificial respiration.

As explained under 'Mechanism of action' above, local anaesthetics can cause cardiac arrhythmias or cardiac arrest if the plasma concentration in the vicinity of the heart is sufficiently high. This situation might arise following an overdose or an inadvertent intravenous injection of the drug. In abnormal individuals, local anaesthetics can precipitate an acute and potentially fatal allergic response called anaphylactic shock which is characterized by asthma, rhinitis, angio (neurotic) oedema or urticaria. These conditions are examples of drug allergy and require emergency treatment. Rarely adverse effects due to intolerance (exaggerated response to a normal therapeutic dose) or idiosyncrasy (a bizarre response not involving allergy) occur and require urgent and appropriate treatment.

Finally, adverse effects which are *not* due to the local anaesthetic may be the result of a simple faint or, alternatively, may be caused by the vasoconstrictor agent, usually adrenaline (tartrate), which has been added to the solution of local anaesthetic for reasons discussed earlier (see above). Adverse effects due to adrenaline include tachycardia (interpreted by the patient as palpitations), apprehension and a rise of blood pressure that may be dangerous in subjects with cardiovascular disease. This problem is treated with reassurance and, if necessary, by the use of drugs that antagonize the pharmacological actions of adrenaline. A suitable emergency box containing resuscitation equipment should always be available wherever and whenever local anaesthetics are administered.

Therapeutic uses of nerve blocks: There are many clinical conditions for which nerve blocks can be used and these are summarized in Table 11.4. It is

Table 11.4 Examples of nerve blocks used to relieve acute and chronic pain

Anatomical site of block	Clinical condition treated with block
Peripheral nerves and plexuses	
Cervical plexus	Neck tumour
Brachial plexus	Operation on upper limb
Phrenic nerve	Intractable hiccough
Intercostal nerve	Postoperative pain; compression or infiltration by tumour
Ilio-inguinal nerve	Postoperative pain,
Ilio-hypogastric nerve	nerve entrapment
Lateral cutaneous nerve of thigh	Meralgia paraesthetica
Sacral and coccygeal nerves	Obstetric analgesia
Sympathetic nerves and plexuses	
Stellate ganglion	Reflex sympathetic dystrophy of arm or hand
Dorsal sympathetic chain	Vascular problems of limb or fingers
Coeliac plexus	Chronic pancreatic pain
Lumbar sympathetic chain	Sympathetic algodystrophy

important for physiotherapists to be aware of the potential therapeutic uses of nerve blocks although details of the techniques used are outside both their domain and the scope of this chapter.

Implications for physiotherapy

The use of local anaesthetic blocks for the management of various acute and chronic pain conditions has three important implications.

1. To facilitate physiotherapy by removing pain and muscle spasm: For example, the acute pain of a fractured rib can be relieved by one or more intercostal nerve blocks. When this has been achieved it makes it possible for the physiotherapist to instruct the patient in breathing exercises much more effectively. A similar situation pertains to the treatment of painful myofascial trigger points in muscles of, for example, the neck following which the physiotherapist is much better able to obtain the patient's cooperation over exercises for the neck and shoulder girdle. (It should be noted here that myofascial trigger points can often be treated just as effectively by dry needling these with an acupuncture needle, i.e. without the use of local anaesthetic.) A third example is the striking facilitation

of back movements that follow a lumbar epidural injection (or infusion) of local anaesthetic in patients with certain types of chronic, low back pain.

2. To mark a cautionary note and to remind the physiotherapist that blocking nociception with a local anaesthetic is to treat only the symptoms and not the cause of a painful condition such as low back pain: thus, both patient and physiotherapist must be aware of the dangers of carrying out excessive physical exercises under local analgesia which could result in dangerous mechanical trauma to the lumbar spine.

3. To be aware of adverse effects that can be induced by local anaesthetics, including those that might be induced by the vasoconstrictor present: Although it is not the duty of the physiotherapist to perform nerve blocks, he or she could well be a member of a team where these procedures are carried out and where an adverse effect might develop. Under these circumstances, the physiotherapist might be the first person to recognize such an occurrence and therefore to seek medical aid and also to give valuable assistance to the doctor who arrives on the scene to treat the problem.

Stimulation Induced Analgesia

Modulation of the nociceptive input by different forms of peripheral (and also central) nerve stimulation forms the basis of so-called stimulation induced analgesia (SIA), already described in Chapter 9. The forms of SIA in common use are included in the classification of methods of pain relief given in the introduction to this chapter (see p. 68). With the exception of counter-irritants, these methods are described fully in other chapters of this book, as indicated below, and to which the reader is referred:

Method	See chapter
Massage and vibration	18, 19
Heat and cold	16
Transcutaneous electrical nerve stimulation (TENS)	14
Acupuncture and electroacupuncture	13

Ablation

Ablative or destructive methods used to relieve pain include neurolytics and surgery and radiotherapy. Since these methods are not strictly pharmacological, they will be discussed here only briefly.

Neurolytics

These are agents used to destroy nerve tissue whether irreversibly (phenol, ethanol) or reversibly (cryoprobe = freezing probe). These methods are used mainly for the treatment of chronic pain. Although they can be very effective, great caution is needed when making a decision to use methods of nerve destruction. Some chronic pains are the result of damage to the nervous system (neurogenic pain, neuropathic pain). It is therefore hardly surprising that to try to treat these pains by causing further nerve damage may result in producing worse pain than that from which the patient suffered originally!

Surgery and Radiotherapy

In general, surgery is used to treat pain when the causal lesion can be removed completely; and radiotherapy is used when this goal is unattainable. There are exceptions to this rule, and in some instances both methods are combined and frequently need pharmacological support to control various symptoms, particularly pain. However, these topics are outside the scope of this book and will not be discussed further.

Implications for physiotherapy

These will obviously depend upon many factors, including the nature and site of the lesion (e.g. traumatic, infective, inflammatory, neoplastic), the prognosis and so on. Each and all of these factors will need to be taken into consideration when planning a programme of physiotherapy for a particular patient. Once again, the physiotherapist must bear in mind that pain control does not necessarily indicate causal control and that excessive attempts to mobilize tissues that remain mechanically unsound may do considerably more harm than good.

II. SECONDARY ANALGESIC AGENTS (SYNONYMS: SPECIFIC ANALGESICS, CO-ANALGESICS)

Pharmacological agents

Selected psychotropic drugs

Since the 1950s selected antidepressants, anti-psychotics, anxiolytics and anticonvulsants have been used for the management of chronic pain conditions.

Main uses: Selected antipsychotics, anxiolytics and anticonvulsants are used singly, or in combination, in order to produce one or more of the following effects (Budd, 1982; Thompson and Tyrer, 1992)

1. Analgesia.
2. Antidepressant action.
3. Hypnotic action.
4. Anxiolytic action.
5. Suppression of abnormal nociceptive impulse generators.

It may seem surprising that psychotropic drugs can be of use for the relief of pain and especially for chronic pain. However, the results of a substantial number of clinical trials attest to the value of these drugs, especially antidepressants in sub-antidepressant doses, for the relief of chronic pain. In this situation, the analgesic efficacy is independent of whether the patient is depressed (Watson et al., 1982).

Mechanism of action: Experimental and clinical evidence suggest that several mechanisms are involved. The first is due to activation or reinforcement of pain controlling systems in the brain and spinal cord which depend upon certain neurotransmitters. The most likely candidates are noradrenaline (NAd) and 5-hydroxytryptamine (5HT) which have been discussed already in Chapters 9 and 10. A major pharmacological action of tricyclic and related antidepressant drugs is to facilitate transmission at synapses where NAd and 5HT are the neurotransmitters and these include those in the descending pain inhibitory pathways from the periaqueductal grey area (PAG) to the spinal cord (see Chapter 10). It seems likely that it is by this means that these drugs increase pain control. It should be noted that this effect is separate from the antidepressant action of these drugs because (a) it occurs more rapidly and (b) it requires a smaller dose than that needed for the psychotropic effects.

The second action is by altering the emotional response of the patient to pain; and the third is by reducing the patient's anxiety. Most psychotropic drugs possess these actions.

The fourth mechanism of action is confined to drugs with anticonvulsant properties. This group suppress abnormal nociceptive impulse generators

Table 11.5 Psychotropic drugs used in the management of chronic pain

Class of drug	Official or approved name	Proprietary name	Mechanism of analgesic action	Adverse effects
Anti-depressants	amitriptyline dothiepin doxepin	Domical Lentizol Tryptizol Prothiaden Sinequan	Selected antidepressants, anti-psychotics, anticonvulsants and anxiolytics are used singly or in combination to produce one or more of the following effects: analgesia; antidepressant action; hypnotic action	Anticholinergic: dry mouth, constipation, blurred vision, urinary retention (with prostatism) Cardiovascular: postural hypotension, arrhythmia, oedema CNS: sedation, stimulation, sleep disturbance; appetite and weight increased, extrapyramidal effects Organ damage: liver, bone marrow Drug interactions
Antipsychotics	chlor-promazine	Largactil		Anticholinergic: dry mouth, constipation, tachycardia CVS: postural hypotension CNS: sedation, extrapyramidal (Parkinsonism and tardive dyskinesia) Metabolic/endocrine, allergy
Anti-convulsants	carbamazepine sodium valproate	Tegretol Epilim	Anxiolytic action Suppression of abnormal nociceptive impulse generators (see text for further details)	CNS: dizziness, drowsiness, ataxia, dysarthria, paraesthesia, weakness, diplopia CNS: tremor, ataxia, sedation/aggression (rare) Organ damage: liver, pancreas, bone marrow, hair loss
Anxiolytics	diazepam	Valium	Enhances GABA inhibitory mechanism at spinal cord level and also in reticular formation	CNS: drowsiness, dizziness, confusion, fatigue, blurred vision NB: All benzodiazepines are drugs of dependence and should only be administered for a short course of 10–14 days. (If needed a course can be repeated after an interval of several weeks)

that have developed in damaged or severed nerves, for example, in a neuroma such as is found in an amputation stump.

Implications for physiotherapy

Patients who are achieving pain relief through medication with psychotropic drugs may also be able to achieve greater benefit from concurrent physiotherapy. The reduced pain, anxiety and improved sleep pattern are likely to result in both mental and physical improvement which will facilitate physiotherapy rehabilitation programmes. Nevertheless it is important for the physiotherapist to be aware of and take into consideration, where necessary, certain adverse effects of psychotropic drugs which may limit the capabilities of the patient. For example, a patient might suffer from drug-induced sedation, dizziness or postural hypotension and these could well place a limit on certain physiotherapeutic exercises or manoeuvres.

Antispastics

Official name	Proprietary name
dantrolene	Dantrium
baclofen	Lioresal
diazepam	Valium

Main uses: Dantrolene, baclofen and diazepam are

Table 11.6　Antispastic drugs

Official name	Proprietary name	Mechanism of action	Adverse effects	Comments
dantrolene	Dantrium	A peripheral action directly on skeletal muscle where it interferes with calcium release	Drowsiness (usually transient); dizziness, weakness, fatigue and musculoskeletal disturbance; malaise, diarrhoea, rashes	Caution should be observed in presence of impaired pulmonar cardiac and hepatic function. Normally liver function should tested before and during treatment
baclofen	Lioresal	Enhances GABA inhibitory mechanism at spinal cord level probably by stimulating GABA receptors which inhibits release of excitatory amino acids (glutamate and aspartate)	Nausea and vomiting (avoid in peptic ulcer); drowsiness, fatigue, confusion, hypotension; muscle hypotonia	Interactions: CNS drugs, includ alcohol, may cause increased sedation; with antidepressants baclofen may be potentiated to cause muscular hypotonia
diazepam	Valium	Enhances GABA inhibitory mechanism at spinal cord level and also in recticular formation	Drowsiness; dizziness, confusion, ataxia (especially in the elderly); impairment of skilled tasks, e.g. driving a vehicle; dependence. Sometimes headache, giddiness, hypotension, rashes, gastrointestinal disturbances	Drug interactions: when prescribed with other drugs which have sedative effects, e.g. opioi antidepressants, antihistamine (H1 blockers), alcohol (ethanol anaesthetics; all of these are likely to increase the degree of sedation produced by diazepan

three useful secondary analgesics for treating chronic pain caused by prolonged spasm or spasticity of skeletal muscle, for example in multiple sclerosis. These drugs are often used in combination with primary analgesics. However, the use of diazepam should be restricted to 2 weeks because of the considerable risk of dependence. (See also **Selected psychotropic drugs**, above.)

Mechanism of action: These drugs act either on the muscle directly (dantrolene) or by interfering with muscular control mechanisms at spinal cord level (baclofen) or both there and in the reticular formation (diazepam); they do not affect neuromuscular transmission. For further details see Table 11.6.

Adverse effects: As might be expected, these three drugs may cause muscular weakness combined with sedation. Fuller details are given in Table 11.6.

Implications for physiotherapy

The use of antispastic drugs to reduce spasm and pain in skeletal muscles will obviously facilitate physiotherapy designed to mobilize such muscles.

Nevertheless, the reduced spasticity may well have been achieved at the cost of hypotonia, reduced muscle power together with sedation and possibly other adverse effects (see Table 11.6). These possibilities must be taken into consideration by the physiotherapist when planning and executing a programme of physiotherapy for such patients.

Anti-inflammatory steroids (*corticosteroids*)

The British National Formulary lists more than ten corticosteroids for therapeutic use. However, only selected ones are suitable for the treatment of acute and chronic pain conditions by systemic and/or local administration.

Official name	Proprietary name
Systemic use	
prednisolone	Deltacortril Enteric
	Deltastab
	Precortisyl
	Prednesol
	Sintisone
dexamethasone	Decadron
	Oraclexon

Official name	Proprietary name
Local use	
hydrocortisone	Hydrocortisyl
methylprednisolone acetate	Depo-Medrone
triamcinolone acetonide	Adcortyl

Main use: Corticosteroids can be used for three purposes: (i) **replacement therapy**, e.g. hypoadrenalism; (Addison's disease); (ii) **anti-inflammatory and immunosuppressive therapy**, e.g. rheumatoid arthritis, bronchial asthma, ulcerative colitis, to prevent transplant rejection; (iii) **palliative medicine**, e.g. cerebral oedema, nerve compression, euphorigenic action. In the context of the relief of acute and chronic pain, we are concerned only with those corticosteroids used for (ii) and (iii) above. As indicated above, corticosteroids can be used either systemically, e.g. rheumatoid arthritis, or by local injection, e.g. for a painful joint. In every instance the corticosteroid is not curative but simply suppresses the symptoms and signs of the pathological condition for which it is being used. In order to achieve this suppression, unphysiological and high doses may be required which lead inevitably to some adverse effects (see later) which may have to be accepted if control of the disease is to be maintained. Local treatment of, for example, a painful joint, often produces rapid and useful pain relief with less likelihood of adverse systemic effects; but with repeated local therapy absorption of the steroid into the general circulation may, of course, ultimately lead to the same adverse effects as occur with systemic therapy.

Mechanism of action: The adrenal cortex secretes two principal corticosteroids: (i) **aldosterone**, a so-called mineralocorticoid concerned predominantly with the important regulation of sodium (Na^+) ions and potassium (K^+) ions in the body; (ii) **hydrocortisone** (cortisol) a so-called glucocorticoid, concerned with important effects on protein, carbohydrate and fat metabolism. In higher concentrations, hydrocortisone also has anti-inflammatory and immunosuppressant actions which have been exploited therapeutically by using synthetic derivatives of hydrocortisone in which these actions predominate. These anti-inflammatory glucocorticoids are thus used to suppress the humoral (chemical messenger) and cellular processes that produce the classical signs of inflammation which include swelling, heat, redness, pain and loss of function. Inflammation is, of course, a protective reaction of the tissues in response to many different forms of noxious stimuli, e.g. microbial, chemical, radiation etc.

At a cellular level, corticosteroids pass through cell membranes to combine with protein receptors in the cytoplasm. This complex then passes into the cell nucleus where it binds with the chromatin and, following a chain of reactions which involve RNA (ribose nucleic acid) and mRNA (messenger RNA), new proteins are synthesized in the ribosomes. It is thought that these proteins then control the activities of various cells to induce the changes described above. Complete details of the mechanisms involved are not yet known but what is clear is that anti-inflammatory (and other) steroids are powerful pharmacological agents that must always be used with great care and never inappropriately (see also Adverse effects, below).

Adverse effects: Many of the adverse effects that may occur are predictable because they represent an exaggeration of the physiological actions of corticosteroids. Thus they may be listed as follows:

Tissue, organ or system involved	Adverse effect
Glucocorticoids:	
Infected skin and other tissue	Spread of infection, e.g. septicaemia, tuberculosis
Carbohydrate	Glucocorticoid-induced diabetes mellitus
Protein	Osteoporosis and vertebral collapse
Fat	High doses – Cushing's syndrome: moon face, striae, acne
Brain	Euphoria and other mental disturbances
Skin	Skin atrophy: spread of infection (see above)
Pituitary	Adrenal suppression (due to negative feedback mechanism). (NB: Acute adrenal stress such as administration of general anaesthesia may lead to severe hypotension, collapse and death)
Children	Suppression of growth

Tissue, organ or system involved	Adverse effect
Mineralocorticoids	
Kidney	Sodium (Na$^+$) + Water (H$_2$O) retention; increased (K$^+$) potassium output; muscle weakness

Implications for physiotherapy

The fact that a patient has been prescribed a glucocorticoid has several important implications for physiotherapy. First, it indicates that the patient suffers from, and requires treatment for, a major medical problem, for example, rheumatoid arthritis, polymyalgia rheumatica, bronchial asthma or certain blood disorders. The particular medical condition has, of course, its own implications for any physiotherapy programme that may be deemed necessary either for it or for some incidental and unrelated problem.

Secondly, medication with a glucocorticoid, for whatever reason, carries its own implications for physiotherapy as is evident from the list of possible adverse effects. Thus before starting such a patient on a vigorous programme of physiotherapy, the physiotherapist must consider the possibility of, for example, fragile readily infected skin, osteoporosis with risk of pathological fractures, especially vertebral collapse and the sequelae of adrenal suppression. Other problems that might arise include sodium and water retention with oedema or muscle weakness.

Sympathetic nerve block

Background

The autonomic or involuntary nervous system may be divided into (i) the sympathetic nervous system and (ii) the parasympathetic nervous system.

Some pain conditions, particularly those which follow nerve damage, appear to be maintained by abnormal activity of the sympathetic nervous system and these are referred to as **sympathetically maintained pains** (SMP). On the other hand, many pain problems are independent of the sympathetic nervous system and pains which belong to this category are therefore referred to as **sympathetically independent pains** (SIP). Analogous pain conditions dependent upon the parasympathetic nervous system are not readily apparent although damage to parasympathetic nerves, for example those in the chorda tympani, may be followed by the development of bizarre phenomena such as

gustatory sweating (sweating in response to the stimulus of taste). This phenomenon is probably due to collateral sprouting of parasympathetic nerves fibres in response to injury (Murray and Thompson, 1957).

A very brief summary of the anatomy and physiology of the sympathetic nervous system relevant to pain problems now follows.

Anatomy and Physiology

The outflow of the sympathetic nervous system from cells in the lateral horn of the spinal cord at the levels of T1 to L3 pass out in the ventral root and then synapse in the paravertebral ganglia from where they are distributed through mixed spinal nerves to innervate vascular smooth muscle (e.g. blood vessels of skin), non-vascular smooth muscle (e.g. gut) and cardiac muscle. The nerve supply to each structure consists of two sets of nerves, preganglionic and postganglionic neurons. The chemical transmitter released from the preganglionic nerve endings is acetylcholine whereas that from the postganglionic nerve endings is noradrenaline – except in the adrenal gland where it is a mixture of noradrenaline (for blood pressure regulation) and adrenaline (for fight and flight), the ratio depending on the predominant need at the moment.

The noradrenaline released from the postganglionic nerve endings stimulates adrenoceptors (an abbreviation of adrenergic receptors) which are of two main types, alpha and beta. To complicate matters, there are two sub-types of each main type (alpha$_1$, alpha$_2$, beta$_1$ and beta$_2$) and since these are of considerable clinical importance these also need to be considered. The effects mediated by activating the different types of adrenoceptors are set out in Table 11.7 (the list is not exhaustive).

Alpha- and beta-adrenoceptor blockers

This group of drugs is used to reduce those effects which result from the excessive action of the sympathetic nervous system on certain organs or tissues. In the context of pain control, this may involve angina pectoris (acute pain) or pain resulting from nerve damage (neurogenic or neuropathic, chronic pain). Owing to the extensive distribution of tissues and organs upon which the sympathetic nervous system exerts control, the effects of these drugs tend to be widespread and in some instances it may be difficult to achieve selective control of the pain problem without producing unacceptable adverse effects (see Table 11.8).

Table 11.7   Distribution of adrenoceptors and their actions

Tissue	alpha₁	alpha₂	beta₁	beta₂
Smooth muscle				
Blood vessels	*Constrict*	Constrict		Dilate
Bronchi	Constrict			Dilate
Uterus				*Relax*
GI tract				
Non-sphincter	Relax		Relax	
Sphincter	Contract			
Bladder				
Detrusor				Relax
Sphincter	Contract			
Eye				
Radial muscle of iris	Contracts causing pupil to dilate			
ciliary muscle (controls accommodation of eye)				Relax
Heart			*Increase rate and force*	
Liver	Glycolysis and potassium release			Glycogenolysis
Skeletal muscle				tremor*
Adrenergic nerve terminals		*Decrease release of noradrenaline*	*Increase release of noradrenaline*	

Italic denotes those effects especially relevant to pain problems.
* hence β2 antagonists can be used to control some tremors.

Table 11.8   Adrenoceptor blocking drugs

Class	Official name	Proprietary name	Mechanism of action	Adverse effects
Alpha-adrenoceptor blockers Unselective (α1 + α2)	phenoxyben-zamine prazosin	Dibenyline Hypovase	Compete with noradrenaline at postsynaptic (α1) or presynaptic (α2) adrenoceptors	Vasodilatation is common and leads to compensatory tachycardia, angina pectoris and postural hypotension causing dizziness and headache. Nasal congestion; depression; failure of ejaculation
Beta-adrenoceptor blockers Non-cardioselective (β1 + β2) Cardioselective (β1)	propranolol atenolol	Inderal Tenormin	Compete with noradrenaline at postsynaptic adrenoceptors in the heart (β1) or bronchial and other smooth muscle (β2)	Bradycardia (slow heart rate). May depress myocardium and precipitate heart failure. Bronchoconstriction (especially with non-cardioselective β-blocker) which in asthmatics can precipitate an attack. Peripheral vasoconstriction (Raynaud's phenomenon) especially in cold weather. Depression. Sleep disturbances and hallucinations

Mechanism of action: Alpha- and beta-adrenoceptor blocking drugs act by competing at alpha and beta receptors, respectively, with noradrenaline released from adrenergic nerve endings. Table 11.8 gives details of a selected list of these drugs.

Adverse effects: Details of these are given in Table 11.8.

Rationale for inducing autonomic block

When a particular condition is caused by, or is dependent upon, abnormal activity of the sympathetic nervous system, it is rational to treat it by taking steps to reduce the nervous activity to a normal state. This can be achieved through the action of drugs designed to modulate synaptic transmission in the autonomic nervous system. Consider, for example, pain in a limb that is due to inadequate blood flow (and hence inadequate oxygen tension) secondary to intense vasoconstriction caused by excessive discharge in the sympathetic vasoconstrictor nerves supplying the arterioles in the affected part. As can be seen in Table 11.7, the autonomic control of blood vessels involves activation of alpha receptors (primarily $alpha_1$). From this fact it follows that a drug, for example prazosin, which blocks $alpha_1$ receptors, will block vasoconstriction induced by discharge of the sympathetic nervous system.

The pain of angina pectoris occurs when the oxygen demand needed for an increase of cardiac work, signified by increased rate (tachycardia) and force of cardiac contraction, cannot be met owing to an impaired coronary circulation caused by arterial disease. Since the increase in rate and force of cardiac contraction are controlled by increased sympathetic discharge to the heart, this painful condition can be relieved by prescribing a beta-adrenoceptor blocking drug. This reduces the sympathetic drive to the heart and so reduces cardiac work to a level at which the oxygen demand can be met adequately by the compromised coronary circulation. The beta-adrenoceptor blockers available are either cardioselective ($beta_1$ antagonists) or non-selective ($beta_{1+2}$ antagonists).

Sympathectomy

This is an alternative and invasive method of producing sympathetic blockade. It can take the form of a reversible nerve block using an injection of local anaesthetic or of an irreversible nerve block using a neurolytic agent such as phenol. Alternatively, it is carried out using an ablative surgical technique.

Sympathectomy is used in the following situations:

1. When drugs have failed to control the pain problem;
2. When drugs are only able to control the pain problem if administered in doses that produce unacceptable adverse effects;
3. When a selective block without the use of continuing medication is desired.

Examples of sympathectomy (nerve blocks) used to relieve acute and chronic pain conditions are shown in the lower half of Table 11.4.

Implications for physiotherapy

Patients with sympathetically dependent pains (SMP) which have been controlled by means of adrenoceptor blocking drugs or sympathectomy often require appropriate physiotherapy. In planning a programme for such patients, the physiotherapist will need to take into account the following points (more particularly in patients on adrenoceptor blockers):

1. Cardiovascular effects: postural hypotension causing dizziness; an inadequate response to exercise (due to beta-blockade) and the possibility of precipitating heart failure. Peripheral vasoconstriction (due to unopposed alpha effect in presence of beta-blockade) causing Raynaud's phenomenon (most likely in cold weather); sleep disturbances and depression.
2. Respiratory effects: bronchoconstriction causing wheeziness.

Vasodilators

These are drugs or other agents that produce relaxation of vascular smooth muscle by acting either (i) indirectly via modulation of its sympathetic nerve control or (ii) directly on control mechanisms within the smooth muscle. The first group have been discussed already in the section on sympathetic nerve block. The second group is composed of a heterogeneous collection of drugs. There are four drugs used most commonly. Details of these are given in Table 11.9

Table 11.9   Vasodilators

Type	Official name	Proprietary name	Mechanism of action	Adverse effects
Antihistamine (H1 blocker)	cinnarizine	Stugeron Forte	This H1 antagonist acts as a vasodilator via a calcium channel blocking action	Drowsiness, fatigue, blurred vision. Rarely extrapyramidal effects, allergic reactions
Direct acting vasodilator	nicotinic acid derivatives	Hexopal	Inositol nicotinate is the active principle	Flushing, dizziness, hypotension nausea, vomiting
Calcium channel blocker	nifedipine	Adalat	Reduces availability of intracellular calcium ions $[Ca^{2+}]$ thereby reducing electro-mechanical coupling which results in weaker contractions	Flushing, dizziness, lethargy, headache, peripheral oedema, gum hyperplasia, eye pain
?	oxpentifylline	Trental	?	Flushing, dizziness, nausea, vomiting, diarrhoea. Rarely tachycardia, hypotension. Very rarely, allergic reactions; thrombocytopenia

Main Uses: These drugs are used principally to try to improve an inadequate peripheral circulation as occurs in peripheral vascular disease and vasospastic disorders, e.g. Raynaud's syndrome. They are usually to be found prescribed in combination with other drugs acting on the cardiovascular system, for example, hypotensive drugs.

Mechanism of action and adverse effects: See Table 11.9.

Implications for physiotherapy

Patients who have been prescribed vasodilator drugs are likely to suffer from an impaired peripheral circulation due to vascular disease. It is probable that they also suffer from cardiovascular disease. As a consequence, their exercise tolerance will be reduced, possibly grossly so. In addition, they may be prone to dizziness, flushing, postural hypotension and lethargy, all of which will affect their ability to adhere to a physiotherapy programme. Caution must also be given to any physiotherapy procedure which might jeopardize the patient's peripheral circulation, especially of the hands and feet.

Psychosocial factors

As stated earlier in Chapters 4 and 6, pain has been defined by the International Association for the Study of Pain (IASP) as:

> an unpleasant sensory and emotional experience associated with actual or potential tissue damage, or described in terms of such damage.

In other words, **every pain has an emotional component** and this needs to be considered and treated with as much care and attention to detail as the concomitant sensory component. Unfortunately, one of the most neglected areas in pain management is that of communication between health professionals (especially doctors) and patients concerning the explanation of pain problems! More often than not, nobody thinks it necessary (or bothers) to explain to a patient the reason for their pain, the implications of it and the proposed treatment plan. As a consequence, patients suffer a great deal of unnecessary anxiety about their pains which, in turn, lowers their pain tolerance and so aggravates the situation.

Counselling is a means whereby the patient can be helped to cope with their pain, irrespective of how well it may be controlled by pharmacological and/or physical treatments. The meaning of pain to a patient has a powerful influence on their subsequent experience and reaction to it. Simple counselling forms part of good practice by all health professionals; when needed, more advanced counselling is available from trained counsellors such as a social worker, priest, clinical psychologist or psychiatrist.

Cognitive-behavioural techniques are used to help patients cope with pain that has failed to respond to pharmacological and/or physical treatments. It is normally given by someone with special training who is most likely to be a clinical psychologist. The approaches used include special techniques for **relaxation**, possibly utilizing **biofeedback** techniques. In addition **hypnosis** is often used with a view to teaching the patient **self-hypnosis** so that the locus of pain control can be handed over to the patient with many obvious advantages.

Rehabilitation must obviously be the ultimate aim for every patient with a pain problem. In essence this means the maximum possible improvement in the quality of life. The more fortunate patient will be able to achieve a return to near or full normality. The less fortunate, particularly those with untreatable cancer, will clearly be unable to attain such a goal, but the aim of all treatment continues to be the same, namely to achieve the maximum possible improvement in the quality of life that remains.

Implications for physiotherapy

Like every other health professional involved in the care of patients with pain problems, the physiotherapist must always ensure that the emotional, as well as the physical (sensory), component of a pain is receiving adequate care and attention. This concerns not only that part of the treatment for which the physiotherapist is responsible, but also the whole treatment plan for a particular patient. The physiotherapist, through opportunities for physical and psychological contact with a patient, is well placed to monitor a patient's reaction to a pain problem and their response to treatment of it. But in addition to the specialized treatment which the physiotherapist contributes, he or she can make other valuable contributions by acting as an observer who can provide feedback on the patient's progress to other members of the pain management team. Indeed, no member of the pain management team is better placed than the physiotherapist to carry out this important and valuable role.

Acknowledgements

The author wishes to thank his colleagues for their helpful discussions during the preparation of this chapter. In particular, he is indebted to Mrs Lydia Gillham, Senior Physiotherapist, St Oswald's Hospice, and to Mr Robert Packham, Superintendent Physiotherapist, Royal Victoria Infirmary, Newcastle upon Tyne, who strongly encouraged him to write a more detailed account of pharmacology and its implications for physiotherapy than that originally envisaged by the editors. He also wishes to express his grateful thanks to Mrs Anne Nicholson for her excellent secretarial help

References

Budd, K. (1981) Non-analgesic drugs in the management of pain. In *Persistent Pain*, vol. 3. (ed. S. Lipton and J. Miles), Academic Press, London, pp. 223–40

Murray, J.G. and Thompson, J.W. (1957) Collateral sprouting in response to injury of the autonomic nervous system, and its consequences, In *Autonomic Nervous System* (ed. W.S. Feldberg), British Council, London. *Brt. Med. Bull.*, **13**, 213–19)

Thompson, J.W. (1984) Pain: mechanisms and principles of management. In *Advanced Geriatric Medicine 4* (eds J. Grimley Evans and F.I. Caird), Pitman, London, pp. 3–16.

Thompson, J.W. (1990) Clinical pharmacology of opioid agonists and partial agonists. In *Opioids in the Treatment of Cancer Pain* (ed. D. Doyle), Royal Society of Medicine Services International Congress and Symposium Series No. 146, London, Royal Society of Medicine Services, pp. 17–38

Thompson, J.W. and Tyrer, S.P. (1992) Psychotropic drugs. In *Psychology, Psychiatry and Chronic Pain* (ed. S.P. Tyrer), Butterworth Heinemann, Oxford, pp. 95–106

Watson, C.P., Evans, R.J., Reed, K. et al. (1982) Amitriptyline versus placebo in postherpetic neuralgia. *Neurology*, **32**, 671–3

Bibliography

Foster, R.W. (ed.) (1991) *Basic Pharmacology*, 3rd edn, Butterworth Heinemann, Oxford

Grahame-Smith and Aronson, J.K. (1992) *Clinical Pharmacology and Drug Therapy*, 2nd edn, Oxford University Press, Oxford

Rang, H.P. and Dale, M.M. (1991) *Pharmacology*, 2nd edn, Churchill Livingstone, Edinburgh

Tyrer, S.P. (ed.) (1992) *Psychology, Psychiatry and Chronic Pain*, Butterworth Heinemann, Oxford

12 *The neuromuscular facilitation of movement*

A.J. GUYMER

Introduction

Patients who seek medical assistance for musculoskeletal problems will almost always do so because of pain, either acute or chronic. The fact that they have loss of joint range and hence functional limitation is not usually of sufficient importance, by itself, for them to ask for treatment.

The origin of painful or noxious stimuli may be in the skeletal, soft tissues of joints, contractile or nervous tissue, or as is sometimes hypothesized, from venous distension or a combination of these. The fascia and connective tissue surrounding musculoskeletal structures may also give rise to pain. The noxious stimuli will reflexly affect the degree of excitation occurring in the muscle fibres around the damaged structures. This reflex effect is explained in Chapter 6, Table 6.1 (p. 4.1).

Because proprioceptive neuromuscular facilitation (PNF) techniques can alter the degree of muscle excitation and inhibition they can sometimes be used very effectively when treating benign musculoskeletal problems.

Muscular Function

The musculoskeletal system has to be able to respond to the needs of an individual in terms of postural control and coordinated movement. Unless there is good control of the background posture, i.e. joint position and muscle origins controlled, it is not possible to produce movement that is smooth and efficient. In normal situations muscles must be able to perform in the following ways:

1. Low threshold tonic muscle fibres (Type I) should control the position of one or more joints against any reasonable force. This means that muscles must be able to work isometrically at any length in the available joint range.
2. Activity in high threshold phasic muscle fibres (Type II) should produce coordinated movement, either through large or minute ranges, at varying speeds and against different forces. Movement will occur in any number of joints at one time. This requires exquisite coordination of the surrounding musculature for the agonists, synergists and antagonists to work isotonically while lengthening or shortening.

To function normally muscles must have:

1. Normal nerve supply.
2. Full passive physiological length.
3. Strength in tonic muscle fibres sufficient to control joints in all possible positions.
4. Strength in phasic muscle fibres sufficient to move average loads in any direction.
5. Endurance sufficient to maintain all postures and movements during a reasonable length of time.

In order to have full range in the physiological movements of a joint there must be a full range in the accessory movements. During active movement the accesory movements are brought about by:

1. The contours of the cartilage at the articular interface.
2. The architecture of the ligamentous fibres which will limit movement in specific directions while allowing freedom in others (Evans, 1988).
3. Normal coordination of all muscles concerned – this means excitation of the agonists and synergists, together with inhibition of the antagonists.

The central nervous system should coordinate the

activity in the motor neuron pools so that the necessary precision and punctuality of movement can occur at any normal speed. For the sportsman, of course, the efficiency of the cardiorespiratory and cardiovascular system in relation to muscle function is of vital importance.

In normal circumstances muscles may have a role in limiting joint range, particularly the two- or multi-joint muscles. In the presence of abnormal hypermobility, muscle strength is most important to prevent joint structures from becoming overstretched and possibly painful.

Much research has been carried out on the plastic adaptation of muscle fibres to their environment and how their form, i.e. having the physiology of a phasic or tonic muscle fibre, will adapt according to the type of neurological stimulus on the motor neurone pools. Plastic adaptation in the muscle fibres occurs in response to their environment, e.g. during overuse or disuse, or when the muscle is held in a lengthened or shortened position for a long period of time, and of course during the ageing process (Rose and Rothstein, 1982). When the patient presents for treatment, there is no way of identifying clinically whether any changes have occurred at cellular level (Kidd et al., 1992), but the physiotherapist needs to be very clear about the existing conditions under which the muscles have been working.

Pain and Musculoskeletal Dysfunction

When considering treatment of patients by physiotherapeutic techniques, reference will only be made to the treatment of the benign musculoskeletal disorders. In such patients, all or some of the muscles may be functioning abnormally. Most patients who have had a movement malfunction for some time will have, due to disuse, weakness in all or part of the available range, loss of extensibility and endurance. These effects may be local or more extensive in a limb or quadrant of the body. Following trauma, or due to a disease process, a patient may suffer pain which is either acute or chronic in type. Consequently, and over a period of time, they may develop antalgic postures or abnormal movement patterns so that the muscle fibres will be working either at an abnormally longer or shorter length. The movement abnormalities will also be of speed, coordination and strength and in addition the reversal of antagonists will be very slow. Over a period of time the muscles will

adapt physiologically to their changed environment.

In the presence of pain, many patients have an understandable reluctance to move, while in others there is such a high level of cocontraction in the muscles that movement cannot occur. The normal response to movement in any one area of the body is a reflex irradiation of activity into other muscle groups. In acutely painful conditions, it is almost impossible for the patient to inhibit excessive irradiation into the adjacent normal joints. This mechanism may be the basis for perpetuating symptoms from a muscular system which is working at a permanently hyperactive level. There are situations in which the pain is so severe that the response is a neurological inhibition of muscle activity. One hypothesis is that this mechanism minimises the approximation or compression of the articular surfaces and thus prevents exacerbation of pain if this is of intracapsular origin. When any of the conditions exists for a period of time, plastic changes will occur in the neuromuscular system.

The healing and repair process which occurs after tissue damage (Evans, 1980) results in the formation of new collagen tissue which eventually contracts. There may be scarring or adhesions within the contractile, articular or nervous structures, as well as at their mechanical interface with adjacent tissues, thus causing decreased extensibility in these structures as well as preventing the normal mobility occuring between the structures and the different layers of tissues in the area of damage. It is hypothesized that these collagenous adhesions may be one of the causes of pain.

Stretching, compressing or putting tension on to tissues in which there are adhesions or scarring may give rise to pain and other symptoms. A very clear explanation of what may happen within the nervous system is given by Butler (1991).

When there has been trauma to the muscle or tendon itself, the formation of adhesions may cause pain when the muscle contracts. Symptoms may be reproduced during the examination by placing the muscle in its lengthened and/or shortened range, adding a strong isometric contraction plus local palpation.

When considering how pain and other symptoms may arise from the muscular system, we should remember the effects of denervation in muscle fibres. In this situation they become supersensitive to circulating chemicals (Gunn, 1980) and so may give a clinical presentation of muscle tenderness. 'It is known that re-innervation may

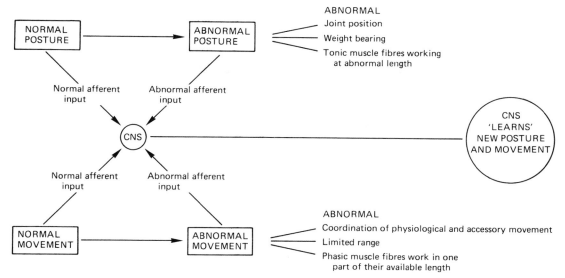

Fig. 12.1   Sensory feedback mechanisms and their effect on the CNS.

be facilitated through increased activity and irradiation from the surrounding normal motor neurons, i.e. axonal sprouting.

Janda (1986) put forward the concept that symptoms within the musculoskeletal system may occur because of habitual bad posture. These abnormal positions may lead to plastic changes within the muscles due to the fact that they are functioning over a period of time, at an abnormal length, either shorter or longer, than in the normal posture. The consequence of this is that the underlying joints may become hypomobile in some directions and may start to be symptomatic.

The abnormal sensory feedback from muscles, tendons and joint structures will, if continued for long enough, 'convince' the central nervous system that this particular pattern of activity must be accepted as 'normal' (Figure 12.1). Thus in re-education not only must pain be reduced, passive joint range and muscle extensibility be restored, but the normal coordination of muscle fibres must be facilitated and the central nervous system re-trained through appropriate biofeedback. Once pain is reduced, the strength and endurance can be developed.

Physiotherapists, knowing the effects and uses of PNF techniques, can use these skills when treating painful musculoskeletal problems, providing that they select the appropriate facilitating factors and techniques carefully in accordance with each patient's clinical picture.

Muscle Spasm

A patient with a painful musculoskeletal problem may also have a varying degree of protective muscle spasm. The latter can be divided into three causes:

1. Mishandling the patient. So often people are already tense, anxious and perhaps frightened by the hospital or treatment environment and have often heard 'true' stories about 'treatment' from their friends and acquaintances.
2. Mishandling of the painful structures by the physiotherapist so that protective muscle activity is provoked (Figure 12.2).
3. Reflex muscle spasm protecting the joint. This is unlikely to be affected until the cause of the pain is treated successfully. It may be possible temporarily to reduce the muscle spasm by extremely precise positioning of the affected part, but with the true reflex muscle spasm the patient often has so much pain that he may want to frequently change positions.

Assessment

When considering the use of muscle techniques for the treatment of pain of musculoskeletal origin it has to be presumed that the patient has been

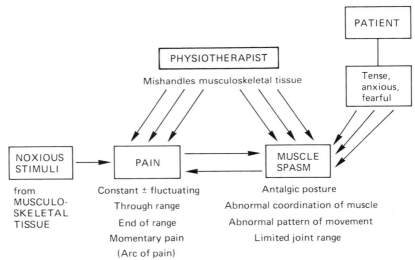

Fig. 12.2   Factors producing pain during physiotherapy.

given a very full, detailed examination in order to ascertain the local and distant sources of the symptons and the direction of movement causing the pain. The final decision about treatment using PNF techniques involves choosing the type of muscle work, isometric or isotonic, the pattern, and so the muscle groups to be facilitated, the amount of resistance and therefore irradiation which can be used.

The manner in which the treatment is modified will be guided by continual re-assessment of the patient's symptoms and signs which should be carried out both during treatment and between each attendance. The author uses Maitland's concept for examination, assessment and treatment, and so abnormalities of movement can be defined very precisely in movement diagrams (Maitland, 1986: 365–72) (see also Chapter 3, p. 8). The diagrams enable the physiotherapist to record the different characteristics and behaviour of pain resistance and spasm in relation to available joint range. As a consequence, it is possible to decide up to what point of pain and where in range the therapist will facilitate movement. The physiotherapist will then decide the response to treatment by identifying the changes in the movement diagram and will modify treatment accordingly.

In this concept pain can be described as having severity (from low to high) and the condition may be irritable (from low to high). This latter defines whether the symptom is easily stirred to a high severity and then takes a long time to die down

(irritable), or the opposite, being a symptom which may still be easily stirred up but which goes away *at once* when the provocation stops (non-irritable) (Maitland, 1986: 49).

PNF Techniques

The only effect that these techniques can have on muscle activity is to facilitate the excitation or inhibition of muscle fibres (Type I or Type II) to a greater or lesser extent. The muscle techniques used by the author are proprioceptive neuromuscular facilitation (PNF) techniques and these are very completely described elsewhere (Voss *et al.*, 1985: 298–306).

The facilitating factors used when applying PNF techniques must be carefully adapted when treating patients with pain. The main factors are as follows (Voss *et al.*, 1985: 291–7):

1. **Patterns of movement**   Movement occurs in diagonal patterns which are established along the line of fibres in the main agonist muscles. In the presence of pain the initial pattern chosen should use the least painful combination of muscles and therefore the least painful direction to start with. When working with an arm or leg it is important to clarify whether the patient works more efficiently with the middle joint flexed or extended.

2. **Hand holds**   These must be on the surface of

the muscles working at all times, but particularly in the presence of pain these hand holds should avoid using fingertips and should be very large, comfortable hand holds avoiding painful bony points. The inability to place hand holds on one surface of a limb may make the physiotherapist modify the choice of pattern and technique to be used, e.g. hyperalgesia, hyperaesthesia.

3. **Stretch stimulus** Starting position – normally with isotonic techniques, the pattern of movement starts when the agonist muscles are fully stretched, including rotational component, in order to facilitate activity. In the presence of pain, the starting position often has to be modified and one or all of the component directions will be released slightly. The quick facilitating stretch technique uses the monosynaptic reflex arc and cannot usually be used when there is pain.

4. **Traction and approximation** The former is used to facilitate activity in flexor muscles and the latter for the extensor muscles. It is often far too painful to approximate the joint surfaces of these patients – similarly, traction for the acute pain problem is generally not used. Both could be used, with care, in the chronic pain stage.

5. **Appropriate resistance** Where pain is the main limiting factor then both isotonic and isometric techniques are performed by facilitating a degree of muscle activity which will not provoke any pain. When aiming for inhibition of antagonists the same limiting criteria apply.

6. **Timing / Irradiation** The order in which the muscle groups are brought into action can be varied by the physiotherapist's skills. When using isometric techniques, the muscles far away from the problem area are facilitated first and then irradiation into the local muscles can be exquisitely controlled up to the point of pain.

   Isotonic techniques are not usually chosen where symptoms are severe and the condition is irritable, but can be used in a clinical situation involving chronic pain. It should be possible to use normal timing from proximal to distal or distal to proximal and to keep the irradiation of muscle activity to an acceptable level. This may be totally without pain or to an acceptable low level of pain.

7. **Verbal comments** For isometric techniques the command word should be 'Stay', 'Don't move', 'Don't let me move you', etc. For isotonic techniques the command should be for movement, e.g. 'Pull', 'Push', 'Lift', or more detailed as appropriate to each patient. The better the hand-

ling skill of the physiotherapist the fewer words will be needed by the patient. In theory, PNF techniques can be used where there is a total language barrier! Naturally, the quality of the command is adapted to the acutely painful situation.

The Use of PNF Techniques for Acute and Chronic Pain

Before giving details of treatment it is worthwhile considering some of the hypotheses supporting the selection of muscle techniques for treatment, and to do this it is simplest to keep to two categories of patients:

1. **Acute pain** – may be severe and the condition is irritable. The behaviour may vary as shown in Figure 12.2.
2. **Chronic pain** – may also be severe but usually the condition is only slightly irritable or non-irritable.

Acute pain

If the cause of this is trauma, then the tissues will go through the normal cycle of repair and healing (Evans, 1980) and the physiotherapist will therefore have some indication as to whether the repair collagen is still being laid down, or whether it is likely to have started contracting. The pain is often severe and it may manifest itself as a through-range pain, or an end-of-range pain.

In acute pain, it is usually accepted that an increase in venous return from the part and blood supply to the area is therapeutic, and certainly muscle activity is known to help both these actions. Sometimes the severity of the pain indicates that only a very small amount of muscle excitation should be facilitated.

If the patient attends for treatment while the new collagen is being laid down, there may be a lot of protective muscle spasm. The aim of treatment is to reduce pain and muscle spasm and so regain a full range of movement as quickly as possible by gently facilitating inhibition in the antagonistic muscle of the required movement followed by gently facilitating excitation in the agonist muscles. This brings about further reciprocal inhibition in the antagonists, and it may then be possible to achieve the desired movement passively or by coordinated activity in the agonist muscles. This normal coordination of muscles may produce the correct accessory movements at the articular interface, and so allow more physiological movement to occur. If isometric techniques are used it is possible for the physiotherapist to keep the inevitable irradiation of muscle activity below the pain threshold. This is more difficult to do with isotonic techniques and so the latter should be used with great caution. The result is to stress the newly formed collagen in all directions, so that at the time when collagen contraction starts to occur it will not interfere with the restoration of full function.

If the cause of the acute pain is an intra-articular problem, then the approach may be as above or the aim of treatment may be to enable the patient to relax the muscles around the relevant joint in a position of minimum pain. It would seem a sensible hypothesis that this category of patient does not want to increase muscle activity and so cause greater compression at the articular interface. Similarly, this aim applies to the patient who has had plastic surgery and must remain in a very abnormal position for several weeks. They should be treated with techniques aimed at relaxing all muscles around the joints and so helping to reduce their postural ache. By using the reflex phenomenon of irradiation from other normal areas of the body, it is possible to produce minimal muscle activity around the affected joint, and this can be followed by relaxation throughout the body. The physiotherapist merely applies her techniques as far away as possible from the area of acute pain. Needless to say there are always many situations in which acute pain is made worse by facilitation techniques, and then extremely gentle passive mobilizing techniques or other pain-relieving modalities must be used.

Chronic pain

When this is the clinical situation following trauma, it is likely that the healing and repair of the tissues will have resulted in the formation of scar tissue and adhesions in various structures. Any limitation of movement may be due to pain more than resistance in the tissues, or resistance more than pain. Depending on the severity of the pain and irritability of the condition, muscle spasm may be provoked in some part of the available range.

The aim of treatment is as before, to increase movement without increasing the pain or provoking muscle spasm. The muscle techniques which are most effective are the same as those used for patients with acute pain, but it may be possible to produce greater irradiation of muscle activity within the limitations of pain and spasm and therefore greater excitation of agonists and inhibition of antagonists.

The question as to whether to develop strength in the presence of pain is difficult to answer out of the clinical setting. In the patient with acute pain, it is usually impractical to attempt to strengthen muscles until the condition is no longer irritable and severity is low. However, in the patient with chronic pain, where the physiotherapist is treating resistance of the tissues and where the pain is not severe or irritable, the aim of treatment is to re-educate muscle activity so that the agonists will have strength in their inner, shortened range. In the chronic pain patient, with the resistance as the main problem together with some end-of-range pain, manipulative techniques will be necessary to increase the range first and then facilitation techniques can be used to consolidate the passive range gained and so avoid any regression over a 24 h period.

Application of PNF Techniques

The techniques of PNF can be applied to many different combinations of muscles (i.e. patterns), but when treating patients with a pain problem, the author uses patterns which are non-painful or least painful for that patient, and starts with isometric techniques as it is then possible to control the extent of recruitment and irradiation of muscle activity and to keep within pain. However, in the patients with less pain, it is possible to progress to isotonic techniques, but only with great care. Eventually it is important to use the isotonic techniques, so that the movements in the affected joint may be coordinated again with all other joints on that limb, or between the limb and trunk.

The three most useful techniques are:

1. Hold relax.
2. Rhythmical stabilizations.
3. Repeated contractions.
4. For final re-education, slow-reversal and hold will be needed.

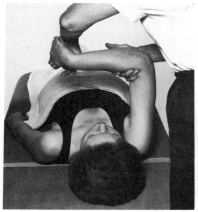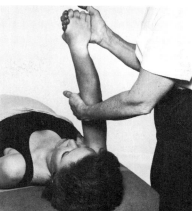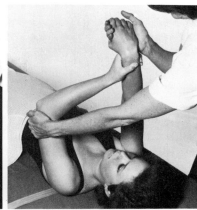

Fig. 12.3 Hold–relax technique showing three different methods used to relax the fibres of the pectoralis major muscle: *a*, hold–relax to sternal fibres of the pectoralis major using unilateral pattern with elbow flexion (method A): *b*, hold–relax to sternal fibres of the pectoralis major using unilateral pattern with elbow extension (method B): *c*, hold–relax to sternal fibres of the pectoralis major using bilateral pattern (method C).

Hold relax

This technique (Voss *et al.*, 1985: 298–306) facilitates isometric muscle activity in the antagonistic muscle of the required movement so that this may be followed by complete inhibition and relaxation of the same muscles. In the presence of severe pain, which is then the limiting factor to the irradiation, only a very small muscle contraction should be produced.

The affected joint is placed at the maximum range possible before pain, and then the technique is performed at this point on the muscle that is required to eventually lengthen out, i.e. the antagonist. Having achieved the relaxation of all muscles in that pattern, there are three alternative ways of gaining increased range:

1. The physiotherapist **passively** moves the joint further.
2. The patient gently and **actively** moves the joint further.
3. The physiotherapist gently **resists** the agonist pattern in order to produce greater reciprocal inhibition in the antagonists.

In Figure 12.3 this hold relax technique is being performed on the right shoulder, and there are examples of three different patterns being used to relax the sternal fibres of the pectoralis major:

1. Unilateral arm with elbow flexed so there is a short lever and irradiation from biceps and wrist flexors.
2. Unilateral arm with elbow extended – patients sometimes get less pain when the biceps is *not* so dominant in the pattern.
3. Bilateral arm pattern when the command to the patient relates to the left arm (the normal arm) whereby irradiation to the right is smoother as the patient is not thinking of the affected joint.

Figures 12.4 and 12.5 demonstrate the alternative hand holds when the physiotherapist gently resists the agonist muscle – namely the middle fibres of the deltoid. In both instances, this is chosen to attempt to facilitate further relaxation of the sternal pectoral by reciprocal inhibition.

It will, of course, be necessary to carry out a similar technique on a pattern involving the latissimus dorsi as this muscle must fully lengthen to enable a painful shoulder to move into full flexion, adduction and external rotation range.

Rhythmical stabilizations

This technique (Voss *et al.*, 1985: 298–306) is based on the neurological phenomenon of the reversal of antagonists in order to build up the cocontraction between agonists and antagonists. The cocontraction is built slowly to the maximum

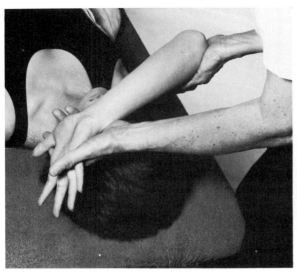

Fig. 12.4   Repeated contractions for inner range work to the middle fibres of the deltoid muscle (method A).

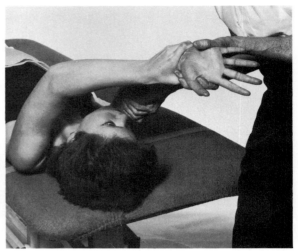

Fig. 12.5   Bilateral pattern using repeated contractions for inner range work to the middle fibres of the deltoid muscle (method B).

possible before the onset of pain by alternating between agonistic and antagonistic patterns with *no* relaxation during the change over, thus the cocontraction continues to build isometric strength until limited by pain. This is then followed by total relaxation of all muscles around the joint. The other effect of this technique is thought to be an increase in circulation by alternating the muscle activity, with the result that waste products are removed and healing is promoted. Thus it is a useful technique for pain problems which result from tissue damage, but with acute, severe and irritable symptoms it needs to be performed with great gentleness. In fact, the physiotherapist may often get the desired result of relaxation by applying the technique as far away from the painful area as possible, e.g. at the feet of patients who have just had surgery around the hip joint.

Figures 12.6, 12.7 and 12.8 show rhythmical stabilizations performed at the maximum range of hip flexion. An isometric contraction for the gluteus medius (extension, abduction, internal rotation), hamstrings and dorsiflexors is followed by an isometric contraction for the psoas (flexion, adduction, external rotation). There is no relaxation of activity while changing from antagonistic to agonistic patterns. These two actions are continually alternated and the strength of the cocontraction built up to the point *before* pain starts.

When the resultant muscle relaxation occurs

the physiotherapist can passively take the joint through further range, or with the patient suffering from chronic pain it is often possible to finish with repeated contraction to facilitate inner range activity of the agonist patterns (see Figure 12.8).

Repeated contractions

This is a series of isotonic contractions through-range facilitated by gentle rotational stretch at the point where the contraction starts to diminish.

Figures 12.9, 12.10 and 12.11 show rhythmical stabilization followed by repeated contractions being used to gain knee flexion beyond 90°. The aim here is to facilitate inner range work of the biceps femoris as a knee flexor and external rotator of the tibia, while producing inhibition and relaxation of the quadriceps muscles, especially the vastus lateralis.

Repeated contractions and slow reversal hold are most effective techniques when treating patients with habitually dislocating shoulders (Mathews *et al.*, 1991). Due to constant misuse of the shoulder complex, there is gross abnormality in the coordination of the muscle groups around the joint so that eventually symptoms develop. By treating the scapula dysfunction and re-coordinating the muscle action around the upper quadrant surgery may be avoided and asymptomatic function restored. Strengthening into inner range of all scapu-

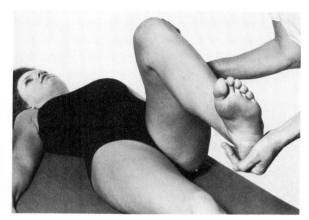

Fig. 12.6 Rhythmical stabilization to the gluteus medius muscle (approximation through calcaneum).

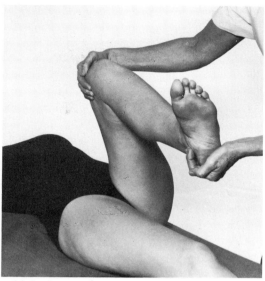

Fig. 12.8   Repeated contractions to the inner range of psoas-iliacus muscle.

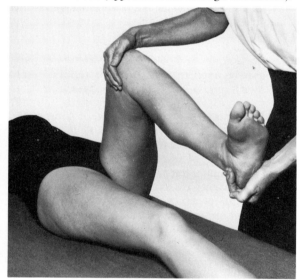

Fig. 12.7   Rhythmical stabilization to the psoas-iliacus muscle.

lar muscle is a prerequisite for the re-education of normal shoulder movement.

Slow reversal and hold

This is an isotonic contraction through-range of the stronger, more normal, or less painful pattern, finishing with an inner range isometric hold. This is then followed by an isotonic contraction through-range of the antagonistic pattern plus another inner range hold.

This technique may be useful with some patients when they are starting treatment immediately following trauma, as the healing tissue may respond to *very gentle* facilitation and minimal excitation without any appreciable increase in pain.

With the patient who has chronic pain, this technique is used as a means of coordinating the joints of one limb again so that function may become normal.

In all muscle techniques used for re-education there is inevitably a greatly increased sensory, afferent feedback from the muscle and joint receptors and it is important that this should be an exaggeration of the norm for the central nervous system to relearn (Morris and Sharpe, 1993). PNF techniques are so useful in painful musculoskeletal disorders because there is a great variety of patterns of movement to choose from, and so the physiotherapist is able to 'tailor' the choice to the needs of each individual clinical situation. Similarly, the techniques available are very varied and although the author has suggested the use of certain techniques in this chapter, it is often the case that other patterns may produce better results in specific clinical situations.

The 'dosage' of each application of a technique is represented by:
1. The extent of the irradiation which is allowed to develop.

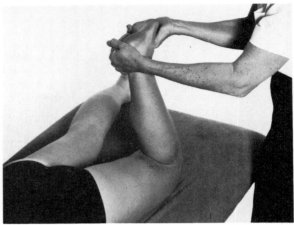

Fig. 12.11   Repeated contractions to the inner range of the hamstrings stressing the biceps femoris as the external rotator of the tibia.

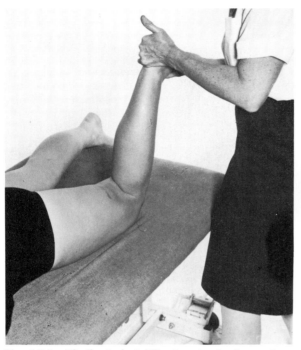

Fig. 12.9   Rhythmical stabilization to the hamstrings stressing the biceps femoris as an external rotator of the tibia.

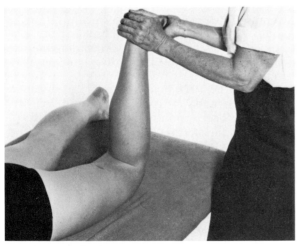

Fig. 12.10   Rhythmical stabilization to the quadriceps stressing the vastus lateralis muscle.

2. The amount of resistance given which will result in a desired level of muscle activity.
3. The time for which each technique is applied before re-testing the result.

These techniques and principles for treatment may, of course, be applied to any joint or series of joints in the body.

All the examples mentioned so far are on peripheral joints; a review of the use of PNF for spinal problems can be found in Grieve (1986).

The principle of applying these techniques to spinal problems is the same, but the patterns used may be bilateral extremity patterns to irradiate into the trunk or direct trunk patterns, e.g. patients who have lumbar spinal canal stenosis syndrome need to learn to maintain a degree of lumbar flexion in order to minimize the pain. Thus, using bilateral leg patterns, the physiotherapist develops middle range strength in the abdominal and gluteus muscles.

A second example is the patient with a 'dowager's hump' in the upper thoracic level, with compensating hyperextension of the mid cervical area giving rise to the characteristic symptoms. These patients need to learn a correct posture and the muscles need to have their strength and endurance built up in their realigned position.

Another example is when a patient has had spinal surgery, then PNF techniques can be used to increase lumbar movement in all directions in a non-weight-bearing position in bed, as well as regaining full lengthening of the spinal canal structures.

Most musculoskeletal problems have abnormalities in both systems as well as in the nervous system. The spinal canal structures and the peripheral nerves can be mobilized and extended using PNF techniques. Cadaveric research is needed to identify which of the patterns affect the elongation of specific nerves. The best results are usually obtained by using these PNF techniques in close conjunction with manipulative techniques for the joint dysfunction. They can also be combined very effectively with such modalities as ice and TENS, but it must be remembered that such pain-relieving treatments do not give the physiotherapist licence to overdose with these highly potent PNF techniques!

References

Butler, D. (1991) *Mobilizations of the Nervous System*, Churchill Livingstone, Edinburgh

Evans, P. (1980) The healing process at cellular level. *Physiotherapy*, **66 (8)**, 256–9

Evans, P. (1988) Ligaments Joint Surfaces, Conjunct Rotation and Close Pack. *Physiotherapy*, **74 (3)**, 105–14

Grieve, G.P., (ed.) (1986) *Modern Manual Therapy of the Vertebral Column*, Churchill Livingstone, Edinburgh, Ch. 58, pp. 622–39.

Gunn, C. (1980) 'Prespondylosis' and some pain syndromes following denervation and supersensitivity. *Spine*, **5 (2)**, 185–92

Janda, V. (1986) Muscle weakness and inhibition (pseudo paresis) in back pain syndromes. In *Modern Manual Therapy*, Churchill Livingstone, Edinburgh

Kidd, G. Laws, N. and Musa, I. (1992) *Understanding Neuromuscular Plasticity*, Edward Arnold, London

Maitland, G.D. (1986) *Vertebral Manipulation*, 5th edn, Butterworths, London

Mathews, H.J., Damrel, U.D. and Sibilia, K. (1991) *The Recognition and Treatment of Habitually Dislocating Shoulders*. Proceedings of WCPT

Morris, S.L. and Sharpe, M.H. (1993) PNF revisited. *Physiother. Theory Pract.*, **9** (1), 43–51.

Rose, S.J. and Rothstein, J.M. (1982) Muscle mutability. Part I: General concepts and adaptation to altered pattern of use. *Phys. Ther.*; **62**(12), 1773–87

Voss, D., Ionta, M. and Myers, B. (1985) *Proprioceptive Neuromuscular Facilitation*, 3rd edn, Harper and Row, Philadelphia

13 Acupuncture

JON ALLTREE

Introduction

Acupuncture developed as part of Traditional Chinese Medicine, a system of medicine based on different concepts, language and practices to those widely used in the West. These differences have complicated the introduction of acupuncture into countries practising modern Western medicine and it is often regarded as unconventional, unscientific or even mystical. Today many methods of practice are subsumed under the title acupuncture. Authors such as Mann, Baldry and Gunn (see Bibliography) have described approaches which are explained in Western neurophysiological terms. There remains, however, common ground with traditional acupuncture. Even if the West has difficulties with its theories, traditional acupuncture's long empirical heritage cannot be ignored and nowadays many practitioners draw their practice from both traditions (Alltree, 1993; Rickards, 1979).

Physiotherapists and acupuncture

In 1973 the use of acupuncture by physiotherapists in New Zealand was a disciplinary issue, but by 1983 it was an accepted part of practice (Drok, 1983). In the UK the scope of practice of the Chartered Society of Physiotherapists was amended in 1982 to include acupuncture as a 'form of pain relief'. A clinical interest group, the Acupuncture Association of Chartered Physiotherapists, was formed in 1984 and campaigned for the scope of practice for acupuncture to be widened. In 1988 it was changed to allow acupuncture to be used to treat 'any condition normally treated by physiotherapists'. The primary concerns of the World Health Organization are that those trained to practise acupuncture should have a knowledge of anatomy, physiology, pathology, pharmacology and medicine, as well as diagnostic skills, in order to ensure safety and competence (Akerele, 1991). These requirements are incorporated into the training of physiotherapists and supplemented by excellent manual skills, and therefore it is no surprise that acupuncture has become incorporated into physiotherapy practice in many countries.

This chapter will outline the history of acupuncture as well as Traditional and Western theory. A brief impression of traditional practice will be followed by more detailed descriptions of Western approaches to pain relief.

The history of Traditional acupuncture

Traditional acupuncture is one of the two main therapeutic branches of Traditional Chinese Medicine, the other being herbalism. It dates back to around 2000 BC. Although the exact origins are unclear, it is believed to have been developed from two observations made by the ancient Chinese. First, they realized that there was a relationship between injury to certain parts of the body's surface and beneficial effects elsewhere. Secondly, they understood that diseased organs could cause pain at distant sites. They began to define a relationship between surface points and certain organs. The Chinese already used stone knives or sharp edged tools to drain abscesses and in time such implements were used to stimulate the points that had become recognized as helpful. Stones were replaced by metals such as copper, gold, silver and chrome when they became available.

The many points that had become known were eventually categorized in groups. This may have been because certain points appeared to have similar properties, but it was also a helpful method for remembering the large number of points which had been identified. The groups were developed into the system of channels, known as 'the meridians', which were believed to act as a connection between the major organs and the body surface. In fact, Chinese knowledge of anatomy was not particularly accurate as it was largely based on observations of bodies on the battlefield. Formal anatomical studies were banned until this century because the Chinese believed that their bodies belonged to their ancestors and had to be returned to them intact.

At this point the two main philosophies in ancient China should be mentioned as they played a considerable role in acupuncture's subsequent development into a sophisticated system for the prevention and treatment of disease. Confucianism defined a rigid social structure, with every person part of a complex hierarchy. Acupuncture developed a very complex system of rules and relationships, reflecting this influence. The Taoists, on the other hand, sought harmony between man and the natural world in order to achieve good health. They believed that everything had a 'Yang' component and a 'Yin' component. Yang was associated with heaven and the sky, warmth and dryness, while yin was associated with things of the earth, coldness and dampness. Each organ needed correct proportions of yin and yang in order to remain healthy and this balance was regulated by the flow of chi, or 'vital energy' around the body via the meridians. If the balance was disturbed for too long, or the overall level of chi in the system was wrong, illness resulted. It was believed that needling, and other forms of stimulation such as moxibustion, corrected deficiencies or excesses of chi and restored function to the organ.

Traditional acupuncture enjoyed increasing popularity in China until early in the seventeenth century. It then began a slow decline before falling into disrepute in the nineteenth century and in 1929 it was officially outlawed in China. Implementation of this ban was only practical in the coastal cities and the huge rural population still had access to traditional techniques. The communists, who took power in 1949, were suspicious of traditional acupuncture because of its links with the philosophies of the past. The need to provide health care for the huge population and the dearth of Western doctors necessitated a compromise. United clinics, where practitioners of both systems could work together and learn from each other, were set up. Although cooperation was poor at first, the situation improved in 1955 when both parties were officially accorded equal status. In recent years two major Chinese Institutions, the Chinese Traditional Medical Research Institute and the Acupunc- ture Research Institute, have attempted to describe and explain the effects of acupuncture in terms of Western neurophysiology and morphology.

Traditional practice

Traditional practitioners will take a detailed and systematic history about various aspects of the patient's life which are believed to cause imbalances of chi. They will ask about environmental factors, including wind, cold, heat, dampness, dryness and fire which are believed can invade the body if it is weak. Details of diet, physical and sexual activity are ascertained as deficiencies or excesses are considered potentially harmful. They will assess the influence of the 'seven emotions' – joy, anger, fear, sadness, grief, pensiveness and fright. Each emotion is considered to have a relationship with a particular organ and it is believed that problems with a particular organ manifest themselves with certain emotional disturbances, and vice versa. A physical examination, including tongue and pulse diagnosis, follows. The tongue's colour, shape and the quality of its coating are all noted. Twelve pulses, six at each wrist, are taken. Each pulse is associated with one of the major organs and its quality is said to reflect the state of the organ.

The above examination will help the practitioner to make a traditional diagnosis. It may identify a blockage of chi in a particular meridian, which would result in disharmony in the related organ. Alternatively, dysfunction in the organ would disrupt the flow of chi in the related meridian. Each organ is associated with one of the Taoist's natural elements and five element theory could be used to help determine where needles should be placed and how vigorously they should be stimulated.

This assessment is holistic and recognizes the two-way relationship between body and mind. It also elicits information about aspects of lifestyle over which patients have the potential to take responsibility and influence their health. Traditional diagnoses, however, raise two problems for the West. First, they use different terminology. Large bowel obstruction, for example, might be termed 'spleen weak and loses its movement; empty evil becomes accumulated' (Macdonald, 1989). Secondly, because they apply different diagnostic criteria, a group of patients with the same Western diagnostic may each receive different traditional diagnoses (Vincent and Richardson, 1986). Nowadays many practitioners in China use Western methods of diagnosis alongside their traditional methods (Aakster, 1986) and have discarded pulse diagnosis and five element theory (Rickards, 1979).

The history of acupuncture in the West

The practice of acupuncture began to spread to China's neighbouring countries in the 6th century AD when a monk named Zhi Cong introduced it to Japan. Around the same time it was introduced into Korea and from there spread to Viet-Nam. It reached Europe in the seventeenth century when Willem ten Rhijne (1647–1700), a Dutch physician, visited China and described his encounter with acupuncture to the West. By the nineteenth century many doctors were practising acupuncture in Europe, but there was considerable scepticism for the traditional Chinese theories and methods, alien to Western medical thought. Anatomical studies, of the kind banned in China, had been conducted since the sixteenth century and did not support the models put forward by the Chinese. Practitioners often ignored the complexities of traditional practice and favoured needling tender points.

The first practitioner of acupuncture in Britain is reported to have been J.M. Churchill, who published a series of case histories in 1828. Although he admitted he did not know how it worked, his paper caused an upsurge of interest in England. In time, however, acupuncture fell into disuse. There was a brief resurgence of interest later that century as physiologists and microscopists began to postulate that the reflex arc or hyperaemic effects were implicated. Ultimately, however, these hypotheses did not satisfy the doctors of the day. The lack of explanation, coupled with the widespread use by charlatans and the links with Taoism, resulted in acupuncture falling into disuse in Britain once more (Editorial, 1973).

There has been renewed Western interest in acupuncture over the past two decades. One reason for this was President Nixon's visit to China in 1972, which ended its four decades of isolation. A second factor was the publication of the 'gate theory of pain' by Melzac and Wall in 1965. This theory gave some respectability to the idea of needles influencing pain and the revival has been characterized by a particular interest in pain relief.

The interest in pain was further stimulated by Chinese demonstrations of subjects undergoing surgical procedures without general anaesthesia. In fact, acupuncture analgesia of this kind was not as impressive as perceived because the procedures were usually accompanied by Western premedication and analgesics, and were suitable only for a highly selected group of patients (Skrabenek, 1984).

Western practices

Classical acupuncture

While practitioners of Traditional acupuncture select points on the basis of a traditional diagnosis, the term 'classical acupuncture' has been used to describe the practice of using traditional points in conjunction with Western diagnoses (Vincent and Richardson, 1986). Practitioners may rely on selecting a 'prescription' of points to match the diagnosis. Alternatively, they may employ local points, distant points, points in line and points in opposition (see below). Although there are clear links between classical acupuncture and its traditional origins, it does not rely on some of the more controversial elements, such as pulse diagnosis and five element theory. This blend of Eastern and Western approaches evolved over many years and represents a pragmatic compromise.

Trigger point acupuncture

Western observation that certain muscles develop tender points in association with either pain or visceral problems, such as appendicitis, are long-standing. Trigger point acupuncture involves the needling of 'trigger points'(TPs) in muscle in order to deactivate them and relieve the pain referred from them. It has its theoretical background rooted in the Western medical tradition, yet it has much in common with the Ah Shi school of acupuncture dating back to the China of the seventh century AD. The phrase 'myofascial trigger point' (MTP) was first used in the 1940s by Travell who, with her colleague Rinzler, mapped out the typical patterns of pain referral from a variety of muscles. Further work on this subject culminated in two comprehensive texts, in which an MTP is defined as a 'hyperirritable locus within a taut band of skeletal muscle, located in the muscular tissue and/or its associated fascia. The spot is painful on compression and can evoke characteristic referred pain and autonomic phenomena' (Travell and Simons, 1983, 1992).

Characteristics of trigger points

MTPs refer pain to a predictable site. This has two clinical implications. First, because MTPs are distant from where the pain is felt, patients are often unaware of their presence. Secondly, the distribution of pain can guide the therapist to the MTP.

MTPs are tender on palpation. A transient contraction of the muscle, known as a 'twitch sign', may be elicited on palpation. The patient may even flinch or cry out – a 'jump sign'.

Muscles with active MTPs shorten and weaken. Resisted isometric contraction is frequently painful, as is stretching the muscle.

MTPs may be 'active' or 'latent'. An exquisitely tender MTP which refers symptoms is in an active phase. One that is tender, but not causing symptoms, is in a latent phase. Symptomless subjects may have latent MTPs which can become active following relatively minor trauma.

TPs can be found in skin, ligaments and periosteum. In skin they are frequently associated with scar tissue. Likewise, ligamentous TPs are often found at the sites of old injuries. Periosteal TPs may be amenable to periosteal pecking (see below).

Aetiology of myofascial trigger points

Muscles appear to develop active MTPs due to primary or secondary causes. Primary causes include direct trauma, strains, excessive or unaccustomed exercise and the accumulated effects of repeated minor trauma or loading. Secondary causes include pathological events that typically cause referred pain or spasm. Disc disease may refer pain to the leg, in a similar area to that referred by a trigger point in the buttock. Travell and Simons (1983) suggest that the muscle containing this trigger point will now react as though it is in pain, and become active. As muscles learn movement patterns and habits very quickly the MTP can remain active and become the primary source of pain even if the disc pathology resolves. Visceral disease, for example cardiac problems, can activate MTPs in the same way.

Neurophysiological aspects of acupuncture

Mechanisms of pain relief by acupuncture, the effects of acupuncture on the autonomic nervous system (ANS) and the nature of acupuncture points and meridians have all been investigated. Apparently conflicting reports do occur (e.g. Mayer et al. 1977; Chapman et al., 1980). This is due, in part, to the many methods of point selection and stimulation that have been used by different researchers. Some of the main areas of research are highlighted below.

Pathways

A summary of the nervous pathways probably involved in acupuncture pain relief follows.

In the periphery, needling stimulates A-delta mechanoreceptors, which typically respond to pin prick. At spinal level, enkephalinergic interneurons from the A-delta fibres inhibit pain transmission. Meanwhile, the A-delta input continues on its path towards the thalamus via the spinothalamic tract. This pathway sends a major collateral branch to the periaqueductal grey matter, which then produces descending inhibition (Bowsher, 1988). The involvement of the spinothalamic tract is supported by the clinical observation that patients with syringomyelia destroying that part of the cord do not experience needle sensation (see below), whereas those with the dorsal columns destroyed, as in tabes dorsalis, do (Shanghai First Medical College, 1973).

Humoral factors

The first suggestion that acupuncture analgesia may be mediated by a humoral mechanism came from a controlled experiment when transfer of cerebrospinal fluid (CSF) from rabbits having acupuncture produced pain relief in recipient rabbits (*Research Group of Acupuncture Anaesthesia, Peking, 1974*). On subsequent investigation on human subjects CSF showed raised betaendorphin levels after 30 minutes of low frequency electroacupuncture (Clement-Jones et al., 1980). The involvement of endogenous opioids is also supported by studies showing that acupuncture analgesia is at least partly reversed by naloxone, an opiate antagonist (Sjolund and Erikson, 1976; Mayer et al., 1977). Not all work, however, has shown naloxone reversibility (Chapman et al., 1980). That author noted that his method of electroacupuncture was not painful whereas that of Mayer's team was. He concluded that a painful stimulus may have been necessary to stimulate endogenous opioids. A study of the effects of electroacupuncture found that opioid requirement for 2 hours postoperatively was significantly reduced in patients receiving acupuncture (Christensen et al, 1989). As the half life of beta-endorphin is approximately 2 hours, these results may also be consistent with its release.

The autonomic nervous system

The influence of acupuncture on the autonomic nervous system has been investigated. A controlled study of normal subjects demonstrated increased skin temperature, from head to toe and bilaterally, following manual needle stimulation to a point (colon 4) on the left hand (Ernst and Lee, 1985). Electroacupuncture to real acupuncture points for treating hypertension produced a transient reduction in blood pressure which was not found in a control group treated with sham points (Williams et al., 1991). Sympatholytic effects may well be of use in treating sympathetically maintained pain, such as reflex sympathetic dystrophy, and problems which are aggravated by stress, such as muscle contraction headaches.

Placebo response

Acupuncture, with its mystique and 'hands on' nature, certainly has the potential to generate a placebo response. A placebo component cannot be discounted entirely, especially as endorphin release has been implicated in the placebo effect (Gielen, 1989). It is difficult to believe that this is the only factor involved. Long's review (1991) of the literature suggested that a placebo response is usually sustained in about 10–12% of patients only, and Beecher's review (1955) of many trials suggested a mean of 32% of patients are placebo responders. Long- and short-term success rates with acupuncture are generally higher than these figures (e.g. Fox and Melzack, 1973; Coan et al 1980; Hansen and Hansen, 1983).

Other hypotheses

The sections above provide insight into acupunc-

ture providing transient relief of pain. Pain relief in the clinical situation may last much longer, or even indefinitely, and additional explanations are required.

Melzack et al. (1977) postulated that pain associated with muscle TPs may be maintained by low level pathological input causing abnormal reverberating circuits of CNS activity. Needling may provide massive input disrupting the circuits for a long time or permanently. Moreover, as pain often results in altered motor patterns, temporary pain relief could permit more normal motor activity leading to more normal afferent input, which in turn would help prevent further abnormal central activity (Melzack, 1989).

It has also been proposed that the local trauma of needling produces a sterile inflammatory reaction. The response to trauma includes the release of nervous system mediators, such as histamine, which would promote healing and reduce pain by triggering the body's defence mechanisms (Kim, 1981).

Acupuncture points, trigger points and motor points

Although anatomical studies have failed to demonstrate a Western equivalent of the meridians, acupuncture points do have some anatomical characteristics. Most appear to be sites intimately related to superficial nerve endings, intramuscular and visceral nerve endings and musculotendinous junctions (Gunn et al., 1976; Wu, 1990). A double-blind experiment found many, but not all, acupuncture points to have locally low skin impedance (Liu et al., 1975), which is indicative of increased sweating and vasomotor activity. This characteristic underpins many of the electrical point finders available commercially.

Work by Melzack et al. (1977) demonstrated that all Travell and Rinzler's MTPs had corresponding acupuncture points and overall there was a 71% correspondence between the pain syndromes associated with a particular acupuncture point and the equivalent MTP.

Many trigger points also correspond with motor points.

A study by Miehlke et al. (1960) suggested that active MTPs showed dystrophic changes and alterations in lipid content. Other studies supported the idea that MTPs' local blood supply was impaired (Fassbinder, 1975; Popelianskii et al., 1976).

Travell and Simons's (1983) hypothesis for the mechanism underlying the MTPs physiological contracture is summarized below.

Initial muscle overload could disrupt the sarcoplasmic reticulum, releasing free calcium ions which would cause local muscle contraction. The muscle fibres would normally relax as the calcium was returned to the sarcoplasmic reticulum by energy released from ATP. If, however, the local circulation was compromised by metabolite build-up and sustained muscle contraction, the demand for ATP might not be met. Persisting levels of calcium in the muscle fibres, without ATP to remove them, would result in an energy-deficient activation, as in McArdle's disease or rigor mortis. This would continue even after the sarcoplasmic reticulum repaired. The authors acknowledge this is not a complete explanation as the calcium would eventually disperse allowing the muscle to relax and they speculate that another mechanism is probably involved.

PRACTICAL ASPECTS

Indications

Acupuncture is used in the management of a wide range of painful conditions. A recent survey of UK physiotherapists found that respondents perceived acupuncture to be useful for treating a variety of soft tissue and degenerative disorders of the type seen in a typical outpatients department. Low back, head, neck, shoulder and knee pain all received strong support. Many other musculoskeletal conditions were also being treated (Alltree, 1993). Neuropathic pains, including neuralgia and phantom limb pain, may respond. Pain clinics frequently use acupuncture for managing chronic pain problems, refractory to other forms of treatment. Its role in the management of acute pain, including perioperatively (Christensen et al., 1989), must not be forgotten.

It is likely that conditions with substantial pathological changes, or with longstanding symptoms, will be more difficult to treat. Symptoms are more likely to recur and such patients may benefit from further courses of treatment in the future. As with any long-term pain problem, self-help strategies, such as exercises and relaxation training, should be considered. They may help the patient to make best use of their own coping strategies and reduce the risk of dependence on the therapist.

Acupuncture is often used as a treatment of 'last resort'. This can happen because it is not as widely available as other forms of treatment and is used only when the patient encounters a therapist who practises acupuncture. Even then, some therapists are reluctant to use it until they have exhausted other modalities. There is no sound reason why acupuncture should be relegated to this status. Any therapist skilled in its use should consider whether its effects would prove beneficial to the patient from the outset of treatment.

Assessment

A comprehensive musculoskeletal assessment should be made prior to treatment, together with regular reassessments during the care episode. The objectives of the initial assessment include identifying, where possible, the structures responsible for the patient's signs and symptoms; obtaining a baseline measure against which progress can be judged; and identifying any contraindications or precautions.

Many therapists choose to use acupuncture in conjunction with manual therapy, exercises or other physiotherapeutic modalities (Wigram, 1989; Alltree, 1993) and a comprehensive clinical assessment, such as that advocated by Maitland (1991), is recommended. This section discusses only those aspects of the examination that are of particular relevance to acupuncture.

Pain

Pain distribution is very important as it can direct the therapist to search for trigger points known to refer to that area. It can also help identify the segmental level involved, which may in turn direct stimulation to the related dermatome, myotome or sclerotome.

Previous treatment

A previous good response to acupuncture is a promising sign, although a previous poor response need not preclude treatment. Asking about the number of treatments and where the needles were inserted may reveal a different approach from your own has been used.

Drug history

Anticoagulants may suggest altered clotting times. High dose steroid use may result in areas of fragile skin, necessitating extra caution.

Past medical history

Ask the patient specifically about pacemakers or heart valve implants, other cardiac problems, epilepsy, diabetes and allergy.

Special questions

Special questions about general health, weight loss and neurological symptoms should always be asked. As with any form of pain relief, it is imperative that acupuncture is not used to mask symptoms of undiagnosed, potentially serious pathology.

Range of movement

Restricted passive movement may be secondary to muscle spasm. An awareness of the muscles responsible for specific physiological restrictions can direct the therapist to those muscles for further investigation. A muscular restriction of cervical rotation, for example, would probably be due to tightness of the contralateral splenius capitus and cervicus and the ipsilateral upper fibres of trapezius. Stretches may well be used to complement the acupuncture.

Palpation

Careful palpation of soft tissues is especially important if acupuncture is being considered as a treatment option. The distribution of pain will guide the therapist to potential sites of referral. Suitable points to needle, whether MTPs or Traditional points, are often tender or feel knotted.

Needling

Needle selection

Reusable needles are employed much less often nowadays as they require a rigorous procedure to ensure adequate sterilization by autoclave. They tend to blunt with repeated use and patients are often concerned about the risk of infection (even if adequate precautions ensure none exists). The use of presterilized, disposable needles is recommended.

The length of needle used will be determined largely by the site to be needled, as different areas require different depths of insertion. Short, fine needles are good for points in delicate or bony areas such as the hand and face. Longer needles, which are usually thicker, allow adequate penetration in areas where fat or musculature is thicker. The needle should be long enough so that no more than two-thirds of its shaft needs to be inserted.

Depth of insertion

The depth of insertion usually depends on the area being needled. If muscles are being needled, subcutaneous tissue, which varies in thickness, will have to be penetrated first. It is imperative that therapists have a good knowledge of the underlying anatomy because incorrect needling can do damage. Needles are usually advanced from 0.5 cm to 2.0 cm into the patient, the therapist gaining feedback from the patient about the sensation experienced, as well as feeling the transition from tissue to tissue via their fingers. Both these types of feedback are important. Many therapists use the patient's report of needle sensation as an indication that the depth and site of penetration are correct. Others prefer to feel for the resistance associated with local spasm and the subsequent release of needle grasp to be their guides to correct needling. Some therapists favour very superficial needling, where at times the needle may only be advanced into the subcutaneous tissues. Even such shallow needling may produce needle sensation.

Type of stimulation

Insertion/withdrawal only

Inserting the needle into the acupuncture point and leaving it for a period of time is known in traditional terms as sedating. The period of time is usually about 20 minutes, although some practitioners leave them in for much less. Other practitioners believe that correct needling of an active trigger point will be met with resistance and needle grasp. They advocate withdrawing the needle as the needle grasp lessens, which may be within 30 seconds or so.

Manual stimulation

Once the needle has been inserted to the correct depth, the tissue can be stimulated manually. A typical technique is to roll the needle between the thumb and forefinger, simultaneously moving it in and out. This is usually performed for about a minute, during which time needle sensation may occur or increase (to an acceptable level only). The needle is then withdrawn. This is known as supplying or tonifying in traditional terms. It can be combined with the sedating method above, in which case the needle is inserted and left for about 5 minutes; it is then manually stimulated for up to a minute and again left in place. This cycle is repeated until approximately 20 minutes has passed, at which time the needle is withdrawn.

Periosteal pecking

Certain points are amenable to periosteal pecking. The needle is advanced to impinge on the periosteum, gently tapped against it for a short time and then withdrawn. The needle must not be pushed through the periosteum.

Electroacupuncture

Needles may be inserted and then connected to a purpose-built electrical stimulator, which is known as electroacupuncture. Stimulation may last for 20 or so minutes, and a low frequency of 2–3 Hz is often chosen. A visible muscle contraction may be evident. An allied technique (e.g. Frampton, 1985) uses a probe, rather than a needle, to stimulate points transcutaneously. These probes usually act as point locators as well (see Chapter 14, p.134).

Moxa

Some practitioners heat the ends of special needles, or stimulate the skin directly, by burning the herb moxa. This traditional practice is termed moxibustion.

Other methods

The points may also be stimulated with manual pressure (acupressure), TNS electrodes, laser, and ultrasound. As none of this group uses needles, they have been more correctly termed 'physical therapy on acupuncture points' (Zhuo, 1988), rather than acupuncture.

Effects of acupuncture

Needle sensation

Acupuncture often causes a variety of sensations which radiate from the point being needled. The feeling(s) may be described as aching, numbness, fullness, heaviness, warmth, or tingling. Known as techi ('the arrival of chi') in traditional practice, it is considered by many to be essential for effective treatment. Beneficial results can, however, occur without it.

Local erythema

A small erythema usually develops around the needle.

Needle grasp

The tissue will sometimes grip the needle for a short while. This is presumed to be contraction of muscular fibres. Occasionally it can be very strong, making the needle difficult to withdraw. If this happens, leaving the needle for a few minutes usually allows sufficient relaxation to withdraw the needle. Gently rolling the area around the needle between thumb and index finger may also help.

Altered mood

The patient may feel lightheaded, sleepy, intoxicated or even euphoric, possibly due to the release of endorphins. If this happens, it is usually short-lived, but occasionally persists all day.

Fainting

Vasovagal reactions do happen and it is difficult to predict which patients may be susceptible. It is therefore wise to treat the patient lying down for their first few treatments, until their response has been gauged. If a patient does faint, remove the needles at once, lie them down and elevate their legs.

Bleeding

Occasionally the needle site will bleed when the needle is withdrawn. It usually stops very quickly following digital pressure. Warn the patient that a small bruise may appear.

Exacerbation of symptoms

Sometimes the patient will experience a temporary exacerbation in symptoms. This should not be a cause for concern unless it is severe and prolonged.

Progression of treatment

Treatment regimes are best kept simple at first. For the initial treatment a maximum of, say, five points should be used and it is probably better to use the 'insertion only' technique outlined above. Using this gentle technique may be enough, and therefore be in keeping with the idea of using the least intervention to produce the required therapeutic result. In addition, a more vigorous technique is more likely to exacerbate symptoms, especially if the patient reacts particularly strongly, as some do.

Three outcomes may result:

1. The patient will improve. If the patient improves following the treatment, it may be reasonable to continue in this way, spacing treatment sessions out until the problem resolves.
2. There may be no change. In this case additional points may be incorporated, or existing ones stimulated more vigorously. This may take the form of manual stimulation, electroacupuncture or periosteal pecking (in appropriate areas) As with any therapy that may not show an instant change, it is better to change one variable rather than two.
3. The patient may be worse. If the patient is worse after a treatment, it may be helpful to treat fewer points, use points further away from the pain or use a gentler form of stimulation.

As with many physiotherapeutic techniques, patients may be seen from one to three times in the first few weeks, treatments being spaced out as the problem resolves. The effect of acupuncture is not always appreciated at once, and patients may need several treatments before improvement is noted. It is worth persevering for three to six treatments before abandoning this modality.

Point selection

Although Traditional methods are often criticized in the West, the classical methods outlined in the first five sections below deserve serious consideration by therapists. A knowledge of the meridians opens up a wealth of potential treatment points, as well as providing a useful method of recording where has been treated. For those therapists primarily following the trigger point approach, there will be times where an appropriate myofascial trigger point cannot be found and the meridians may provide a treatment option.

Prescriptions

Recognizing that certain points were used regularly for particular clinical presentations, the Chinese developed prescriptions for choosing appropriate points. Originally developed from traditional ideas about illness, these points can be used by people who do not subscribe to traditional theories (Vincent and Richardson, 1986). Compilations of prescriptions can be found in many texts (e.g. Chaitow, 1983; Mann, 1987). A typical prescription for headache is shown in Figure 13.1.

Local points

Acupuncture points located in the area the pain is felt are called local points and are a good choice in the first instance. In the case of referred pain, points near the origin of the symptoms should also be considered.

Distant points

Certain distant points are believed to reinforce the effect of local points. For example, Colon 4 (in the web between the thumb and index finger) can be used in conjunction with local points for the treatment of toothache or facial pain. Other points, known as *ho* points, are located around the knees and elbows. Each meridian has one *ho* point, and it may be used to enhance treatment if local points on its meridian are being used. In traditional practice it is common to use opposite forms of stimulation for local and *ho* points. Thus if a local point is sedated, the *ho* point will be supplied and vice versa. Figure 13.2 shows local and distant points for the treatment of elbow pain.

Points in opposition

Local points are not always suitable for needling. An area may be so tender that needling it is unacceptable to the patient. Alternatively, in the case of phantom limb pain, the pain will be felt in a non-existent area. In these circumstances the equivalent points on the opposite side of the body may be used and are termed points in opposition. Alternatively, distant points could be used on their own.

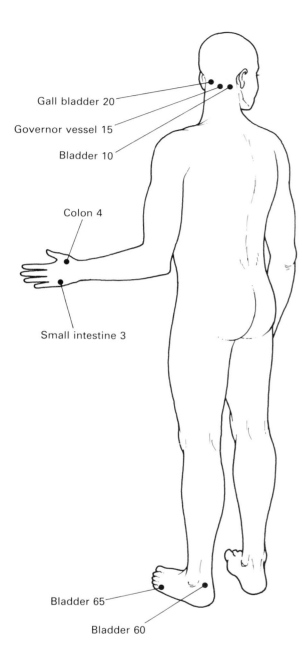

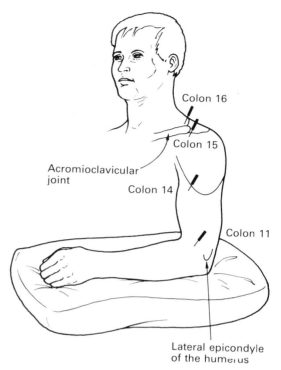

Fig. 13.2 Local acupuncture and the points for the treatment of a painful shoulder.

Fig. 13.1 A typical presentation for the treatment of occipital headache.

Points in line

A series of adjacent points on one meridian passing through the painful area, points in line, may be used.

Trigger points

Trigger points in muscle, fascia, skin, ligament and periosteum may all be used for treatment. They may be found in the painful area, or at some distance from it. Active MTPs may be found by palpating and stretching muscles known to refer symptoms to the painful area. Figure 13.3 shows typical patterns of MTP referral, as described by Travell and Rinzler (1952). Patients with back and referred leg pain frequently have active MTPs in the leg and acupuncture points around the ankle may also be tender. Areas of tenderness are valuable guides for point selection. Loh *et al.* (1984) found that acupuncture for migraine and headache was much more likely to help if the patient had locally tender trigger and acupuncture

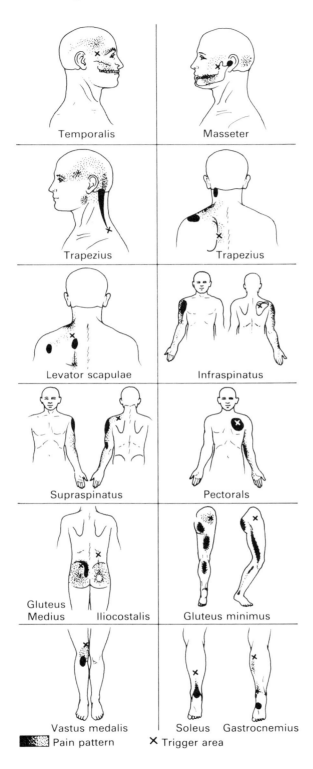

Temporalis

Masseter

Trapezius

Trapezius

Levator scapulae

Infraspinatus

Supraspinatus

Pectorals

Gluteus
Medius   Iliocostalis   Gluteus minimus

Vastus medalis   Soleus   Gastrocnemius

▬ Pain pattern   ✕ Trigger area

Fig. 13.3 A selection of trigger points and their typical pattern of referral. (Adapted from Travell and Rinzler, 1952, by kind permission of Williams and Wilkins)

points. Therapists must always satisfy themselves that tender points are not suspicious in any way.

Auricular points

The use of ear points can be traced back to the ancient Egyptians, but in the 1950s a French doctor, Paul Nogier, developed a coherent system for their use (Lewith, 1985). A fuller description is beyond the scope of this chapter.

Safety aspects

Hygiene

Acupuncture has the potential to transmit bacterial or viral infections in the same manner as other invasive procedures.

Risks to therapists

Risks are reduced by avoiding needlestick injury and contact with blood, especially if your skin is broken. Health service employees who have a needlestick injury should be managed in accordance with health authority guidelines. Independent practitioners should consult their own doctor or local casualty department. Owing to the prevalence of HIV and hepatitis B, some practitioners advocate wearing sterile gloves, while others use these only in the case of blood spillage, or if they have abrasions on their hands. Therapists should consider immunization against hepatitis B. Whether to treat or not to treat patients known to be carrying these infections is a personal decision. Many carriers may be unaware of their status and utmost care is always needed. If good procedures are followed, risks are minimal.

Risks to patients

The risks to patients are minimized by the use of disposable needles and scrupulous aseptic technique, including clean hands and work surfaces.

Situations where patients should not be needled

Heart implants

Patients with implanted valves or pacemakers should not be needled, due to the risk of developing bacterial endocarditis.

Pregnancy

Proponents of Western methods usually consider pregnancy to be a contraindication to treatment, due to the risk of abortion.

Uncontrolled movements

Patients who may not be able to keep reasonably still during treatment should not be needled. This may include people with poorly controlled epilepsy, athetoid problems, agitated patients and children.

Overanxious patients

Patients who are extremely anxious, particularly those with a fear of needles, are not suitable for acupuncture.

Areas that should not be needled

The following areas should not be needled:

- Anywhere near the carotid bodies.
- Lungs or pleura. Take extra care needling near the apex of the lung and the chest wall.
- The eyeballs, nipples and gonads.
- Any lump or bumps that may harbour infection.
- Areas of poor skin. Avoid using peripheral points in people with diabetes and peripheral vascular disease.
- Skin which exhibits eczema or psoriasis.
- Veins, arteries, nerves and tendons.
- Joint capsules and periosteum (except periosteal pecking).

It may be as well not to needle those points described in traditional practice as 'forbidden points'.

Situations where additional care is required

Other cardiac problems

It is advisable to avoid using the heart, heart constrictor and triple heater meridians in patients who have had a heart attack, stroke or other cardiac disease.

Allergy to stainless steel

Do not use stainless steel needles for patients allergic to this substance. Treatment with gold or silver needles may be possible.

Bleeding disorders

Haemophiliacs and patients taking anticoagulants may be treated with care, following consultation with the referring doctor. It may be necessary for clotting times to be checked.

Immunosupressed patients

Consult with the referring doctor about patients with SLE, AIDS or who are taking immunosupressive drugs as they are at increased risk of infection.

Patients with, or carrying, infectious diseases

These patients pose a risk to the practitioner. As many such people may be unaware of their status, the body fluids of ALL patients should be treated with utmost care.

Other safety considerations

1. Do not push the needle up to its hilt. The weakest part is the junction of the shaft and handle.
2. If a needle breaks while in a patient, mark the spot immediately. This is very rare, but if it happens, surgical removal may be necessary.
3. If the needle causes pain, withdraw it at once. Be aware of the difference between pain and an acceptable needle sensation.
4. Do not allow the patient to move around after the needle has been inserted.
5. Warn patients not to overexert themselves if the treatment greatly reduces their level of pain.
6. Warn patients that they may feel drowsy, light-headed or even 'high' after treatment, and that they should not drive or operate dangerous machinery straight afterwards, at least until they have found out how they respond.

Consent

Any treatment should be carefully explained to a patient to obtain their informed consent prior to carrying out the treatment. This means that the patient should have potential benefits and risks explained and alternative treatments outlined in a manner that they can understand.

Patients who intend to donate blood should check with the Blood Transfusion Service as to what their current guidelines are before having acupuncture.

While it is not currently general practice to obtain written consent, all practitioners should obtain consent explicitly, and note this in the treatment record.

The Way Forward

This chapter has outlined practical aspects of classical acupuncture and trigger point acupuncture for pain relief. Even though the traditional principles from which classical acupuncture evolved have not satisfied Western scrutineers, its methods are based on a vast empirical heritage. It would seem prudent not to reject this too quickly.

Although research has started to unravel the mechanisms underlying acupuncture, further work is required. A more complete understanding of humoral, autonomic and reflex mechanisms will help therapists in terms of point selection and type of stimulation as well as explain treatment in purely Western terms. More clinical studies are required to identify the response to acupuncture of different conditions. As therapists frequently use acupuncture in conjunction with other modalities, combinations should be investigated to determine where the therapeutic effects lie and which combinations are most effective.

Acupuncture has always been used for the treatment of disease. Although initially used for pain relief only, physiotherapists now use it for the management of a variety of neurological, dermatological, respiratory and stress-related conditions (Wigram, 1989; Alltree, 1993). This expansion of practice should be welcomed, but physiotherapists must be aware of the responsibilities it brings and of any limitations inherent in their own training.

Finally, acupuncture should not be seen as a treatment of 'last resort'. Its appropriateness should be considered alongside other modalities from the outset of treatment.

Acknowledgements

In the first edition of this text, the chapter on acupuncture was written by David Jackson. I am particularly grateful to him for letting me use parts of that work without specifically referencing it. The books written by the other four authors mentioned in the Bibliography were most helpful for background reading.

Bibliography

Policy for the Practice of Acupuncture by Chartered Physiotherapists (1990) Chartered Society of Physiotherapists, London

Baldry, P. (1989) *Acupuncture, Trigger Points and Musculoskeletal Pain*, Churchill Livingstone, Edinburgh

Gunn, C.C. (1989) *Treating Myofascial Pain: Intramuscular Stimulation [IMS] for Myofascial Pain Syndromes of Neuropathic Origin*, University of Washington, Seattle

Jackson, D. (1988) Acupuncture. In *Pain: Management and Control in Physiotherapy* (eds P.E. Wells, V Frampton and D. Bowsher), Butterworth Heinemann, Oxford, pp. 71–88

Macdonald, A. (1982) *Acupuncture from Ancient Art to Modern Medicine*, George Allen and Unwin, London

Mann, F. (1987) *Textbook of Acupuncture*, William Heinemann Medical Books, London

References

Aakster, C.W. (1986) Concepts in alternative medicine. *Soc. Sci.Med.*, **22** (2), 265–73

Akerele, O. (1991) WHO and the development of acupuncture nomenclature: overcoming a tower of Babel. *Am. J. Chin. Med.*, **19** (1), 89–94

Alltree, J. (1993) Physiotherapy and acupuncture: practice in the UK. *Comp. Ther. Med.*, **1**, 34–41

Beecher, H.K. (1955) The powerful placebo. *J. Am. Med. Assoc.*, **159**, 1602–6

Bowsher, D. (1988) Modulation of nociceptive input. In *Pain: Management and Control in Physiotherapy* (eds P.E. Wells, V. Frampton and D. Bowsher), Butterworth Heinemann, Oxford, pp. 30–6

Chaitow, L. (1983) *The Acupuncture Treatment of Pain*, 2nd edn, Thorsons Publishers Inc., New York

Chapman, C.R., Colpitts, Y.M., Benedetti, C. *et al.* (1980) Evoked potential assessment of acupuncture analgesia: attempted reversal with naloxone. *Pain*, **9**, 183–97

Christensen, P.A., Noreng, M., Andersen, P.E. and Nielsen, J.W. (1989) Electroacupuncture and postoperative pain. *Br. J. Anaesth.*, **62**, 258–62

Clement-Jones, V., Tomlin, S., Rees, L.H. *et al.* (1980) Increased beta-endorphin but not met-enkephalin levels in human cerebrospinal fluid after acupuncture for recurrent pain. *Lancet*, **2**, 946–8

Coan, R.M., Wong, G., Su Liang Ku *et al.* (1980) The acupuncture treatment of low back pain: a randomized controlled study. *Am. J. Chin. Med.*, **8**, 181–9

Culpan, S. (1983) Clinical update on the art and science of acupuncture. *NZ J. of Physiother.*, August, pp. 19–21

Drok, E. (1983) The New Zealand Physiotherapist's Acupuncture and Pain Modulation Association. *NZ J. Physiother.*, August, p. 21

Editorial, (1973) When acupuncture came to Britain. *Br. Med. J.*, **5894**, 687–8

Ernst, M. and Lee, H.M. (1985) Sympathetic vasomotor changes induced by manual and electrical acupuncture of the Hoku point visualised by thermography. *Pain*, **21**, 25–33

Fassbinder, H.G. (1975) *Pathology of Rheumatic Diseases.* Springer-Verlag, New York

Fox, E.J. and Melzack, R. (1976) Transcutaneous electrical stimulation and acupuncture: comparison of treatment for low back pain. *Pain*, **2**, 141–8

Frampton, V.M. (1985) A pilot study to evaluate myofascial or trigger point electroacupuncture in the treatment of neck and back pain. *Physiotherapy*, **71** (1), 5–7

Gielen, F. (1989) Discussion of the placebo effect in physiotherapy based on a noncritical review of the literature. *Physiother. Can.*, **41** (4), 210–16

Gunn, C.C., Ditchburn, F.G., King, M.H. and Renwick, G.J. (1976) Acupuncture loci: a proposal for their classification according to their relationship to known neural structures. *Am. J. Chin. Med.*, **4** (2), 183–95

Hansen, P.E. and Hansen, J.H. (1983) Acupuncture treatment of chronic facial pain – a controlled cross-over trial. *Headache*, **23**, 66–9

Kim, S.S. (1981) The mediator theory of acupuncture and its practical application in bronchial asthma and myasthenia gravis. *Am. J. Acupuncture*, **9** (2), 101–16

Lewith, G.T. (1985) Acupuncture and transcutaneous nerve stimulation (TENS). In *Alternative Therapies* (ed. G.T. Lewith), Heinemann, London

Lewith, G.T. and Kenyon, J.N. (1984) Physiological and psychological explanations for the mechanism of acupuncture as a treatment for chronic pain. *Soc. Sci. Med.*, **19** (12), 1367–78

Liu, Y.K., Varela, M. and Oswald, R. (1975) The correspondence between some motor points and acupuncture loci. *Am. J. Chin. Med.*, **3** (4), 347–58

Loh, L., Nathan, P.W., Schott, G.D. and Zilkha, K.J. (1984) Acupuncture versus medical treatment for migraine and muscle tension headaches. *J. Neurol. Neurosurg. Psych.*, **47**, 333–7

Long, D.M. (1991) Fifteen years of transcutaneous electrical stimulation for pain control. *Stereotact. Fucnt. Neurosurg.*, **56**, 2–19

Macdonald, A. (1989) Acupuncture analgesia and therapy. In *Textbook of Pain* (eds P.D. Wall and R. Melzack), Churchill Livingstone, Edinburgh, pp. 906–19

Maitland, G.D. (1991) *Peripheral Manipulation*, 3rd edn, Butterworth Heinemann, Oxford

Mayer, D.J. Price, D.D. and Rafii, A. (1977) Antagonism of acupuncture analgesia in man by the narcotic antagonist naloxone. *Brain Res.*, **121**, 368–72

Melzack, R. (1989) Folk medicine and the sensory modulation of pain. In *Textbook of Pain* (eds P.D. Wall and R. Melzack), Churchill Livingstone, Edinburgh, pp. 897–905

Melzack, R., Stillwell, D.M. and Fox, J.F. (1977) Trigger points and acupuncture points for pain: correlations and implications. *Pain*, **3**, 3–23

Miehlke, K., Schulze, G. and Eger, W. (1960) Klinische und experimentelle Untersuchungen zum Fibrositis-syndrom. *Zeit. Rheumaforsch.*, **19**, 310–30

Popelianskii, I., Zaslavskii, E.S. and Veselorskii, V.P. (1976) Medicosocial signifcance, aetiology, pathogenesis and diagnosis of nonarticular disease of soft tissues of the limbs and back (Russian). *Voprosy Revmatizma*, **3.**, 38–43 (in Baldry, 1989, see Bibliography).

Research Group of Acupuncture Anaesthesia, Peking (1974) The role of some neurotransmitters of brain in finger acupuncture analgesia. *Sci. Sin.*, **17**, 112–30

Rickards, F.S. (1979) A fresh appraisal of an ancient science. *Update*, February, pp. 301–10

Shanghai First Medical College, Department of Physiology (1973) Preliminary observation on needling sensation affected by certain diseases of the central nervous system. *Bull. Sci.*, **2**, 90–2

Sjolund, B. and Erikson, M. (1976) Electroacupuncture and endogenous morphines. *Lancet*, **13**, 1085

Skrabanek, P. (1984) Acupuncture and the age of unreason. *Lancet*, 26 May, 1169–71

Travell, J. and Reizler, G.H. (1952) The myofascial genesis of pain. *Postgrad. Med.*, **11**, 425–34

Travell, J. and Simons, D.G. (1983) *Myofascial Pain and Dysfunction: The Trigger Point Manual*, Williams and Wilkins, Baltimore, Md

Travell, J.G. and Simons, D.G. (1992) *Myofascial Pain and Dysfunction*: vol. 2, *The Trigger Point Manual – The Lower Extremities*, Williams and Wilkins, Baltimore, Md

Vincent, C.A. and Richardson, P.H. (1986) The evaluation of therapeutic acupuncture: concepts and methods. *Pain*, **24**, 1–13

Wigram, J. (1989) Acupuncture and physiotherapy. *Comp. Med. Res.*, **3** and (3), 49–53

Williams, T., Mueller, K. and Cornwall, M.W. (1991) Effect of acupuncture-point stimulation on diastolic blood pressure in hypertensive subjects: a preliminary study. *Phys. Ther.*, **71** (7), 523–9

Wu, D-Z. (1990) Acupuncture and neurophysiology. *Clin. Neurol. Neurosurg.*, **92** (1), 13–25

Zhuo, D.H. (1988) Traditional Chinese rehabilitative therapy in the process of modernization. *Int. Disabil. Stud.*, **10** (3), 140–2

14 *Transcutaneous electrical nerve stimulation and chronic pain*

VICTORIA FRAMPTON

Introduction

The ancient Egyptians were the first to apply electric currents therapeutically, using electric eels in the treatment of headaches and gout. Throughout the centuries there have been references to the use of electrical stimulation for pain relief, though these were not taken seriously by the medical profession. By the late 1950s and early 1960s, research into the pathological changes which occurred in nerves after injury indicated that there might be a scientific justification for applying electrical impulses to such nerves to modify their response. These and other findings led Melzack and Wall (1965) to formulate their hypothesis of **gate control** to explain pain modulation. Although this has been revised since, it still remains the basis for much of our understanding of pain mechanisms and may explain the therapeutic value of electrical nerve stimulation.

When fast-conducting, large diameter afferent sensory fibres are stimulated they produce some form of presynaptic inhibition, which effectively blocks further transmission in the smaller, slower-conducting afferent fibres (the nociceptive afferents) which may be carrying noxious information.

Electrical stimulation can be given transcutaneously or by directly implanting an electrode on the nerve. Direct implantation requires a difficult invasive procedure with many possible complications. Cutaneous nerve stimulation or transcutaneous electrical nerve stimulation (TENS) is much easier to apply and less hazardous. An electric current is transmitted to the body through the skin by means of electrodes on the skin surface. This technique exploits the concept of the gate control theory in that long-term stimulation produces presynaptic inhibition of noxious information in the small diameter afferent nerves. Similar inhibition can, of course, be produced by rubbing and vibration, but these modes are not easy to use for the prolonged periods necessary to achieve good results.

The application of TENS

Despite the extensive use of TENS over the past 20–30 years, there still remains a great deal of work to be done to establish this inexpensive, non-invasive technique as a widely used, accepted modality for pain relief. Clinical trials are often poorly controlled and lack long-term follow-up and the difficulty in establishing conclusive placebo trials still exists. The complexities of the chronic pain sufferer, and the lack of adequate numbers of trials, make it almost impossible to substantiate and identify conclusively the ideal prescription for any particular pain problem. Johnson *et al.* (1991 b) have made a significant contribution by studying in depth the long-term uses of TENS, looking at patient stimulator and outcome variables. Certainly, more recent work on pulse frequencies and patterns, and different stimulation modes (Tulgar *et al.* 1991a and b), have made significant contributions to identifying optimum parameters for electrical stimulation. It is well established that modulation of normal physiological pathways can effect pain relief. Although in many cases application of TENS is very similar, the exact mechanism of how pain is inhibited will depend on an understanding of the pathology. An understanding, not only of the cause of the initial injury, but of the subsequent changes that may take place in the nerve pathway and how these have been damaged or are behaving 'abnormally'.

This chapter discusses the use of TENS in a variety of painful conditions, reflecting the author's personal experience of this modality over 15 years.

Treating inpatients with chronic pain in a rehabilitation setting and working as a physiotherapist in a multidisciplinary pain clinic provided the opportunity for a comprehensive approach to the control of pain by modulation of normal physiological pathways. Monitoring, evaluation short- and long-term follow-up have led to the evolution of the method of application of TENS which will be described here. Sadly, the close monitoring that a specialist in-patient service can provide is not the usual setting in which chronic pain sufferers are normally seen. Based on the experience of close monitoring, the author was able to preserve aspects of in-patient care and translate this to the most frequent treatment setting of the busy outpatient department experienced in most district general hospitals.

Pain mechanisms and pain pathways have already been discussed in earlier chapters of this book. It is obvious, therefore, that pain can be approached in many ways. The technique of using peripheral nerve stimulation to relieve pain is primarily to use the large myelinated circuits to activate local inhibitory circuits within the dorsal horn of the spinal cord. These inhibitory circuits then act to diminish nociceptive transmission through the spinal cord. It is possible that inhibitory processes act to constantly modulate the sensory inflow into the spinal cord; alternatively, the use of TENS may distort the functioning activity of the nervous system by 'jamming' one of its inputs (Woolfe, 1989).

The large myelinated A-beta fibres provide the vehicle for TENS. These large, fast-conducting fibres are highly susceptible to electrical stimulation, and will conduct the electrical impulse quickly to the spinal cord. Slower-conducting, non-myelinated C fibres are thus unable to pass on their message of noxious stimulation; presynaptic inhibition has occurred (Wagman and Price, 1969; Handwerker et al., 1975; Woolfe and Wall, 1982; Chung et al., 1984). This over-simplified summary of the gate control theory (Melzack and Wall, 1965), as already described in Chapter 9 allows the logical application of TENS as, obviously, the closer to the damaged area TENS can be applied, the more likely it is that inhibition of noxious stimuli will be effected at the appropriate level. The arrangement of inhibitory circuits mediated by A fibres is segmental. Therefore, low intensity segmental stimulation is required, such as that which is produced by TENS. Other polysegmental inhibitory circuits require higher intensity stimuli to activate them, as these inhibitory mechanisms are mediated by A-delta and C afferents. For example, techniques such as myofascial or trigger point acupuncture are extrasegmental and use painful stimuli (Woolfe, 1989). TENS may also produce analgesia by the effect peripheral stimulation has on endogenous opioid peptides. Eriksson et al. (1977) and Salar et al. (1981) demonstrated increases in opioid peptides in lumbar CSF.

Damaged peripheral nerves

When peripheral nerves are damaged, there are profound peripheral and central pathophysiological effects, a summary of which can be seen in Figure 14.1a. One might argue that the barrage of abnormal peripheral discharges leads to the consequent changes and effects that occur at spinal level and higher centres. These central changes may, in themselves, produce further abnormal peripheral nerve discharges. The cycle of events has to be interrupted at more than one point to modify chronic pain (Figure 14.1b).

Experimental work (Wall and Gutnik, 1974) has shown that proximal application of vibration or electrical stimulation 'dampens', or stops the abnormal firing that occurs at the damaged end of the nerve or neuroma and along the length of that nerve. So TENS may have a 'mechanical' effect on damaged nerves to 'subdue' or lessen the abnormally firing, excited damaged nerve. This hypothesis can be compared with the pathology that may be occurring in a damaged nerve root. Long-term irritation or pressure on, for example, the L5 root can lead to chronic firing at the site of irritation and along its length (Wall and Devor, 1981). TENS may also play a part in restoring an artificial input when the normal afferent supply is cut off.

Deafferentation

Previous experiments (Loeser and Ward, 1967) have demonstrated that following severance of the trigeminal nerve of the cat, the cells in the dorsal horn fired spontaneously. The frequency of this abnormal firing increased over a 3-week period until the cells were firing almost continually. This barrage of abnormal firing could result from the

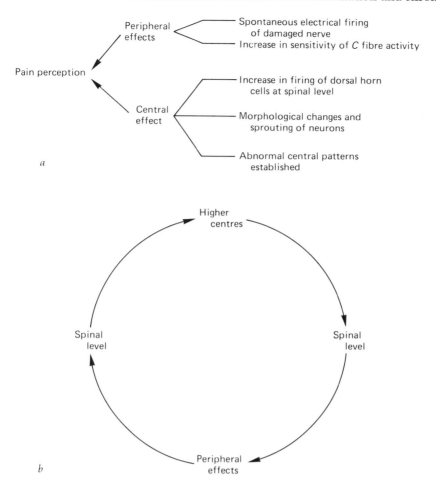

Fig. 14.1 *a*, A summary of peripheral and central effects following nerve damage. *b*, The autonomous cycle of peripheral and central effects of nerve damage.

loss of normal afferent input from the nerve that has been divided. After all, much of the input to the spinal cord results in central inhibition, and its loss leads to the unsuppressed firing of cells in the dorsal horn. In the author's clinical experience, many patients with avulsion lesions of the brachial plexus complain of severe pain of a characteristic nature (see Wynn Parry, 1980); however, the pain does not necessarily occur immediately but up to 2–3 weeks after injury (Wynn Parry, 1981). This clinical observation is certainly compatible with the experimental findings. One might argue that application of TENS artificially restores an afferent input to the spinal cord. Thus TENS may be working in one of several ways to inhibit or relieve pain:

1. by presynaptic inhibition;
2. by direct mechanical inhibition on an excited, abnormally firing nerve;
3. by restoring an artificial afferent input;
4. by the role played by endogenous opioid peptides.

The aetiology of chronic pain involves changes, both in the central nervous system and peripheral nervous system. It is vital that the role played by both must be understood in order to manage chronic pain (Devor, 1989). A lack of understanding of the ways in which TENS may work to inhibit or relieve pain has led to its random application. A greater understanding of these mechanisms provides the physiotherapist with a more logical

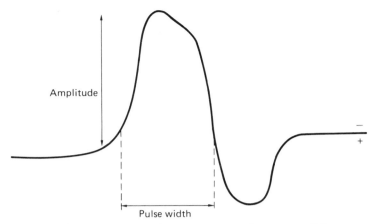

Fig. 14.2 Biphasic asymmetrical square wave with a zero net DC component.

baseline from which to apply TENS, and from the examination and assessment of the patient how best to judge where to focus treatment.

TENS can only form part of the whole treatment programme for patients suffering from chronic pain (Frampton, 1982). As has been described by Withrington and Wynn Parry (1984), central changes that have occurred must be reversed or modified. A full programme of normal functional activities must be employed in conjunction with TENS, so that normal use can be restored to the affected part once the pain has been reduced or relieved. Many clinics have reported poor results with TENS for pain relief. This may be due to their failure to consider the management of pain as part of a comprehensive rehabilitation programme. Short-term treatment with TENS may be inadequate to modify the complex changes that result in a chronic pain state, whereas shorter periods may be adequate for more acute pain.

The apparatus and working of TENS

Since the introduction of TENS approximately 25 years ago, a wide variety of machines are commercially available. Many of these have similar fixed parameters and vary only in size, colour, durability, reliability and mode of operation. Although a great deal of work has demonstrated the efficacy of TENS for pain relief, the ideal parameters required have not been established. Recent work has shed some light on the effects of different pulse patterns and frequencies and these will be discussed.

The wave form

This may be described as an asymmetric biphasic modified square output waveform. There is a zero net DC component (Figure 14.2), the area of the positive wave portion is equal to the area within the negative portion. Therefore, there are no net polar effects to cause long-term positive – negative ion concentrations within the tissues beneath each electrode (Mannheimer and Lampe, 1984), and adverse skin reactions to polar concentrations are avoided.

Amplitude of the current output (OP)

This can be adjusted between 0–50 mA (milliamperes) into an electrode impedance of 1 kΩ (kiloohms). This range is standard for almost all TENS machines and does not vary from one manufacturer to another. It must be noted that amplitudes (i.e. current strengths) producing only a mild paraesthesia are required (see p. 121).

The Pulse Width (PW)

This is fixed in many machines, usually at 200 μs (microseconds); however, other machines provide a variable pulse width ranging usually from 50–300 μs. The relationship of the pulse width and amplitude dictates the net potential output or strength of stimulus that is produced (Mannheimer and Lampe, 1984). That is, the strength of the stimulus can be increased either by increasing the

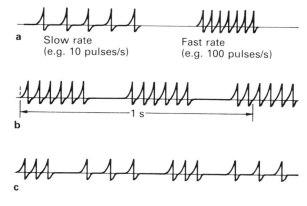

Fig. 14.3 *a*, Impulse frequency or rate of impulse expressed in 1 s (not drawn to scale). Note: The pulses demonstrated do not necessarily represent 10 pulses/s or 100 pulses/s. They merely represent the difference between fast and slow. *b*, Burst wave form low frequency additional 'burst-type' output. In this example 2.3 burst/s are shown. Note: Amplitude, pulse width and rate of individual impulse does not alter from the initial settings (the impulse has just been interrupted). *c*, Frequency modulated output wave form. Constant stimulus with a variable frequency.

amplitude of the current or the pulse width. However, by increasing the pulse width, motor nerves are more likely to be recruited, and this is not desirable. The greater the intensity of the current the more nerve fibres will be recruited. As the objective of the stimulation is to activate large diameter, fast-conducting afferent fibres, high intensities or long pulse widths are not necessary. This is often misunderstood by patients, and occasionally physiotherapists, who mistakenly assume that the stronger the current the better the pain relief. Although high intensity currents may provide a 'counter-irritant' effect, this is achieved by different physiological mechanisms, e.g. 'hyperstimulation analgesia' (Melzack and Wall, 1982) or the recruitment of polysegmental inhibitory circuits (Woolfe, 1989).

Pulse frequency or rate (R)

This is variable on almost all machines, varying from 1–150 pulses per second or Hz (Hertz). The sensation of the variable rates can be expressed as a slow 'ticking' pulse (slow rate) and a continuous buzz (high rate) (Figure 14.3*a*).

Burst Type Stimulation and Variable Frequency

One of the criticisms of TENS in the management of chronic pain is that the benefits of TENS tend to fall with time (Loeser *et al.*, 1975; Eriksson *et al.*, 1979; Long *et al.*, 1979; Taylor *et al.*, 1981; Bates and Nathan, 1980). It has been suggested that this might be due to the adaption of the nervous system to regular repetitive stimuli (Thompson, 1987; Pomeranz *et al.*, 1987). Many clinical studies have been carried out to investigate the effects of different parameters (Anderson *et al.*, 1976; Linzer and Long, 1976; Mannheimer and Carlsson, 1979; Wolfe, *et al.*, 1981; Sjolund, 1985; Omura, 1987; Johnson *et al.*, 1991; Tulgar *et al.*, 1991a,b). Confusion still exists as the results of these different trials are not consistent. A double blind controlled long-term clinical trial by Tulgar *et al.* (1991b) validated their earlier pilot study (1991a) which indicated patients preferred burst (Figure 14.3*b*) and frequency modulated (Figure 14.3*c*) stimulation. Four stimulation modes were tried:

Conventional constant stimulation.
Burst stimulation.
High rate frequency modulated stimulation.
Low rate frequency modulated stimulation.

They concluded most patients in their study preferred high rate frequency modulated and burst type stimulation. Johnson *et al.* (1991a) looked at the analgesic effects of different pulse patterns of TENS on cold-induced pain in normal subjects. Five frequencies of pulse delivery, four patterns of pulse delivery and two sizes of electrodes were examined. Their results concluded that frequencies of 20–80 Hz produced the greatest analgesia and the greatest statistical reliability was observed at 80 Hz. A continuous pulse pattern was shown to be optimal. Sjolund (1985) found 80 Hz, out of a range of peripheral nerve stimulating frequencies, produced the maximal suppression of the C fibre evoked flexion response in the rat. Eriksson *et al.* (1979) showed that 'bursts' at high intensity and low frequency (acupuncture-like TENS) were more effective in pain relief than continuous TENS. Burst mode TENS was, therefore, introduced. It is thought that burst mode TENS mimics acupuncture in producing analgesia by stimulating the release of endogenous opiod peptides (Sjolund and Eriksson, 1979). High frequency continuous mode TENS is thought to relieve pain by activating gating mechanisms (Melzack and Wall, 1965; Wall and Sweet, 1967).

An in-depth study of long-term users of TENS with a variety of chronic pain problems (Johnson *et al.*, 1991b) concluded that there was a remarkable lack of correlation between patient, the site or cause of pain with the stimulator and outcome variables, an observation consistent with other authors (Bates and Nathan, 1980; Woolfe, 1981). A subsequent study by Johnson *et al.* (1991c) recorded the consistency of pulse frequencies and pulse patterns of TENS used by chronic pain patients during a series of treatment sessions. The results suggested that individual patients used specific pulse frequencies but the pulse frequency varied significantly from patient to patient. The majority preferred a continuous pulse pattern. The author of this study concluded that the patients use specific pulse frequencies and pulse patterns (unique to the individual) to control their pain. It would appear in this study that patients turn to such frequencies and patterns for reasons of comfort which may be unconnected with specific pain control mechanisms.

Clearly patients should be encouraged to try a variety of different frequencies and modes of stimulation to find their optimum parameters for pain relief. If TENS is successful at first and then ceases to be of any effect burst mode should be tried to combat accommodation and adaptation.

Lead wires and electrodes

The stimulus from the machine is delivered to the patient transcutaneously via lead wires (or cables) and conductive electrodes. Some machines have single leads with separate output sockets, others have a single output socket and bifurcated leads into a single plug. Most units are issued with a pair of black silicon rubber carbon-impregnated electrodes. Although these are available in several sizes, manufacturers issue the small 4 × 4 cm electrodes as standard. The efficacy of larger pads is said to be less due to a fall off in current density in length (Brennan, 1976; Woolfe, 1989). In the author's experience, the use of larger pads 4 × 8 cm² has proved to be more effective in relieving pain caused by deafferentation or central pain. Little clinical work has been done to establish the efficacy of different electrode sizes and more studies are required. It may be that the use of a large pad requires a higher intensity stimulation than a smaller pad.

There are a variety of different electrodes available. Those of most note are the self-adhesive electrodes. The carbon rubber electrodes require an electroconductive gel (which is supplied as standard) to transmit the current through the skin, and they have to be fixed in place with tape or adhesive patches. Self-adhesive electrode pads dispense with gel and tape but ususally incur greater cost as they are not indefinitely reusable and some only last for one application. As electrodes often provide the greatest problems in TENS application owing to allergic responses to the tape or gel, it is important to familiarize oneself with the available alternatives, such as electroconductive gum pads which provide another medium to electroconductive gel and tape. Other available electrodes are small button electrodes for stimulation of small difficult areas.

It is essential to emphasize the importance of using the correct electroconductive gel. Experience has shown that the use of EMG gel has produced severe allergic responses, as it was designed only for short-term use. Other mediums, such as KY jelly, are also unsuitable as they do not possess the cohesive properties of the TENS gel, and following a relatively short period, the gel contracts to cover only the centre of the electrode pad. The electroconductive TENS gel has high-conductive, non-allergic and cohesive properties which make it suitable for use with the TENS equipment.

Although many manufacturers are now producing a wide range of accessories, adaptability and improvization are still necessary skills of the physiotherapist. The use of the 'Prembaby butterfly' ECG electrodes provides an excellent solution for the treatment of areas with uneven or difficult contours, such as the fingers, where conventional carbon rubber electrodes are inadequate on account of the inability to maintain a good fixed contact with the skin.

Single and Dual Channel Units

There are many different manufacturers producing single and dual channel units. A single channel unit has a single amplitude parameter and one pair of electrodes. Alternatively, a dual channel unit will have two amplitude parameters and two pairs of electrodes. In most cases where one site of pain is identified, a single channel is adequate; the rationale of treatment must include ease of application and operation and cost-effectiveness.

Why complicate the situation with a dual channel machine (which is more expensive) if a small unit is effective in providing adequate pain relief? Indications for use of a dual channel unit are when two sites of pain need to be treated or the pain is widespread and a single unit is not sufficient, e.g. a patient suffering with back and leg pain may find that a single channel unit will only relieve one pain, in either his leg or back, but not in both depending on where the pads are placed (Figure 14.4, 11c and d). In this case a dual output machine would enable back and leg pain to be treated to maximal effect (Figure 14.4, 11g and h). Burst and sophisticated variable frequency machines are now available, a direct development from recent clinical studies. Among these Neen Pain Management Systems introduced a new range of machines, 'Xenos', with greater variability. These models provide an auto-scanning for frequency and pulse width. It is also fitted with a reset facility which automatically returns the machine back to a frequency of 80 Hz and a pulse width of 210 μs. These models also provide a multi-frequency (random) output mode to overcome 'accommodation'. The frequency spectrum spans from a minimum of 8 Hz to the maximum preset by the frequency setting when on the continuous mode. The burst facility utilizes 320 μs on and 180 μs off (two bursts per second).

Operation of TENS

The concept of an electric current is sufficient to prevent many people using TENS. It is essential to explain to patients the working of the machine, what the stimulus feels like and that the current can do no harm regardless of the intensity used. Accidental knocking of the OP dial can give a strong jolt but no personal permanent damage!

Once the site of stimulation and the size of the pad have been selected, one surface of the pad is completely covered with electrode gel and secured well to the skin and connected to the stimulator via the lead wires. All dial settings must be on zero, or the lowest setting; the amplitude is then switched on and increased until a mild buzzing or a pulsation sensation of the impulse is felt. The rate (R) should then be altered from the minimum setting to the maximum to demonstrate the range to the patient; this should then be set at mid-range and any further alterations in R or OP should be monitored so that the optimum settings for comfort and pain relief are obtained. It is important to explain to the patient that he will feel a slow pricking or ticking sensation on a low rate, whereas on maximum pulse frequency the sensation is one of continuous buzzing. It should be emphasized that only a mild sensation of the stimulus is required and that the stimulation should not be strong or painful, that TENS is effective only with mild stimulation and is not a counter-irritant. There is a tendency for patients to feel that the stronger the stimulus the more pain relief they will obtain. However, the objective is to stimulate the large, fast-conducting low-threshold A-beta afferent fibres, and higher amplitudes are not necessary.

As mentioned previously, the PW is often fixed; the author has found limited use of a variable PW, the exception being in the management of brachial plexus lesions when areas of diminished skin sensation may require higher pulse widths in order for the patient to perceive the impulse (Frampton, 1982). Many of these patients have denervated muscles and, therefore, stimulation of motor nerves at these higher PW settings does not result in muscle contraction, which in normally innervated areas would be contraindicated and unpleasant.

Fig. 14.4 1–11 (see pages 122–3) Some examples of electrode placements in certain conditions. (The electrodes are either placed in position *a* or *b*, etc.) 1*a–b* Median nerve injury. 2*a–b* Ulnar nerve injury. 3*a–b* Sudeck's atrophy. 4*a–g* Brachial plexus injuries. 5*a–f* Phantom limb and stump pain in above knee amputations. 6*a–f* Phantom limb and stump pain in below knee amputations (position similar to 5 can be used). 7 Painful neuroma following amputation of digit demonstrating the use of the butterfly electrode. 8 Painful menisectomy scar. 9 Post-herpetic neuralgia involving the T4 dermatome. 10 Trigeminal neuralgia and facial pain – two alternative positions. 11*a* and *b* Low back pain (single channel unit). 11*c* and *d* Low back pain L5 root pain (single channel unit). 11*e* Low back pain S1 root pain (single channel unit). 11*f* Back pain following laminectomy and painful scar over bone graft donor site. 11*g* Low back pain and left leg pain (dual channel unit). 11*h* Low back pain and bilateral leg pain (dual channel unit).

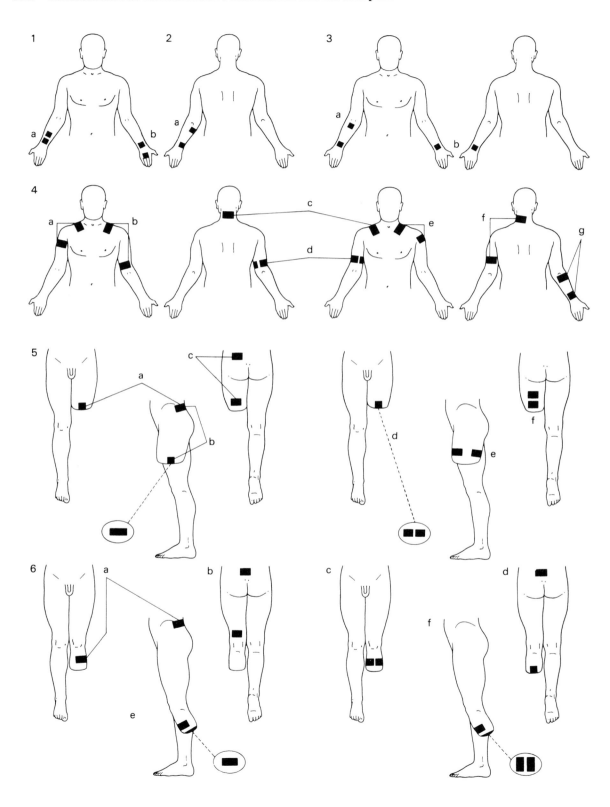

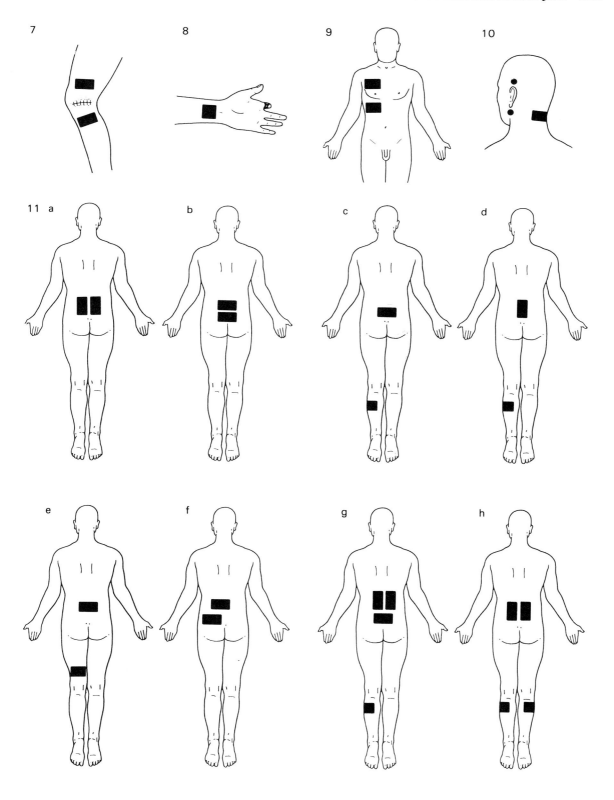

Principles of electrode placement

These are based on an understanding of the physiological pathways and of the pain mechanisms involved; if deafferentation is the predominant feature, then one large pad should be placed over the appropriate damaged dermatome (provided there is some residual afferent input). The other pad may be placed over the nerve trunk of the appropriate root level of damage (Figure 14.4, 4a,b,c and e). Alternatively, with peripheral nerve damage, such as carpal tunnel syndrome or ulnar nerve neuritis, these may be best treated directly over the affected nerve with one electrode proximal to the site of damage where the affected nerve is nearest the surface (Figure 14.4, 1 and 2). Small pads may be adequate for these stimulations.

The fundamental guidelines to follow are that the pads should be placed:

1. Over the peripheral nerve where it is most superficial proximal to the site of pain.
2. Over the affected dermatome or the adjacent dermatome.
3. Over the nerve root.
4. Above and below the painful area.
5. Not over anaesthetic areas.
6. Over areas which will still allow functional use of the limb or part.
7. Over trigger points (Melzack *et al.*, 1977).

One or more of the above principles of placement may be employed in one treatment, e.g. stump and phantom limb pain, one pad may be placed over a painful neuroma, the other over the adjacent dermatomes to the deafferented limb (Figure 14.4, 6e). As already discussed, little conclusive work has been done to establish ideal electrode placements for specific conditions (Johnson *et al.*, 1991a). However, systematic application of electrodes over successive sessions will lead to a more successful outcome (Woolfe *et al.*, 1981; Frampton, 1982).

Possible reasons for poor results

The reasons for poor results are related to either patient, technique or equipment. A summary of these is:

Patient — inappropriate patient selection, e.g. an hysterical patient, or an unreliable patient.

Technique — inappropriate placement of electrodes, e.g. over anaesthetic areas.
— inadequate coverage or too much electroconductive gel on the pad.
— inadequate securing of electrodes.
— failure to explore different placements of electrodes in systematic consecutive manner or alternative electrode sizes.
— failure to explore various parameters of stimulation comprehensively and sequentially.
— inadequate treatment time.

Machine — application of flimsy cables that break easily.
— the use of flat batteries.
— poor battery connection of the wires with the machine.
— failure to replace the carbon silicon electrode pads when the life of the original pad has expired.
— failure to try a dual output, or variable pulse frequencies or patterns.
— inadequate monitoring of results and documentation for comparative evaluation and follow-up.

It can be seen that poor results can be attributed to many different factors, ranging from patient treatment techniques to basic technical faults. These may seem trivial in isolation, but a combination of these problems is most frequently the cause of the TENS application being abandoned as unsuccessful. It is worth re-emphasizing that poor results may be attributed to failure in considering TENS as part of a comprehensive rehabilitation programme.

Criteria for the Selection of Machines

As already discussed, the parameters vary little between manufacturers. The following suggestions must act as a guide to the physiotherapist, enabling selection of the machine which best suits the patients' needs. Obviously, the ultimate choice is a balance between what the machine offers in relation to its cost. The following features are useful to consider when making a selection:

1. A small compact size.
2. A robust casing.
3. A functional low profile clip.
4. Dials that are easy to operate with a moderate turning resistance to avoid accidental knocking and a consequent sudden increase in current.

5. A unit with a single amplitude output socket with bifurcated lead wires.
6. A variety of electrode sizes and types.
7. Robust leads.
8. A lightweight unit.
9. A good back-up service and maintenance facility.
10. A variable pulse width.
11. A burst, continuous or modulated frequency unit.

Other machines for specialist use are the obstetric TENS units (see Chapter 23), which have been modified to meet the needs of acute spasmodic pain and incorporate a burst facility.

Assessment, monitoring and evaluation

Successful treatment will depend on an accurate assessment of the patient, and whether that patient is a suitable candidate for TENS (see Case histories). All patients with pain must be thoroughly examined. There is a great temptation to omit conventional assessments with chronic pain patients on the grounds that they have been referred for the 'treatment of pain'. There may be many contributing factors associated with the pain and these must be identified. In some cases, however, an effective objective examination is almost impossible and a subjective and functional assessment is the only baseline that can be obtained. The pain charts illustrated in Figure 14.5 provide a quantitative analysis using a 10 cm horizontal visual analogue scale (VAS) (see Chapter 6). In a busy out-patient department a verbal score of 0–10 can be used but loses the advantage that the visual record offers to demonstrate improvement in the relief of pain. A behavioural analysis (Figure 14.6) of pain provides a baseline of information which can be compared with subsequent measures following treatment by TENS. For example, a patient with a brachial plexus lesion has intense shooting pain. Following TENS the frequency of the spasms may be reduced from ten every 5 minutes to once every hour. But the background burning pain that frequently exists may remain unchanged and, therefore, the patient's score on the VAS remains unchanged.

It is the evaluation of both the behavioural and quantitative analysis of pain which assists in the management of TENS, together with other objective signs from the original examination. The chart of the VAS allows a score to be taken before and after stimulation. It is important that records are kept for at least 1 week's trial, as very often pain relief is not immediate due to one of the reasons mentioned on p. 124. A data and body chart (Figure 14.7 and 14.8) record all relevant information regarding the parameters used, type of machine and length of treatment time. The body chart provides a quick way of recording electrode positions, which can be numbered and then recorded in the data chart; thus, on any one treatment session an immediate comparison can be made between the parameters used, the position of electrodes and length of treatment time with the VAS and pain behaviour. The comments column allows information regarding drug intake to be recorded. Frequently large doses of analgesics are taken and a reduction in dose may be another indicator to successful treatment with TENS. Outpatients are not as easily monitored as inpatients. It is necessary to see the patient the next day following initial application of TENS. He should be requested to reapply the TENS himself and this enables a more accurate monitoring of his technique and placement of electrodes. It may be necessary for the patient to attend daily in an attempt to find the most successful position. It is unwise, therefore, to apply TENS on a Friday if review is not possible until the Monday. Failure with the chronic pain patient, even if it is due to poor technique, might dissuade him from continuing with TENS.

Many people have expressed a disappointment in the less dramatic effect of TENS. All too often the chronic pain patient comes in looking for the 'cure', anticipating immediate relief with TENS. Objectives must be clearly set prior to treatment. It must be explained to the patient that TENS may only reduce the pain at first and not obliterate it, and that the overall effect may only be to allow the discontinuation of all analgesics, which in some cases may be narcotic, and if this goal alone is achieved some success of treatment must be claimed. This attitude results in different goals being set for different conditions, e.g. a patient with an 11-year history of back pain is not going to have the same outcome as a patient with postherpetic neuralgia with single root involvement.

Above all, the patient's expectations must be rationalized but without damping their hope, which may already be at its lowest level. The need to encourage and motivate the chronic pain patient is an extremely important facet of treatment and the need to gain the patient's confidence is vital.

Name:. . . . . Medical record number:. . . . . Date:. . . . .

Date:. . . . .

Before stimulation

No pain   Maximum pain

After stimulation

No pain   Maximum pain

Date:. . . . .

Before stimulation

No pain   Maximum pain

After stimulation

No pain   Maximum pain

Date:. . . . .

Before stimulation

No pain   Maximum pain

After stimulation

No pain   Maximum pain

Date:. . . . .

Before stimulation

No pain   Maximum pain

After stimulation

No pain   Maximum pain

Date:. . . . .

Before stimulation

No pain   Maximum pain

After stimulation

No pain   Maximum pain

Date:. . . . .

Before stimulation

No pain   Maximum pain

After stimulation

No pain   Maximum pain

Date:. . . . .

Before stimulation

No pain   Maximum pain

After stimulation

No pain   Maximum pain

Fig. 14.5   Visual analogue scale chart. On a full-sized VAS chart the scale measures 10 cm in length. This enables the physiotherapist to obtain accurate data of the patient's pain after each treatment session.

PAIN

Onset

Increasing/static/decreasing

Nature

Distribution

Frequency of pain in one day

Daily pattern

Aggravates

Eases

Drugs

Sleep disturbance

COMMENTS

Fig. 14.6   Pain behaviour chart.

Date	Tens Make & Number	Time on	Time off	Total h Stimulation	Electrode Position/ Size	Most Effective Position			Comments
						Output	Frequency	Pulse Width	

Fig. 14.7   TENS data chart.

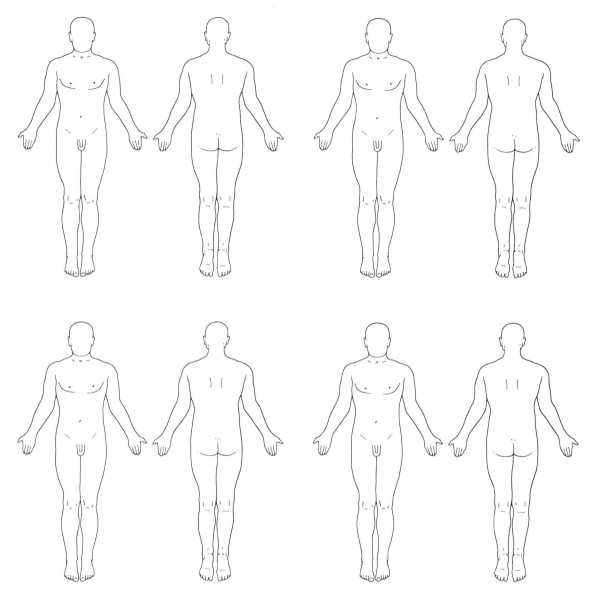

Fig. 14.8 Body chart for the physiotherapist to complete with the electrode positions used. Examples of the completed chart are show in Figure 14.4.

TENS can provide an excellent tool in the total management of these patients who, once pain is relieved to some degree, are encouraged to participate in their own treatment.

Duration of treatment

This is one of the most frequent reasons for poor or unsustained pain relief with TENS. Work has shown that TENS can have a cumulative effect (Sjolund and Eriksson, 1979; Woolfe *et al.*, 1981; Wynn Parry, 1980). Certainly, the need for prolonged periods of stimulation is compatible with the evidence of the profound peripheral and central effects chronic pain has had on the central nervous system. On the basis of a comprehensive rehabilitation programme once pain has been relieved, normal functional stimulation must be fed back into the spinal cord so that abnormal central patterns can be replaced by more normal ones. Exact recommendations are impossible to make as each patient varies considerably, but the following provides a helpful baseline from which to work:

1. Use continuous stimulation for a minimum of 8 h/day.
2. Continue experimenting with TENS for at least 1 week before abandoning it as unsuccessful.
3. Continue a regime of 8 h for 3 weeks and then reduce the treatment gradually if it is helping.
4. If less than 4 h of TENS stimulation a day results in returned or increased pain, return to 4 h a day for a further week or so.
5. Continue to reduce the treatment until no stimulation is required.
6. Keep the TENS machine for a further 2–3 months before returning it to the department.
7. Stimulation for 24 h may be necessary in some cases.
8. Complete cessation may not be possible, and the patient may require 2 h TENS stimulation in the morning or at night.
9. In some cases, such as amputation, the need to wear a prosthesis is obvious not only for function but also to restore afferent stimulation to the stump. In such a case TENS may be used for the required 8 h, either overnight (when pain is often the most intense) or in the evening when the prosthesis is removed.

In a recent study, Johnson *et al.* (1991b) analysed in depth the long-term users of TENS. From 179 questionnaires they ascertained that 47% of patients reported their pain reduced by half or more, 13.7% reported no relief from pain, 15.5% reported total relief of pain. Two-thirds of the patients who reported complete failure continued to use TENS on a daily basis.

Seventy-five per cent of patients used daily stimulation. Patients used TENS between 39.7 and 19.8 hours per week, that is 6.1 days per week for between 6.3 and 2.5 hours each day. In their study, onset of pain relief occurred within 0.5 hours in 75% of patients and within 1 hour in over 95%.

Post-TENS analgesia lasted more than 1 hour in over 30% and less than 30 minutes for 51% of patients. They reported that there was no significant difference between the time of onset or post-TENS pain relief between burst and continuous modes of stimulation.

The authors of the 1991 study hypothesize that those patients in whom pain relief was rapid from onset of TENS but equally short-lived following offset of TENS are demonstrating the gating mechanism. In those patients whose analgesia was more prolonged, the endorphin release mechanism may have been responsible.

Despite these valuable recent studies, it would appear that patients use a pulse frequency and pulse pattern to suit their comfort, which also affords maximum pain relief. Thus, adequate time must be set aside to try different parameters and placement sequentially.

The author is aware that not all physiotherapists are working in the 'ideal' environment and shortage of machines may result in sacrificing the length of treatment for more patients being treated. Evidence of successful treatments on a regular basis will demonstrate and confirm the correct treatment techniques. Some manufacturers offer a free loan service which enables the patient to try the TENS before deciding to purchase their own equipment.

The use of TENS in specific conditions

TENS can be used in acute and chronic pain; the most common use in acute pain is in the management of labour pain (see Chapter 23) and postoperative pain (see Chapter 20). Chronic pain may present most commonly in the following cases (Frampton, 1982):

1. Chronic back, leg or neck pain (see Case history 1).
2. Post-herpetic neuralgia (see Case history 2).
3. Brachial plexus lesions (see Case history 3).
4. Peripheral nerve injuries (PNI), including painful neuromas, reflex sympathetic dystrophy and nerve compression injuries (e.g. carpal tunnel syndrome) (see Case history 4a, 4b).
5. Stump and/or a phantom limb pain (see Case history 5).
6. Trigeminal neuralgia.

Some case histories illustrating the use of TENS in specific conditions are given below.

Case History 1 (Chronic low back and leg pain)

A 34-year-old woman developed acute low back pain. The previous day she had carried her sick child around 'on her hip' all day. She was treated initially with bedrest for 3 months, with only marginal improvement in her pain. She subsequently received two epidural injections weekly for 8 weeks. Over the next 6 months she developed leg pain and was referred for physiotherapy. She received traction and mobilization and finally was put in a plaster-of-Paris jacket. Nine months later EMGs showed denervation in the L4–L5 roots, and the patient proceeded to a laminectomy of L4–L5. Relief of pain lasted 6 weeks and then returned as intensely as before. One year later a spinal fusion was performed and 2 months later the pain was significantly worse. Three years following the onset of her pain, the patient was referred to a pain clinic and from there to an inpatient rehabilitation ward for assessment and management of her pain.

The woman was distressed and depressed; she showed little faith in the prospect of any further successful treatment. She complained of a constant dull ache in her back, with intermittent shooting pain down her right leg. Pain was present at night and was increased when standing for longer than 15 minutes, sitting for 10 minutes and sustained flexion, and walking 18.2 m (20 yd). Pain was relieved by lying flat and painkillers (Diconal × 6 a day; Distalgesic × 8–10). She was stiff and painful in the morning and the pain gradually increased towards the end of the day. Movement was restricted in all directions and she had a bilateral 40° straight leg raise. Her abdominal and back extensor muscles were very weak.

On the visual analogue scale she scored 9 out of 10. She was counselled and encouraged to make a fresh start on treatment. On the following day a single channel TENS unit was tried with large pads, size 4 × 8 cm. As she had both back and L5 root pain into her leg, position 11d (Figure 14.4) was selected. After 2 hours she had some relief from leg pain and noticed an increase in walking distance. Following 1 week of 8 hours TENS a day she had

50% reduction in her leg pain and was walking 91 m (100 yd). Also, in this first week, she had commenced gentle mobilization in the hydrotherapy pool, and Maitland mobilizations to L3–L4 proximal to the fused segment, which was painful. As her back pain continued to be a problem, a dual channel unit was selected in the second week and position 11g (Figure 14.4) was tried, and this successfully relieved her back pain.

Mobilization and monitoring of all activities was continued, and on discharging her 3 weeks following admission her VAS was 3 out of 10 for back and leg pain. She was walking 273 m (300 yd) and could sit up to 1–2 hours, and she had completely stopped all analgesics and felt much happier and 'back to normal'.

At a 3-year follow-up she was still using TENS 8 hours a day; this may seem a limited successful result. However, the patient was very happy not to be taking analgesics; she was leading a normal and full life, and also had a part-time job.

Case History 2 (Post-herpetic neuralgia)

A 71-year-old man developed herpes zoster affecting his right upper quadrant. The visicles remained for 3 weeks and his onset of pain was immediate, which gradually increased. He was treated with carbamazepine with no effect. Nine weeks following the onset of the virus he was referred to physiotherapy.

On examination he complained of a constant, searing, burning pain and was hyperaesthetic over the anterior and posterior area of his neck over his shoulder girdle and anterior chest wall to the level of his nipple. The pain also extended down his arm to the mid part of his humerus. He also complained of a shooting pain three times every hour into a smaller area around the supraclavicular fossa and over the

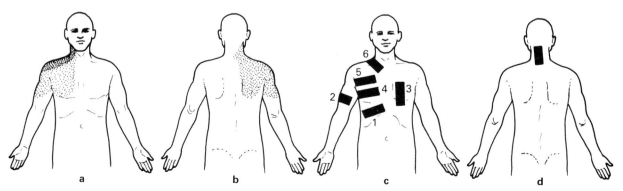

Fig. 14.9   *a–d*, Distribution of pain in Case History 2 and progressive and successive electrode placements.

posterolateral aspect of his shoulder (Figure 14.9, *a* and *b*). He was unable to tolerate light touch or wear clothes on that side. He was unable to sleep or drive his car.

A TENS single channel unit with 4×8 cm² electrodes was applied. The proximal pad was placed over the cervical spine and the distal pad was placed in position 1 (see Figure 14.9, *c* and *d*). On review the following day there had been no relief so position 2 was applied. Three days later there was some relief distally and his shirt was less irritating to wear. At 6 days the area of pain was receding but he was still very painful over the chest wall. Position 3 was applied. At 8 days, as the area of pain continued to diminish, position 4 was applied.

Three weeks from the onset of TENS his sharp pain was less frequent and the area of hyperaesthesia continuing to reduce in area and intensity. Four weeks post TENS he was left with a small area of residual pain at the base of the neck. Position 5 was applied. Six weeks post TENS position 6 was applied. He was wearing the stimulator for 8 hours a day and at this point he began to reduce the hours of stimulation.

Approximately 13 weeks following the commencement of TENS he discontinued stimulation. He was able to wear clothes, drive and his sleep pattern had returned to normal.

In this case it was necessary to change the position of the distal pad regularly, as the area of hyperaesthesia diminished. Constant monitoring was essential to reassess the extent of his pain and pursue different positions.

Case History 3 (Brachial plexus lesion)

An 18-year-old man was involved in a motorcycle accident while travelling at 66 km/h (40 mph). The front wheel of the motorcycle hit a hole in the road and he came off the machine and hit a telegraph pole. The patient sustained a right brachial plexus lesion (BPL) involving roots of C5–T1. C5 and C6 were diagnosed as post ganglionic lesions and C7, C8, T1 as preganglionic lesions. Two weeks later he developed a constant, severe, burning pain in all the fingers of his right hand and the ulnar border of his forearm, with sharp shooting pain in his middle, ring and little fingers occurring every 5–10 minutes. Although the pain varied little, he found that distraction was the only means of providing some degree of relief, as drugs had no effect.

His life was affected dramatically by the pain, preventing him from concentrating on any activity, as he had to stop to grip the arm with every stab of pain. He had been fitted with a flail arm splint (Robinson, 1986; Frampton, 1990) to restore some function

to his paralysed arm but was unable to use it because of the pain.

Following sensory assessment, he was found to have sensation to light touch proximal to the elbow, but no sensation below that level and his VAS score was 10 (the maximum). It was decided to apply TENS and position 4b in Figure 14.4 was used. After only a few hours' stimulation, he had obtained good relief of pain. He was then encouraged to use his flail arm splint to restore some afferent input from the deafferented side. He was discharged 3 weeks later using TENS 8 hours a day. Although he still had the constant burning pain, the frequency of the stab of pain was reduced to once daily and his VAS score dropped to 2. After 2 months he was using TENS one morning per week and had ceased using it altogether at the 7-month follow-up. When seen 2 years after his accident, he was not using TENS and was working full-time as a television engineer.

Case History 4a (Carpal Tunnel Compression)

A 58-year-old night sister had a 10-year history of paraesthesia in her right hand. She had pain at night, had difficulty writing and manipulating small objects. EMG studies demonstrated that she had a moderately severe carpal tunnel syndrome. In July 1990 she had a carpal tunnel decompression. One week post operatively she was complaining of sharp, shooting pain at the wrist and hyperaesthesia in the palm. She continued to have tingling in her hand at night in the median nerve distribution. Two months later she was referred to out patient physiotherapy.

On examination her hand was red and engorged. She complained of hyperaesthesia in the palm, a sharp pain at the wrist and paraesthesia at night and with manual activities, such as writing and opening bottles.

A single channel TENS unit was applied with standard 4×4 cm² pads in position 1a. She was instructed in its use and was requested to leave it on for a minimum of 8 hours and return the following day with the TENS in place so that correct positioning and application could be monitored. She wore the TENS 11–13 hours per day for 3 weeks; she was able to continue working with the TENS in place. At a 3-week follow-up her symptoms were much improved and the hyperaesthetic area reduced by 50%. At 5 weeks after commencement of TENS the area was reduced a further 25%, leaving only a small area of hyperaesthesia around the scar. She reduced the hours of stimulation to 6 hours a day.

Eight weeks following the first application she discontinued TENS and, on discharge, she had no pain or hyperaesthesia. However, she did have some residual clumsiness due to some loss of sensory proprioception.

Case history 4b (A painful scar)

A 60-year-old lady sustained a dislocation of her proximal interphalangeal joint and laceration of the palmar surface of her right middle finger. Five weeks later she was referred for physiotherapy. On examination she had a swollen proximal interphalangeal joint with a range of motion from 20° to 90°. Although the finger was tender, her main symptoms contributing to loss of function of the hand were due to the painful scar of the laceration. She complained of hyperaesthesia over and around the scar with a sharp, stabbing pain when pressure was applied to a nodule that was in the scar. She was unable to use the hand for washing and carrying due to these symptoms.

Single channel TENS was applied in position 1a, using standard 4 × 4 cm² electrodes. She wore the TENS for 6–8 hours a day. She was reviewed the following day for correct positioning and application of the TENS. At one-week follow-up she had minimal relief, so position 1b was applied using a small finger electrode for the distal pad and she continued with the same number of hours of stimulation. Three weeks after application of TENS the pain in the scar had completely resolved.

TENS was discontinued and her range of movement had improved to 15° to 115° with function fully restored except for some residual joint tenderness which limited her ability to carry heavy bags.

In this case it was necessary to move the distal pad closer to the laceration to achieve pain relief. A successful outcome of the dislocation may have been compromised if the hyperaesthesia had not been treated.

Case history 5 (Phantom limb pain)

A 72-year-old diabetic man had undergone a below-knee amputation for gangrenous toes. Preoperatively he had complained of severe continuous pain which was almost intolerable. It had been present on waking and had increased during the day, reaching its peak at night, as a result of which he had difficulty sleeping. Although the pain in his phantom foot decreased over the first postoperative month, as expected, he still had sufficient pain to interfere with mobilization. Therefore, TENS was applied in position 6e in Figure 14.4. The patient used the machine for 8 hours per day and obtained almost immediate relief. After 2–3 weeks, the pain was almost gone and he progressed to wearing his prosthesis all day and only using the TENS machine at night. Eventually he no longer needed to use TENS.

In the category of peripheral nerve injuries (PNI) one may include ulnar neuritis, median nerve neuritis following carpal tunnel decompression or painful digital neuromas (Frampton, 1985b), as previously described. The most common symptom of a painful PNI is one of hyperpathia. This abnormal painful response of the patient to light touch makes normal functional use impossible. TENS must be applied to affect the nerve but allow the hand to remain free to participate in a subsequent desensitization programme. In such cases, combination treatments may be necessary (Withrington and Wynn Parry, 1984). A guide to electrode placements for different conditions and alternative placements can be seen in Figure 14.4.

Other conditions, such as osteoarthritis, rheumatoid arthritis, strains and sprains and other sports-related injuries are not discussed here. There is no doubt that TENS is widely used as a pain-relieving modality on painful joints prior to or in conjunction with other treatments. Other modalities are of course available and may be more appropriate to treat joint conditions, as TENS is most effective in treating conditions of a neurogenic origin. However, if TENS is to be used to treat joint conditions, shorter periods of stimulation would be indicated in these cases.

No reference to acupuncture or the use of TENS on acupuncture points has been made. Although the author uses the Western approach to acupuncture, it is in accordance with myofascial or trigger point methods. However, it is interesting to note that successful treatments have been achieved using TENS by placing electrodes over trigger points (Frampton, 1985a).

Contraindications to the use of TENS

Manufacturers quote several contraindications which are listed here:

1. TENS should not be used to treat patients with pacemakers.
2. TENS should not be used to treat patients with known myocardial disease and arrhythmias (except on the recommendation of a physician following evaluation of the patient).
3. TENS should not be used in the area of the carotid sinus and mouth.
4. TENS appliances should be kept out of the reach of children.
5. TENS should not be used while operating vehicles or potentially hazardous equipment.

6. Application or removal of electrodes should always be carried out with the appliance switched off.
7. Electrodes must not be placed over broken skin sites.
8. One side-effect can be a skin irritation or a rash developing beneath or around the electrode in prolonged application. Care of the skin and electrodes is therefore important. It is necessary to wash the area of application and the electrodes following stimulation, in the first case to prevent skin rash, and also to prevent the rubber perishing.
9. TENS must not be used in/over anaesthetic areas of skin.
10. Some manufacturers state that the safety of TENS during pregnancy has not been established. However, there has been no research, so far, to support this claim. Obstetric physiotherapists feel strongly that its use during pregnancy and lactation is preferable to strong analgesic medication. It appears manufacturers include this to avoid litigation. As a result, it is advisable to avoid placing the electrodes directly on the abdomen, but there is no reason why TENS should not be used for the treatment of limb, back or neck pain (Mannheimer and Lampe, 1984). The use of TENS in pregnancy is an area of research that needs urgent investigation.

Common sense must prevail when considering these contraindications, as many are for the purposes of insurance. For example, when driving a car it is obvious that if the driver knocks the dials the sudden jolt may cause him to have an accident. Apart from cases of skin irritation and allergic responses, there are few reasons why anyone may not use TENS. The allergic response to the tape and gel can be overcome by the use of hypoallergenic self-adhesive pads. It is important to look out for the chronic pain patient who is unobserved at home and returns to the outpatient department with what appears to be an allergic response under the pad itself. Frequently, this can be caused by a current that was too intense and the rash is an electric burn. Patients often deny this, and the only remedy is close supervision with the physiotherapist altering the dials. More often the patient presents with a white unaffected skin area under the pad and a red inflamed area around it. This is the common allergic response from the tape.

Research and follow-up

As has already been outlined in the earlier sections, controlled double-blind trials and reliable evaluations of parameters are not easy (Wynn Parry, 1981). The author has based her method of treatments on retrospective studies over the past 14 years of patients whose records have been maintained through follow-up (Frampton, 1982). Following discharge, all patients must be reviewed and a behavioural and quantitative analysis of their pain taken. Each patient should have their own card with the updated information. All the cards can be filed together and colour coded according to the diagnosis. A separate card system for each TENS machine is kept so that at any time one can see at a glance where any particular machine is and this can be cross-referenced with the patients' cards. This system, although initially time-consuming, is certainly time-saving in the long run, and allows an on-going monitoring system for evaluation.

It is necessary that the valuable work completed by recent researchers (Johnson, Tulgar etc.) should be continued. More work needs to be done to look at specific client groups, for example, painful brachial plexus avulsion lesions, nerve compression injuries, phantom limb pain. As the pathology of different painful conditions has different elements to it, these groups need to be looked at separately. More work needs to be done to establish the effects of different parameters on these client groups, also the effect of different electrode size and placement in relation to the different pathologies.

TENS remains another tool for the physiotherapist in the range of treatments for patient care. Properly used and evaluated, it still provides one of the cheapest, non-invasive modalities available for pain relief. However, on occasions it is still prescribed with inadequate information and instruction and patients are told to go away and try it for a while without proper follow-up and monitoring available. If this is the case, TENS will fail to be considered as part of a complete rehabilitation programme and a valuable piece of equipment will be lost to the chronic pain sufferer.

MYOFASCIAL TRIGGER POINT ELECTRO ACUPUNCTURE

Myofascial or trigger point (MTP) acupuncture can be given by needle, with or without an electrical stimulation, or by a metal probe. Acupressure is another method whereby trigger points are treated via manual pressure through the therapist's own hands. Although the term 'acupuncture' is used, this technique must not be confused with traditional Chinese acupuncture where the philosophy of treatment bears little relationship to traditional Western medicine. Electrical stimulation of myofascial trigger points transcutaneously via a metal probe is a useful non-invasive technique which can be used to relieve pain primarily of musculoskeletal origin. It has a wide application in the physiotherapy department and can be used in isolation or in combination with other treatments. The neurophysiology associated with myofascial trigger point acupuncture is described in Chapter 13. The mode of action of electro-stimulation transcutaneously on MTPs for pain relief is compatible with needle stimulation, but offers the alternative of a non-invasive procedure.

Clinical experience (Frampton, 1985a) suggests that this method of treatment is most effective on neck and shoulder pain. Back pain can also be treated successfully, but without the same sustained relief that is achieved in the treatment of neck and shoulder pain. It is important to emphasize that myofascial trigger points were first described 50 years ago (Travell). Since that time, this subject has been further explored and more literature is now available (Travell and Simons, 1983 and 1992).

Patient selection for MTP electro-stimulation

This technique's most useful application is in acute or chronic neck pain. Muscle spasm associated with acute neck pain can be quickly and significantly relieved. However, it is a painful technique and, for this reason, alternative traditional methods of pain relief, such as ice, heat or a soft collar, might be the method of choice. Patients suffering from chronic neck and back pain, who have not responded to conventional treatment and who present with well localized acutely tender trigger points over the painful area, are good candidates for myofascial trigger point electro-stimulation. These patients frequently have significant muscle spasm. It may be for this reason that they respond well to MTP electro-stimulation, as it is thought to stimulate the A-delta fibres from the muscle stretch receptors in muscle fibres which, in turn, activate presynaptic inhibitory mechanisms, and directly

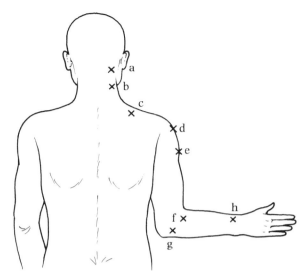

Fig. 14.10 Trigger points. *a*, base of occiput; *b*, C5 transverse process; *c*, upper fibres of trapezius; *d*, greater tuberosity; *e*, insertion of deltoid; *f*, head of radius; *g*, lateral epicondyle; *h*, distal end of radius.

effect muscle relaxation. There are virtually no contraindications for its use.

Patient assessment

Palpation is the most significant part of the examination to evaluate a patient's suitability for MTP electro-stimulation. It is important to locate points of maximal tenderness in order to achieve effective relief of pain from MTP electro-stimulation. This is compatible with other observations, such as those of Lewitt (1979), who observed that effective treatment of pain by the 'needle effect' is related to the intensity of pain produced at the trigger zone and to the precision with which the site of maximal tenderness is located by the needle. It is important to record and map out the painful area on a body chart. Palpation, using the tip of the index or middle finger in and around the painful area, will allow identification of trigger points. Firm, constant pressure must be applied and efforts made not to increase this in pursuit of a trigger spot. True trigger points are immediately identifiable, as the patient instantly reacts by drawing away or flinching (twitch sign). Patients frequently present with consistent characteristic patterns of trigger points (see Figure 14.10.) Frequently, trigger points correspond to Chinese acupuncture points and also to motor points (Liu *et al.*, 1975). The location of the trigger points must be recorded on the body chart. Clearly, full examination of the patient is required, which must include subjective and objective assessment of pain. (see Chapter 6.) When range of movement is reduced or limited by pain, this must also be recorded so that it may be used as another objective measurement to assess the outcome of treatment.

The apparatus

There are several machines available, many of which have a dual facility for TENS and electro acupuncture. It is important that the machine is capable of delivering a strong enough stimulus, which is necessary to achieve pain relief in MTP electro acupuncture (Lewitt, 1979). The Asah El-acupuncture machine has proved to be one of the most effective models. The technical specifications of the machine, as described by the manufacturers are:

> Wave form – monophasic Pulse width – variable, 15–20 Ms Current output – 0–4 mA Frequency – 1–30 Hz.

This machine has an on-switch which has an automatic shut-off, a two-way selector (A - B), for the acupuncture or transcutaneous electrical nerve stimulation (TENS) treatment modes; and an LED scale from 1 to 9. Current consumption is 3–13 mA, voltage, 0.22 volts.

The apparatus has a pair of leads which are connected by one jack plug to the machine. One lead connects to a metal rod which the patient holds in one hand (anode), while the other attaches to a metal probe which the manufacturers call the 'search probe' (cathode). This probe is said to measure skin electrical resistance. The manufacturers advise locating acupuncture points by demonstrating points of lowered skin resistance, that is that the machine's sensor will indicate 9 on the LED scale. In MTP electro-stimulation, points of maximum tenderness are located and the search system is not required. Interestingly, trigger points always register lowered skin resistance on the machine's sensor. The probe is pencil-shaped with a metal tip and it is this part that is used for sensing and delivering the treatment stimulus.

Operation

The patient must be placed in a comfortable position, relaxed and supported. For treatment of the neck the position of choice is either sitting in a chair with the arms supported on a pillow in front of the patient, or side lying. The patient is asked to hold the metal rod in one hand so that good contact with the electrode is achieved. The machine is switched on and set to the acupuncture mode. The output is turned up to halfway. The probe, held in the operator's hand, must be pressed gently and squarely over the trigger spot, at which point the machine emits an audible tone which grows louder until the LED reaches 9 on the scale. Although the output varies from 0 to 4 mA, it is likely that the current will vary depending on the individual skin resistance. The pulse is then switched on to intercept the current, set at approximately 1.4 – 2 Hz, for a duration of approximately 60 seconds. The pulse (or frequency) is then switched off and the probe removed from the patient's skin. A visible red flare is produced similar to that produced with needle acupuncture. Frequently, the patient's pain is reproduced during stimulation and an unpleasant stimulus is experienced. Pain relief, however, can be immediate following cessation of the electrical stimulus. It is advisable to treat only a minimum number of trigger points at the first treatment session. It may be that good pain relief is achieved by treating three trigger points. Distal points can be included if pain relief is not adequate (see Figure 14.10, *d,e,f,g* and *h*).

Duration of treatment

Ideally, treatment should be given daily for one week, then reduced to three, then two times and then once a week, untill the patient is asymptomatic or the symptoms remain unchanged. On average, 11 treatments and approximately six trigger points is a guide to the treatment of neck pain (Frampton, 1985a). Although some back patients experience relief immediately following treatment, in many cases this is not always sustained. However, some patients, despite only temporary relief from symptoms, have bought their own machine and are using it daily at home.

MTP electrical stimulation versus TENS

It is important to appreciate that the mechanism by which MTP electro-acupuncture is thought to act is quite different from TENS. Although both methods promote inhibition of the afferent pathways, it is via different routes. TENS activates a presynaptic inhibitory mechanism by stimulating A-beta fibres to block transmission of nociceptive afferents to the ascending axons. It is thought that stimulation by needle or by myofascial trigger point electroacupuncture activates the medium sized A-delta afferents from the muscle stretch receptors in muscle fibres (Chapter 13). MTP electroacupuncture can be used as a first line treatment, particularly in cases when extreme muscle spasm is a predominating symptom. Unlike TENS, it is a short, sharp treatment with what most patients describe as an unpleasant stimulus. TENS is a prolonged treatment with a tolerable, pleasant stimulus. More often, MTP electro-acupuncture is a useful tool to relieve pain of musculoskeletal origin when other forms of manual techniques have not been completely successful.

MTP electroacupuncture is a safe procedure suitable for use by physiotherapists and effective in the management of chronic pain, particularly in the neck. It is certainly worthy of further evaluation.

References

Anderson, S.A., Hansson, G., Holmgren, E. and Renberg, O. (1976) Evaluation of the pain suppressing effect of different frequencies of peripheral electrical stimulation in chronic pain conditions. *Acta Orthop. Scand.*, 47 149–57.

Baldry, P. (1989), *Acupuncture, Trigger Points and Musculoskeletal Pain*, Churchill Livingstone, Edinburgh

Bates, J.A.V. and Nathan, P.W. (1980) Transcutaneous electrical nerve stimulation for chronic pain. *Anaesthesia*, 35, 817–22

Blumberg, H. and Janig, W. (1984) Discharge pattern of afferent fibres from a neuroma. *Pain.*, 20, 335–53

Brennan, K.R. (1976) Characteristics of transcutaneous stimulating electrodes. *EEG Trans. Biomed-Engin.*, 23, 337–40

Brewart, J. and Gentle, M.J. (1985) Neuroma formation and abnormal afferent discharges after partial beak amputation (beak-trimming) in poultry. *Experientia*, 41, 1132–4

Burchiel, K.J. (1984) Effects of electrical and mechanical stimulation on two foci of spontaneous activity which develop in primary afferent neuroma after peripheral axotomy. *Pain*, 18, 249–65

Devor, M. (1989) The pathophysiology of damaged peripheral nerves. In *Textbook of Pain* (eds. P.D. Wall and R. Melzack), Edinburgh, Churchill Livingstone, pp. 63–81

Eriksson, M.B.E., Sjolund, B.H. and Nielzen, S. (1979) Long term results of peripheral conditioning stimulation as an analgesic measure in chronic pain. *Pain*, 6, 335–47

Frampton, V.M. (1982) Pain control with the aid of transcutaneous nerve stimulation. *Physiotherapy*, 68 (3), 77–81

Frampton, V.M. (1984a) Management of brachial plexus lesions. *Physiotherapy*, 70 (10), 388–92

Frampton, V.M. (1984b) Treatment note: brachial plexus flail arm splint. *Physiotherapy*, 70 (11), 428

Frampton, V.M. (1985a) A pilot study to evaluate myofascial or trigger point electro-acupuncture in the treatment of neck and back pain. *Physiotherapy*, 71 (1), 5–7

Frampton, V.M. (1985b) Conservative management of pain in the upper limb amputee. *Br. Assoc. Hand Therapists Newsl.*, 2, 17–21

Frampton, V.M. (1990) Therapist's management of brachial plexus injuries. In *Rehabilitation of the Hand: Surgery and Therapy* (eds Hunter, Schneider, Mackin and Callahan.), C.V. Mosby, St Louis, pp. 630–9.

Govrin-Lippman, R. and Devor, M. (1978) Ongoing activity in severed nerves; source and variation with time. *Brain Res.*, 159, 406–10

Handwerker, H.O., Iggo, A. and Zimmermann, M. (1975) Segmental and supraspinal actions on dorsal horn neurons responding to noxious and non-noxious skin stimuli. *Pain*, 1, 147–65

Johnson, M.I., Ashton, C.H., Bousfield, D.R. and Thompson, J.W. (1989) Analgesic effects of different frequencies of transcutaneous electrical nerve stimulation on cold-induced pain in normal subjects. *Pain*, 39, 231–6

Johnson, M.I., Ashton, C.H., Bousfield, D.R. and Thompson, J.W. (1991a) Analgesic effects of different pulse patterns of transcutaneous electrical nerve stimulation on cold-induced pain in normal subjects. *J. Psychosomat. Res.*, 35 (2/3), 313–21

Johnson, M., Ashton, C.H. and Thompson J.W. (1991b) An in-depth study of long-term users of transcutaneous electrical nerve stimulation (TENS). Implications for clinical use of TENS. *Pain*, 44, 221–229

Johnson, M.I., Ashton, C.H. and Thompson, J.W. (1991c) The consistency of pulse frequencies and pulse patterns of transcutaneous electrical nerve stimulation (TENS) used by chronic pain patients. *Pain*, 44, 231–4

Koschorke, G.M., Helme, R.D. and Zimmermann, M. (1985) Substance P suppresses the response to brady-kinin and to heat of non-myelinated fibres in experimented neuromas of the cat's sural nerve. *Soc. Neurosci. Abstr.*, **11**, 118

Lewitt, K. (1979) The needle effect in the relief of myofascial pain. *Pain*, **6**, 83–90

Liu, Y.K., Varela M. and Oswald R. (1975) The correspondence between some motor points and acupuncture loci. *Am. J. Chim. Med.*, **3**(4), 347–58

Loeser, J.D. and Ward, A.A. (1967) Some effects of deafferentation on neurons of the cat spinal cord. *Arch. Neurol.*, **17**, 629–36

Loeser, J.D., Black, R.G. and Chirstman, A. (1975) Relief of pain by transcutaneous stimulation. *J. Neurosurg.*, **42**, 308–14

Long, D.M., Campbell, J.N. and Gurer, G. (1979) Transcutaneous electrical stimulation for relief of chronic pain. In *Advances in Pain Research and Therapy 3* (eds J.J. Bonica, J.C. Liebeskind and D.G. Albe-Fessard), Raven Press, New York, pp. 593–9

Low, P.A. (1985) Endoneurial potassium is increased and enhances spontaneous activity in regenerating mammalian nerve fibres – implications for neuropathic positive symptoms. *Muscle and Nerve*, **8**, 27–33

Mannheimer, C. and Carlsson, C. (1979) The analgesic effect of transcutaneous electrical nerve stimulation (TNS) in patients with rheumatoid arthritis. A comparative study of different pulse patterns. *Pain*, **6**, 329–34

Mannheimer, J.S. and Lampe, G.N. (1984) *Clinical Transcutaneous Electrical Nerve Stimulation*, F.A. Davis, Philadephia

Melzack, R. and Wall, P.D. (1965) Pain mechanism: a new theory. *Science*, **150**, 971–8

Melzack, R. and Wall, P.D. (1982) *The Challenge of Pain*. London, Penguin Books

Melzack, R., Stillwell, D.M. and Fox, E.J. (1977) Trigger points and acupuncture points for pain. Correlations and implications. *Pain*, **3**, 3–23

Meyer, R.A., Raja, S.N., Campbell, J.N. *et al.* (1985) Neural activity originating from a neuroma in the baboon. *Brain Res.*, **325**, 255–60

Omura, Y. (1987) Basic electrical parameters for safe and effective electro-therapeutics (electro-acupuncture TES TENMS (or TEMS) TENS and electro-magnetic field stimulation with or without drug field) for pain neuro-muscular skeletal problems and circulatory disturbances. *Acupunct. Electrother.*, **12**, 201–25

Pomeranz, B. and Niznick, G. (1987) Codetron, a new electrotherapy device overcomes the habituation problems of conventional TENS devices. *Am. J. Electromed.*, 22–26

Robinson, C. (1986) Brachial plexus lesion. Functional splintage, part 2. *Br. J. Occup. Ther.*, **49** (10), 331–986

Salar, G., Job, I., Mingrino, S. *et al.* (1981) Effects of transcutaneous electrotherapy on CSF β-endorphin content in patients without pain problems. *Pain*, **10**, 169–72

Scadding, J.W. (1981) Development of ongoing activity, mechanosensitivity and adrenalin sensitivity in severed peripheral nerve axons. *Exper. Neurol.*, **73**, 345–64

Sjolund, B. and Eriksson, M.B.E. (1979) The influence of naloxone on analgesia produced by peripheral conditioning stimulation. *Brain Res.*, **173**, 295–301

Sjolund, B.H. (1985) Peripheral nerve stimulation suppression of C fibre-evoked flexion reflex in rats. *J. Neurosurg.*, **63**, 612–16

Taylor, P., Hallett, M. and Flaherty, L. (1981) Treatment of osteoarthritis of the knee with transcutaneous electrical nerve stimulation. *Pain*, **11**, 233–46

Thompson, J.W. (1987) The role of transcutaneous electrical nerve stimulation (TENS) for the control of pain. In *1986 International Symposium on Pain Control*, (ed. D. Doyle), Royal Society of Medicine Services, London, pp. 27–47

Travell, J. and Simons, D.C. (1983) *Myofascial Pain and Dysfunction: The Trigger Point Manual*, Williams and Wilkins, Baltimore

Travell, J.G. and Simons, D.C. (1992) *Myofascial Pain and Dysfunction*, vol. 2: *The Trigger Point Manual – the Lower Extremities*, Williams and Wilkins, Baltimore

Tulgar, M., McGlone, F., Bowsher, D. and Miles, J.B. (1991a) Comparative effectiveness of different stimulation modes in relieving pain. Part I A pilot study. *Pain*, **47**, 151–5

Tulgar, M., McGlone, F., Bowsher, D. and Miles J.B. (1991b) Comparative effectiveness of different stimulation modes in relieving pain. Part II A double blind controlled long-term clinical trial. *Pain*, **47**, 157–62

Wagman, I.H. and Price, D.D. (1969) Responses of dorsal horn cells of M. Mulatta to cutaneous and sural nerve A and C fibre stimulation. *J. Neurophysiol.*, **32**, 803–17

Wall, P.D. and Sweet, W. (1967) Temporary abolition of pain in man. *Science*, **155**, 108–9

Wall, P.D. and Gutnik, M. (1974) Properties of afferent nerve impulses originating from a neuroma. *Nature*, **248**, 740

Wall, P.D. and Devor, S. (1981) The effect of peripheral nerve injury on dorsal root potentials and on transmission of afferent signals into the spinal cord. *Brain Res.*, **209**, 95–111

Wiesenfeld, Z. and Lindblom, U. (1980) Behavioural and

electrophysiological effects of various types of peripheral nerve lesions in the rat. A comparison of possible
models for chronic pain. *Pain*, **8**, 285–98

Withrington, R.H. and Wynn Parry, C.B. (1984) The
management of painful peripheral nerve disorders. *J.
Hand Surg.*, **9B**(1), 24–8

Woolfe, S.L., Gersh, H.R. and Rao, V.R. (1981) Examination of electrode placements and stimulating
parameters in treating chronic pain with conventional
transcutaneous electrical nerve stimulation (TENS).
Pain, **11**, 37–47

Woolfe, C.J. and Wal, P.D. (1982) Chronic peripheral
nerve section diminishes the primary afferent A-fibre
mediated inhibition of rat dorsal horn neurones. *Brain
Res.*, **242**, 77–85

Woolfe, C.J. (1989) Segmental afferent fibre-induced analgesia. Transcutaneous electrical nerve stimulation
(TENS) and vibration. In *Textbook of Pain* (eds P.D.
Wall and R. Melzack) Churchill Livingstone, Edinburgh, pp. 884–96

Wynn Parry, C.B. (1980) Pain in avulsion lesions of the
brachial plexus. *Pain*, **9** 41–53

Wynn Parry, C.B. (1981) *Rehabilitation of the Hand*,
Butterworths, London

Further reading

Hannington-Kiff, J. (1974) Intravenous regional sympathetic block with guanethidine. *Lancet*, **1**, 1019–20

Loh, L. and Nathan, P.W. (1978) Painful peripheral
states and sympathetic blocks. *J. Neurol. Neurosurg.
Psychiat.* **441**, 664–71

Melzack, R. and Wall, P.D. (1989) *Textbook of Pain*, 2nd
edn, Churchill Livingstone, Edinburgh

Noordenbos, W. and Wall, P.D. (1981) Nerve resection
fails to relieve chronic peripheral nerve pain. *J. Neurol.
Neurosurg. Psychiat.*, **44**, 1068–73

Ochoa, J. and Torebjork, H.E. (1981) Paraesthesiae from
ectopic impulse generation in human sensory nerve.
Brain, **103**, 835–53

Ottoson, D. and Lundeberg, T. (1988) *Pain Treatment by
Transcutaneous Electrical Nerve Stimulation. A Practical
Manual.* Springer-Verlag, Berlin

Rasminsky M. *et al.* (1978) Conduction of nervous impulses in spinal roots and peripheral nerves of dystrophic mice. *Brain Res.*, **143**, 71–9

Symposium on Pain (1979) *Int. Rehab. Med. J.*, **1**(3),
98–116

Wall, P.D. and Devor, S. (1978) Physiology of sensation
after peripheral nerve injury regeneration and neuroma formation. In *Physiology and Pathology of Axons*
(ed. S.G. Waxman), Raven Press, New York

Wall, P.D. and Gutnik, M. (1974) Ongoing activity in
peripheral nerves. The physiology and pharmacology
of impulses originating from a neuroma. *Exp. Neurol.*,
43, 580–93

Wallin, G., Torebjork, E. and Hallin, R.G. (1976) In
Sensory Functions of the Skin (ed. Y. Zotterman), Pergamon Press, Oxford

Wynn Parry, C.B. (1981) Recent trends in surgery of
peripheral nerves. *Int. Rehab. Med. J.* **3**(4), 169–73

Wynn Parry, C.B. and Withrington, R.H. (1984) The
management of painful peripheral nerve disorders. In
Textbook of Pain (eds P.D. Wall and R. Melzack),
Churchill Livingstone, Edinburgh, pp. 395–401

15 Electrotherapeutic modalities

JOHN LOW

Introduction

Most electrotherapeutic modalities have a particular element of mystery about their application. The relief of pain, occasionally dramatic, after the application of ultrasonic energy, or the gentle comforting heat of shortwave diathermy produced from electrodes which do not become hot and do not touch the skin, may seem rather magical. It may, at least, provoke some feelings of awe for the technology and contribute to a placebo effect. How far such beliefs are appropriate for the patient can be a matter of opinion but they are totally and absolutely inappropriate for the physiotherapist applying the treatment, a point emphasized by Scott (1957).

Electrical energy is completely comprehensible and behaves in a predictable way. Its effects, such as the relief of pain, can be explained rationally. In the past electric and magnetic phenomena have been studied from many different standpoints which has led to different ways of expressing the same concepts. Thus radiation may be described in terms of either wave or particle motion; energy released in the tissues by the passage of electric currents may be confused with the energy liberated due to electromagnetic radiations.

Electric and magnetic fields

The electric force exerted between protons and electrons leads to the presence of an electric field between objects and this is measured in volts; the motion of electric charges described as an electric current is measured as the rate of flow in amperes. The motion of charges, be they electrons orbiting atomic nuclei, currents in a wire, or ions moving in a fluid causes a magnetic force (magnetic field) to act at right angles to the direction of motion of the charges.

Direct currents and steady magnetic fields

Steady continuous direct currents have been used for many years, for example, in the treatment of non-united fractures, where it has been considered as effective as bone grafting and safer (Brighton et al, 1981), also for iontophoresis. The d.c. component of several therapeutic currents is considered to contribute to pain relief, diadynamic currents for example. Magnetism has also been used as a treatment for various conditions with rather less justification since magnetic forces pass easily through the tissues and there are no evident effects. Claims of pain reduction being effected by wearing tiny, but powerful, permanent magnets fixed to the skin by adhesive tape have been made in a treatment called biomagnetism or Taki. Various other methods of applying static magnetic fields are available. There seems to be no objective evidence to support the efficacy of such treatments. High intensity magnetic fields do not seem to damage animal or human tissues in any way. There is evidence that some birds can utilize the vertical component of the earth's magnetic field as a navigational aid so that there must be a physiological mechanism for recognizing these extremely weak fields. There have also been suggestions, backed by some evidence, that man has a similar capability.

It must be recognized that the concept of a static magnetic or steady electric field applied to the tissues is rather too simple. Since there is a continuous movement of particles in the tissues, e.g. the blood flow, any magnetic or electric field is bound to interact with moving charges leading to complex effects.

Alternating currents

If the direction of the electric field is repeatedly

reversed a current, which varies in direction and intensity, results and at low rates of reversal is called a **low frequency alternating current**. Such currents produce similar varying magnetic fields. The number of such cycles in each second is referred to as so many **cycles per second** but more properly as **Hertz** (Hz). Thus 1000 cycles/s is 1 kilohertz (kHz) and 1 000 000 cycles/s is 1 megahertz (MHz).

High Frequency Currents

At higher frequencies, over 500 000 Hz or 0.5 MHz, such currents are usually called **oscillating currents**, but may also be referred to as alternating (Figure 15.1).

Electromagnetic Phenomena

Constantly varying electric and magnetic fields generate an electromagnetic disturbance which propagates energy through space and is recognized as **radiowaves** and at higher frequencies as **radiation**. All electromagnetic energy travels in space at a constant velocity of 300 000 000 m/s (3×10^8 m/s) which is the product of the frequency and the wavelength

$$v = f \times \lambda$$

where v = velocity, f = frequency and λ = wavelength. Such radiations differ only in their frequency and wavelength, thus it is only necessary to describe the radiation in terms of either. In the past, many radiations were described by their wavelength, e.g. long, medium and shortwave radio emission, 12.5 cm **microwave**. Nowadays frequencies are often used, and these relationships are shown in diagramatic form in Figure 15.1. The therapeutic modalities are also indicated here and are discussed below. For a more extensive, but simple, explanation of all these phenomena, see Low and Reed (1994).

Therapeutic modalities

Direct Current

Direct current applied to the tissues by electrodes and saline-soaked pads at current intensities of around 0.2 mA per cm² for short periods has been used for pain relief. Similarly this current can be used for the introduction of pain-controlling drugs into the tissues by iontophoresis.

Interrupted and alternating currents of low frequency

These currents are applied to the tissues by means of electrodes, malleable metal or carbon rubber, and saline soaked pads or sponges. The therapeutic currents are confusingly given a variety of names reflecting their pulse length, pulse frequency and mechanism of action in the tissues. The principal effect of them all is nerve stimulation. Strictly speaking all of them are transcutaneous electrical nerve stimulation but the term TENS is customarily reserved for low intensity sensory nerve stimulation specifically for pain relief using relatively short (0.4–0.02 ms) duration. This is described in Chapter 14. Two other currents will be considered here:

1. Diadynamic current, which consists of a series of 10 ms unidirectional pulses.
2. High voltage pulsed galvanic stimulation, which consists of a series of double peaks of short duration at high voltage.

Medium frequency currents

Alternating currents of around 4 or 5 kHz can be passed through the tissues in the same way and made to interfere within the tissues to produce the same effects as the low frequency currents; these are known as **interferential currents** (see Figure 15.1).

High frequency oscillating currents

If evenly oscillating currents at megahertz frequencies are passed through the tissues they will not directly depolarize nerve fibres so that much higher currents can be passed causing local heating. Frequencies around 1 MHz can be passed via wetted pads and were used by physiotherapists about 50 years ago for tissue heating; this treatment was known as longwave diathermy. (Diathermy was a term coined in 1907 from the Greek meaning 'through heating'.)

Higher frequencies around 30 MHz have the advantage that they can be applied to the tissues

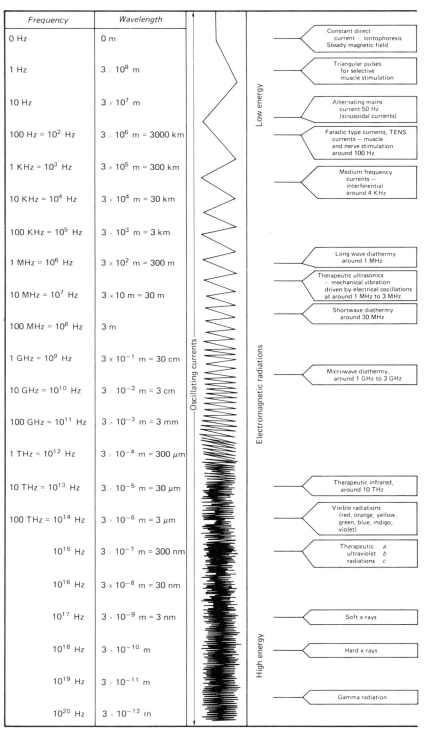

Fig. 15.1 Electric and magnetic fields – electromagnetic radiations. kHz, kilohertz; MHz, megahertz; GHz, gigahertz; THz, terahertz.

to generate heat across an air gap without the need for wet pads. At higher frequencies, and hence shorter wavelengths (see Figure 15.1), such therapies are called shortwave diathermy. By international agreement 27.12 MHz has been designated, with other frequencies (13.56 and 40.68 MHz), for medical and scientific use; most shortwave diathermy machines operate at 27.12 MHz (see Figure 15.1).

Mechanical vibrations

If currents are used to produce mechanical oscillations these ultrasonic vibrations can be passed into the tissues to produce heating and other effects. Various frequencies between 0.5 and 3 MHz are utilized for ultrasonic therapy.

Electromagnetic radiations

Still higher electrical oscillating frequencies lead to the emission of electromagnetic radiations (see Figure 15.1). Microwave (radar) radiations can be 'beamed' into the tissues to cause heating as they are absorbed. A frequency of 2450 MHz is most often used for therapy. Infrared radiations are also used for therapeutic heating and are fully described in Chapter 16. Both infrared and visible radiations in coherent single wavelength beams called lasers are used therapeutically and are described later.

General effects of therapeutic modalities on the tissues

The individual modalities already noted will be fully considered later in this chapter but it is worth clarifying the overall effects of electrical, mechanical and radiation modalities on the tissues.

First, any current passing in the tissues in one direction, continuous or interrupted direct current, will cause local chemical changes at the junction of electrode with the tissues. Secondly, any currents, alternating or unidirectional, changing at relatively low frequencies can stimulate nerve tissue. This can produce tingling and other sensations as well as lead to muscle contractions (under some circumstances muscle contraction can be directly provoked.). All these effects could be pro-

duced at the same time by the same current. If the current is evenly alternating at a higher frequency, say 4 or 5 KHz, it has much less effect on nerves because it is changing too rapidly to allow depolarization of the nerve fibre membrane, thus larger currents can be passed through the surface tissues. If two such currents are passed into the tissue and made to interfere, a resulting low frequency current can produce nerve stimulation deep in the tissues. This is the principle of interferential currents. Clearly, in all cases in which the current is evenly alternating, no chemical effects will be produced.

At still higher frequencies evenly oscillating currents have still less nerve-stimulating effect so that much greater currents can be passed through the tissues. The heating effect of a current passing in a conductor is proportional to the square of the current so that these currents can cause significant heating of the tissues. This is the way in which shortwave (and longwave) diathermy cause the heating. At frequencies around 30 MHz the ohmic resistance of the current pathway becomes much less, so that currents can be generated in the tissues inductively or with the tissues as part of a capacitor.

If current at around 1 MHz is made to cause mechanical vibration at this frequency the mechanical disturbance – sonic waves – can be passed through the tissues as a beam of ultrasound. This can also cause heating. From both these latter modalities there are effects on the tissues due to the mechanical and electrical disturbance – independent of the heating effect – which have therapeutic effects.

Finally, the very high frequency movement of electrons leads to the production of radiations, in increasing frequency microwaves, infrared and visible (see Figure 15.1). When such radiations are absorbed by the tissues they can evoke heating and other effects. Microwave therapy is considered in this chapter and the heating effect of infrared radiations is dealt with in Chapter 16. If visible or infrared radiations are produced in a coherent single wavelength beam, described as a laser source, they have effects on pain and tissue healing and these are also considered later in this chapter.

Direct Current

The use of simple direct current to relieve pain

started in the middle of the nineteenth century but is rarely used in this form at present. Since there can be considerable stimulation of cutaneous sensory nerve endings as a consequence of the electrochemical changes the pain reduction that has been claimed could well be due to the pain gate and opioid mechanisms described in Chapter 9.

Iontophoresis

Direct current can also be used to introduce drugs into the tissues. Thus local cutaneous anaesthesia can be achieved with a drug such as lignocaine combined with adrenaline to cause vasoconstriction which delays dissipation of the drug. This has been used in the treatment of various painful conditions including trigeminal neuralgia, although how successfully is not clear (Boone, 1981). The application obviously needs especial care because the normal protective sensory appreciation is being blunted. Neurogenic pain has also been treated by the iontophoresis of vinca alkaloids which are considered to block transport processes in peripheral nerves (see Layman *et al.*, 1986; Csillik *et al.*, 1982.) For a simple description of the apparatus used for therapeutic application of d.c. and some discussion of the methods and effects see Low and Reed (1990).

Diadynamic Currents

These are basically monophasic sinusoidal currents, rectified mains type current, in various configurations. All are unidirectional. When such currents are applied to the tissues by means of malleable metal electrodes and wet sponges or pads, or by carbon rubber electrodes, they will cause both motor and sensory nerve stimulation as well as provoking chemical changes at the skin surface.

Diadynamic currents are used to relieve pain in many diverse conditions. The mechanism is considered to be both by means of the pain gate pathway and the release of endorphins and enkephalins due to peripheral nerve stimulation, as described in Chapter 9. Not only are cutaneous nerves stimulated directly by the varying current but also the chemical changes produced at the skin surface cause indirect nerve stimulation which may persist for some time in association with the mild cutaneous hyperaemia. Further, an increase in local circulation is claimed to occur not only in the skin but also in the deeper tissues as a consequence of the mild muscle contraction that can be made to occur and perhaps due to altered autonomic activity. This increased circulatory activity, it is postulated, will accelerate the removal of chemical irritants from the area, thus relieving pain. There will also be some placebo effect.

The application of this current at a perceptible, but not painful, intensity starting with a minute or so of DF (diphase fixe—a series of 10 ms sinusoidal pulses at 100 Hz) followed by 5 minutes of some other variation is recommended for pain relief (Rennie, 1988). The reasons for the use of these particular parameters are not made evident.

The possible danger associated with the use of such currents lies in allowing the polar effects to be strong enough to produce tissue damage. This is avoided by reversing the current during treatment; some sources provide automatic alternation of the current, effectively a further modification of the current.

High Voltage Pulsed Galvanic Stimulation (HVPGS)

This current has a twin pulse waveform with very rapid rise and fall providing a pair of high voltage peaks of very short (few microseconds) duration, hence the name. Currents during the brief peaks can be very high but the average current is very small. Such short pulses will pass readily through the tissues but need to be of high voltage to cause nerve stimulation. These currents are reputed to be relatively comfortable because of the wide discrimination between motor and sensory nerves on the one hand and pain nerve on the other to these very short pulses (see Low and Reed, 1990: 47:).

Not only can the current be varied by altering the applied voltage (from 0 to 500 V) but also the frequency of the double pulse from 2 to 100 Hz. The pulses are unidirectional so that polar effects will ultimately occur, this accounts for 'galvanic' in the name. There is provision for reversing the direction.

HVPGS has been recommended for wound healing and muscle stimulation but is also considered an effective current for pain control. It will be noted that both the frequency and intensity can be varied making it possible to produce a high frequency low intensity current for pain gate type pain control and a low frequency high intensity current appropriate for opioid modulation.

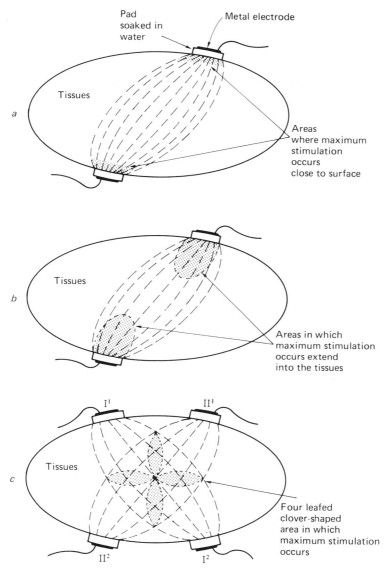

Fig. 15.2 The passage of currents through the tissues. *a*, Low frequency currents. *b*, Low frequency modulation of medium frequency current. *c*, Interferential currents.

Interferential stimulation

Interferential currents, first suggested as a therapeutic modality some 50 years ago, have recently again become popular. This has been partly due to the fact that developments in electronic circuitry have made compact and relatively cheaper machines available.

The currents considered so far have had rates of change suitable for triggering nerve impulses in sensory motor or pain nerves. At such rates the current is markedly affected by the ohmic resistance of the skin.

Compared to the rest of the tissues the skin has a high resistance or impedance, measured in ohms. This leads to a high potential difference across the skin and superficial tissues resulting in maximum stimulation of tissues in this region, illustrated in Figure 15.2*a*.

The impedance offered by the skin depends on the

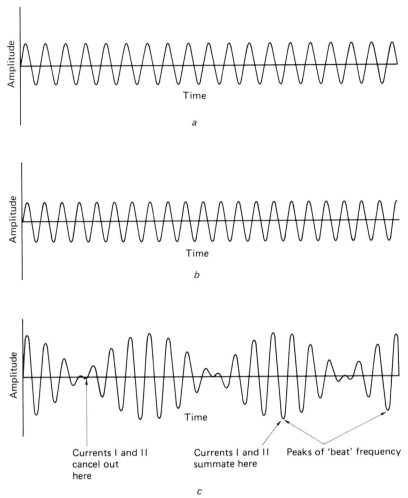

Fig. 15.3   Current frequency. *a*, Medium frequency current I. *b*, Medium frequency current II of slightly higher frequency than I. *c*, Result of combining medium frequency currents I and II.

frequency of the current, the higher the frequency the less the impedance. (This occurs because the capacitance of the skin plays a greater part in transmitting the current at higher frequencies.) Whereas the impedance between a pair of 100 cm² electrodes on the skin was found to be about 1000 ohms for a 50 Hz current, it fell to about 50 ohms for a 4000 Hz (4 kHz) current (Ward, 1980). Currents of 4000 Hz and similar frequencies are known as medium frequency currents (see Figure 15.1), and will obviously pass much more readily through the tissues than low frequency currents. They will not, in a simple regular form, stimulate nerve or other tissue. However, they can be modu-

lated (surged) to give a low frequency current superimposed on the medium frequency (Figure 15.3). The resulting current will pass easily through the tissues because it is a medium frequency current but will stimulate nerve and muscle because of the low frequency variation.

This type of current is produced by some interferential machines and may be called **electrokinesy**. Although the spread of medium frequency current is more uniform than low frequency current it will still have a greater intensity close to the electrodes where maximum stimulation will occur; this is illustrated in Figure 15.2b. Clearly it would be useful if the modulation, and hence nerve stimulation, could be made to occur in the deepest tissues; this is achieved by interferential currents.

Interferential currents

If two medium frequency currents of slightly different frequencies are passed through the tissues they will interfere with one another to produce a combined medium frequency current which varies in amplitude, i.e. it is **amplitude modulated**. This amplitude modulation is regular at a frequency determined by the difference in frequency of the two currents; it is called the 'beat' frequency. The idea is illustrated in Figure 15.3. Thus an interferential machine could deliver one current at a constant 4000 Hz and the other a variable current between 3900 Hz and 3990 Hz which would allow a variable beat frequency of between 100 Hz and 10 Hz. This low frequency variation, the beat frequency, will stimulate nerve and muscle as already described. The great advantage of this method is that the stimulation is not produced close to the electrodes in the skin but near the centre of the four electrode arrangement as indicated in Figure 15.2c.

It will be seen in Figure 15.2c that the area of maximum stimulation is not square as might be expected, but of a four-leafed clover shape. It must be understood that this area merely shows the site of maximum current intensity in an homogeneous medium with small electrodes. The real interference field would pervade all the tissues between the electrodes and would be distorted by the different electrical properties of the various tissues, fat and muscle, etc. The reason for the four-leafed clover shaped area of maximum effect is that the two currents are summated not only in magnitude but also in direction, i.e. vector addition.

While the two medium frequencies remain constant so will the beat frequency, e.g. if the two frequencies differ by 50 Hz then the beat frequency will be a steady 50 Hz sinusoidal current. At suitable intensities, and applied appropriately, it could produce a steady, continuous muscle contraction – a **tetanic contraction**; similarly, it could cause a steady stimulation of sensory nerves. This may lead to a gradually diminished response due to habituation of the tissues to this particular current. It is also considered desirable to stimulate different nerve types and diameters during treatment. Both these deficiencies are corrected by continuously varying the beat frequency. This is called frequency

swing or frequency sweep. The machine can be set to automatically change one of the medium frequency currents continuously to give a continuously varying beat frequency. The variation can be made to occur between specified upper and lower limits, e.g. 20–80 Hz; furthermore, the time taken by each of these swings or sweeps can be controlled on some machines. Thus it is possible to set the machine to swing repeatedly through a preset range of beat frequencies, say 20–80 Hz, during a preset period, say 6 s, followed by another 6 s period during which it swings back from 80 to 20 Hz.

Control of Interferential Output

The intensity of the currents, and hence of the beat frequency current, can be regulated to give more stimulation as required. There is an automatic timer to time the total treatment time, also separate controls for the timing and range of the frequency swing as indicated above. On some machines, provision is made to alter the pattern of the interference field regularly – called **rotating vector systems** or **dynamic interference field systems**. Essentially the four-leafed clover pattern of maximum stimulation shown in Figure 15.2c is made to rotate to and fro through a small angle; this increases the area of effective treatment.

Application of Interferential Therapy

The currents are applied to the skin by means of electrodes which may be either malleable metal or of a special conducting rubber with a water soaked pad (spontex or lint) to pass the current to the skin. The wet pads serve to provide comfort and even current conduction; there is no danger of chemical or heat burns with interferential currents even if the electrode is placed directly on the skin. The electrodes and pads can be held in place either by bandaging or with rubber straps.

An alternative way of holding the electrodes in place is by means of a suction unit. Four flexible rubber cups are connected by tubes to a pump that can produce variable suction; metal electrodes are mounted inside the cups and connected by wires running inside the tubes to the interferential machine. Pieces of dampened spontex are placed inside the cups to provide good conduction to the

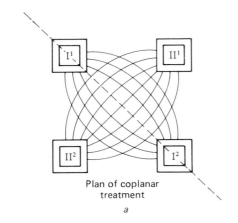

Plan of coplanar
treatment

a

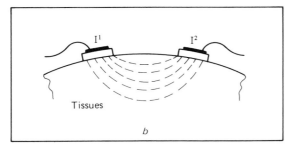

b

Fig. 15.4   A plan of coplanar treatment. *a*, Surface view.
b, A cross-section along the line.

skin. The suction is adjusted to be strong enough to keep the moist spontex in good contact with the skin without being uncomfortable. The suction pressure can be varied regularly during treatment which diminishes any risk of skin damage such as bruising. This is done automatically by the machine with cycles of a few seconds varying the force of the suction; the timing can be altered on some machines. The reasons for using suction are that it is a convenient way to apply the electrodes, it gives good even contact, and the varying suction has a gentle massaging action on the skin. This latter effect may cause mild vasodilatation which can lower the electrical resistance of the skin and may benefit the condition being treated due to the increased blood flow and mild mechanical stimulation of cutaneous sensory nerves.

Application and positioning of the electrodes

The relationship of the electrodes to the tissues is, literally, of crucial importance since the currents must be made to cross in the area being treated –

the **target area**. The common arrangement is shown in cross-section in Figure 15.2*c* in which the current of circuit I is carried by electrodes 1^1 and 1^2, while that of circuit II is carried by electrodes II^1 and II^2. For convenience the wires, or tubes, are usually colour coded. The electrodes can also be positioned in a coplanar arrangement (Figure 15.4) for the treatment of a flat surface, such as the back. In order to ensure a large comfortable current throughout the area of treatment, the largest size of electrodes that can be conveniently applied are normally recommended (Savage, 1984).

The skin must be inspected and may be washed and left damp where the electrodes are to be placed to achieve the best conduction. The nature and effects of the treatment should be explained to the patient and reassurance given that it is a harmless treatment producing no unpleasant sensations.

Effects of Interferential Currents

Different beat frequencies lead to different effects so that regular sweeps through a range of frequencies can lead to multiple effects. This explains why some physiotherapists propose different ranges of frequencies to achieve the same results. In general, the higher beat frequencies, around 100 Hz, are used for their analgesic effect whereas the lower beat frequencies, around 10 Hz, produce contraction of innervated muscle. All the effects appear to be due to stimulation of nerve tissue which leads to various secondary effects, such as muscle contraction and vasodilatation.

Pain relief

This is the most important effect and several mechanisms are thought to be implicated. These are as follows:

1. **Activation of the 'pain gate control' mechanism.** Stimulation of large-diameter afferent nerve fibres closes the 'gate' to nociceptive impulses in the substantia gelatinosa of the posterior horn of the spinal cord (see Chapter 9, Figure 9.2, p. 55). Impulses of very short duration at a frequency of 100 Hz should selectively stimulate these large diameter nerve fibres and this could occur in interferential treatments (De Domenico, 1982).

2. **Activation of nociceptive fibres.** Activation of

the nociceptive fibres themselves can diminish pain by means of the descending **pain suppressor system**. In this system nociceptive impulses passing up to regions in the mid-brain provoke impulses in neurons travelling back down the spinal cord to inhibit nociceptor neurons at the original level. Interferential currents could stimulate these fibres (see De Domenico, 1982).

3. **Physiological block.** It is possible, though not proven, that high frequency electrical stimuli – above 50 Hz – could cause a temporary physiological block in both finely myelinated and unmyelinated nociceptor nerve fibres (A-delta and C fibres).

   This appears to contradict section (2) above, but it is conceivable that both mechanisms could operate at different stages of the interferential current cycle. Both this effect and activation of the 'pain gate' would be expected to occur at a frequency sweep of 80–100 Hz, whereas the descending pain suppressor system is likely to be activated by frequencies in the 10–25 Hz region (De Domenico, 1982).

4. **Increased blood flow.** Pain suppression can also be due to an increased local blood flow and tissue fluid exchange; this may hasten the removal of chemical irritants acting on pain nerve endings and reduce pressure due to local exudate. Vasodilatation may occur as a result of stimulation of the autonomic nervous system (see below), and the regular mild muscle contraction has a pumping effect on vessels. (The varying suction pressure, when interferential current is applied by this method, may contribute to both the vasodilatation and the pumping effect.)

5. **The placebo effect.** Since the placebo effect occurs in all treatments it would be surprising if it did not contribute to pain relief with interferential treatment, especially since the machines are technically impressive and produce an unfamiliar, although not unpleasant, feeling.

In spite of widespread agreement amongst physiotherapists that interferential therapy has a marked pain relieving effect, there is a paucity of objective investigations into this analgesic effect. The time taken to elicit ischaemic pain at a range of pressures before and after interferential therapy was tested in one study (Pärtan *et al.*, 1953). The results showed that an increased pressure was needed to elicit pain after treatment indicating a rise in the pain threshold. A study comparing the conduction velocities of nerve before and after interferential treatment showed no significant difference (Belcher, 1974). A study on jaw pain (Taylor *et al*, 1987) concluded that there was no significant difference between three interferential and three placebo treatments. A pilot study on the relief of experimentally induced pain in normal subjects (Scott and Purves, 1991) found no statistically significant difference between interferential treatment, placebo treatment and control, although a trend towards pain relief due to interferential current was evident which might have been demonstrated with a larger study. Thus the effects of interferential currents on nerves and pain perception are neither quantified nor understood.

Muscle contraction

The lower beat frequencies stimulate motor nerves leading to the contraction of voluntary muscle (mainly at 10–50 Hz) and smooth muscle, via automatic nerves, extending to lower frequencies (Savage, 1984). Muscle contraction can be quite strong without any discomfort because, as already explained, there is little skin effect. When the beat frequency is varied, rhythmic muscle contraction will occur helping to reduce oedema or congestion by the pumping action on soft-walled vessels. It may also aid muscle control as in the treatment of incontinence.

Vasodilatation

Stimulation of the sympathetic ganglia with 100 Hz is claimed to produce reflex vasodilatation and be valuable for the treatment of causalgia (Wadsworth and Chanmugan, 1980). Skin temperature increases of 2–3°C were noted after interferential therapy by Pärtan *et al.* (1953). Other effects due to stimulation of the autonomic nervous system, such as increased rates of tissue healing, have been proposed.

Conditions Treated with Interferential Therapy

Pain

Interferential therapy is widely used for the relief of pain. It is considered to be particularly effective for the treatment of neurogenic pain such as postherpetic neuralgia, causalgia, phantom limb pain; it is also found to be of great value in the treatment of chronic pain both with and without oedema, but it is not considered as effective for the treatment of pain in the acute stage of post-traumatic injury (Wadsworth and Chanmugan, 1980). However, others use it and recommend it at this stage (Savage, 1984).

Muscle spasm

This would be diminished as a consequence of any reduction in pain; strong applications of electrokinesey, modulated medium frequency current through a single path (see Figure 15.2*b*), have also been advocated for the reduction of muscle spasm (Wadsworth and Chanmugan, 1980).

Chronic ligamentous lesions, sprains and strains

Treatment of these lesions to relieve pain and accelerate healing is often recommended in conjunction with other treatments (Wadsworth and Chanmugan, 1980; Nikolova-Troeva, 1967a). Similarly a study on osteoarthrosis (arthrosis deformans), involving treatment with a number of electrotherapeutic agents, found a combination of microwave with interferential therapy to be most effective (Nikolova-Troeva, 1967b).

Gynaecological conditions

Interferential therapy has been applied to various gynaecological conditions, and one report of 300 cases claimed an average 90% improvement (Haag, 1979); swings of 0–100 Hz and 90–100 Hz were used with anterior and posterior electrodes so that the current crossed in the pelvis.

Stress incontinence

Since muscles can be stimulated by interferential currents with little skin effect, it might be expected that this would be a useful way to exercise weakened pelvic floor muscles and this has proved to be the case. Swings of 0–10Hz or 0–100 Hz have been used, with the electrodes positioned anteriorly on the lower abdomen and posteriorly on the upper medial aspect of the thighs, and with the patient half lying. A study of 24 women treated with pelvic floor exercises and interferential therapy showed very convincing improvement (McQuire, 1975).

Chronic oedema

The muscle pumping and autonomic effects are useful in the treatment of postmastectomy or other chronic oedema.

Circulatory disturbances

The vasodilating effect is utilised, but vasoconstricting sympathetic stimulation by 0–5 Hz frequencies should be avoided, and the treatment should not be given if there is any risk of thrombosis (Savage, 1984).

Other conditions

Interferential treatment for asthma and migraine is sometimes given (Savage, 1984), again because of the effects on the autonomic nervous system.

Dangers and contraindications of nerve stimulating currents

1. If the current is sufficiently strong to cause vigorous muscle contraction then diseased joint structures (but not healthy tissue) might be injured by excessive mechanical stress. Where haemorrhage or infection are present vigorous tissue movement may serve to prolong the bleeding or spread the infection. In these circumstances the application of strong muscle-stimulating currents should be avoided. The same constraint also applies to regions in which recent venous thrombosis has occurred in case the clot is disrupted to form an embolus thus initiating further damage.
2. Neoplastic tissue should be avoided in case the currents stimulate growth or encourage metastases. In fact there seems to be no evidence that such changes occur with the application of any of these currents but it is a possibility.
3. Currents should not be applied close to a cardiac pacemaker because there is some risk of altering the rhythm, particularly for a demand-type pacemaker.
4. Since all these currents are applied through the skin variations in the skin resistance, such as spots or open wounds, will cause a local increase in current intensity which could be painful or frightening for the patient. Care in the application is therefore necessary.
5. Perhaps the most likely cause of damage while using these currents is the failure to recognize that unidirectional currents will cause polar effects which are cumulative. This can lead to

irritation and skin damage, especially under the negative pole. This cannot, of course, occur with true interferential currents because they are evenly alternating but will occur with the others.

6. Stimulation of autonomic nerves is often considered a risk in that it might provoke cardiac arrhythmias but, again, there is no evidence for this or other autonomic ill-effects.

7. It is usually recommended that the pregnant uterus be avoided. This is partly due to the reasons given in (1) above and partly an unspecified concern particularly with reference to interferential currents.

Shortwave diathermy

Treatment due to the electric and magnetic fields at radio frequencies between 10 and 100 MHz is traditionally called 'shortwave' because these frequencies are in the shortwave radio band. The patient is placed in the circuit so that energy is released in the tissues by the oscillation of electric charges. The radiation generated by these machines is largely incidental. Virtually all therapeutic sources operate at 27.12 MHz and thus a wavelength of 11.0619 m.

Production of Shortwave Diathermy

High frequency current is generated by a circuit called the *oscillator circuit*, the dimensions of which are such as to allow electrons to oscillate at precisely 27.12 MHz. The part to be treated is included in a separate circuit, either between two electrodes or close to an induction coil, which must be tuned so that it has the same natural frequency as the oscillator circuit. Thus high frequency electrical energy is transferred to the tissues.

Effects of High Frequency Currents on the Tissues

Tissue molecules are influenced in three ways by a varying electric field. Inductothermy causes a varying induced electric field like that produced between the capacitor plates in the condenser field method (below). High frequency currents affect the tissues in the following ways:

1. **Ionic motion.** Masses of positive and negative

ions in the tissues are under the influence of the electric field. As they move rapidly to and fro they collide with other particles and in this way electrical energy is converted to heat. The actual distance moved by each ion is very small at this frequency, more like a vibration, but it is sufficient to generate heat (Figure 15.5a).

2. **Dipole rotation.** Molecules that have a relative positive charge at one end and negative charge at the other (e.g. water) and will orientate themselves appropriately in the field and thus rotate back and forth as the field alternates. The frictional forces generated between these polar molecules and others cause heating (Figure 15.5b).

3. **Distortion of electron 'clouds'.** Molecules that are not polar have the paths of their orbiting electrons distorted by the electric field thus becoming temporarily polarised alternately in each direction. This causes some molecular movement and heating (Figure 15.5c).

All three mechanisms lead to heating but (1) is likely to be the most efficient at converting electrical energy to heat and (3) the least efficient (Ward, 1980).

Application of Shortwave Diathermy

The electric field (electrostatic field) is applied either by rigid metal plates enclosed in plastic cases called **space plates, rigid electrodes** or **plate electrodes**; or by means of flexible metal sheets encased in thick rubber, called **flexible electrodes** or **malleable electrodes**. This is known as the **condenser field** method.

A cable or coil consists of a flexible tubular conductor insulated with thick rubber. When coiled around the part in a helical manner or coiled and laid flat on the skin surface, a so-called **pancake coil**, it generates an electromagnetic field through the tissues which induces eddy currents causing heating as already described. The coil also produces an electric field between the ends and adjacent turns which has been shown to play a major part in heat production. Such treatments are called **inductothermy**. Some machines have a drum-shaped electrode, sometimes called a **monode**, which contains a flat rigid coil and parallel capacitor enclosed in a plastic case. It produces an electromagnetic field like a small pancake coil.

In all these methods the electric field must not

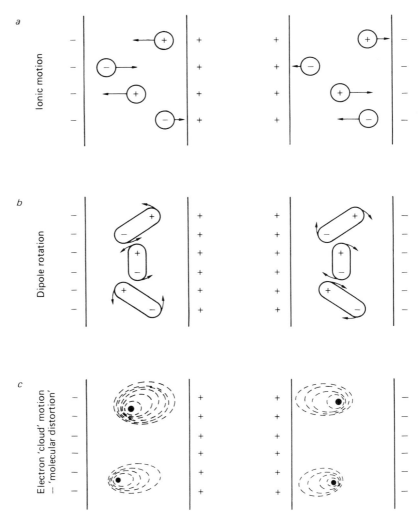

Fig. 15.5 The effects of oscillating high frequency electric fields on the molecules and ions in the tissues. *a*, Ionic motion – positive and negative ions move to and fro under the influence of an oscillating electric field. *b*, Dipole rotation – polar molecules rotate to and fro as the electric field oscillates. *c*, Electron 'cloud' motion (molecular distortion) – the paths of orbiting electrons are distorted first in one direction then in the other as the electric field oscillates.

be concentrated when passing into the tissues so an air gap of a few centimetres is necessary between the metal electrode and the tissues. Air does not become heated by the electric field, similarly the plastic and rubber covers of the metal electrodes have little effect. The gap is usually maintained by felt pads for the malleable electrodes and several layers of towelling with the coil, but other suitable materials can be used.

Controlling and understanding the pattern of the electric field is central to the application of short wave diathermy. Some discussion of the factors involved and description of their application can be found in Low and Reed (1990), Forster and Palastanga (1985) and Wadsworth and Chanmugan (1980).

Application of shortwave diathermy

The part to be treated should be supported in an appropriate and comfortable position. After being given a suitable explanation, the patient is in-structed not to move (since movement may detune the circuit) and to describe both the intensity of heating and the place where it occurs. The patient is also warned to call if any burning or painful sensations are felt. The only information about what heating is occurring comes from the patient so that full communication and normal thermal sensation (which should be tested) are essential to the proper regulation of dosage. At the end of the treatment palpation and the presence of erythema will indicate the degree of heating.

Dosage

Increasing the tissue temperature depends on intro-ducing energy at a faster rate than it is being dissipated but, of course, not at such a rate as to cause damage. As the temperature rises the heat regulating mechanisms of the body react until the heat input is once again the same as the heat loss when a new, higher, local temperature becomes steady (see Figure 15.11a). It usually takes some 15–20 min for these vascular adjustments to take place, although it can take up to 1 h. Most treat-ments are therefore given for periods of 20–30 min (Wadsworth and Chanmugan, 1980). The heating rate can only be ascertained by the pa-tient's perception, as already noted, so that descrip-tions such as: '**comfortable**', '**definite warmth**' for 'normal' heating – moderate heating; '**mild**', '**gentle warmth**' for mild heating; '**I can only just feel the heat**' for minimal perceptible heating and '**I feel no heating**' for no perceptible heating are used to quantify the intensity of heating. (The terms subthermic and athermic are best avoided.) Apparently, similar energy inputs cause widely differing heat perceptions; this is mainly due to differences in blood flow, and Scott (1957) quotes some evidence concerning this point.

Therapeutic Effects of Shortwave Diathermy

The effects of continuous shortwave diathermy are usually considered to be entirely due to the local heating that occurs. The physiological effects of local heating considered below would, of course, pertain to any other form of local heating.
  Local heating produces an interrelated set of physiological responses which occur markedly at temperatures above 40°C and below 45°C; con-tinued heating above 45°C would lead to tissue damage. The direct effects can be summarized as:

1. Increased metabolic activity.
2. Increased blood flow, capillary pressure and permeability of cellular and vessel walls.
3. Decreased viscosity of all fluids, including blood.
4. Increased extensibility of collagenous tissues.
5. Effects on neuronal activity.

All metabolic activity is temperature dependent so that quite small increases in temperature will cause considerable changes in cellular activity, such as greater leucocyte motility and phagocytosis or rates of cell growth. The increase in blood flow is due to reflex effects on arterioles, the consequences of increased metabolism, as well as the reduced viscosity. This is evident on the skin and has been demonstrated in muscle and other tissue (Millard, 1961). This increase may not occur where inflam-matory disease, and hence hyperaemia, are already present (Harris, 1963). A consequence of increased activity and capillary pressure changes is a greater exchange across cell membranes and capillary walls. All these can assist the resolution of acute and chronic lesions. Collagen extensibility has been shown to increase at high, but therapeutic, levels of heating allowing a greater range of joint motion (Lehmann et al., 1970). Similarly joint stiffness is reduced by heating (Wright and Johns, 1961).
  Stimulation of sensory nerves by heat can lead to activation of the axon reflex as well as pro-voking the sensation of heat. Afferent nerve stimulation by heat may have an analgesic effect due to the gate control mechanism (see Chapter 9), such an effect was formerly described as a counter-irritation mechanism (Gammon and Starr, 1941). Some evidence has been produced to show that stimulating heat receptors has an inhibitory effect on neurons conveying nociceptive impulses in rats, and it is believed that this mechanism may account for the analgesic effect of local heating (Kanui, 1985). Muscle spasm is reduced by heating and it has been suggested that this is due to the heating of secondary afferent muscle spindle nerve endings and Golgi tendon endings (Lehmann and de Lateur, 1982). Patients have been found to sleep easily during and after heat treatment, a sedative effect. This could be due to pain relief but it is pointed out that skin temperature rises just before the onset of sleep so that the sedative effect could be a reflex phenomenon (Lehmann and de Lateur, 1982).

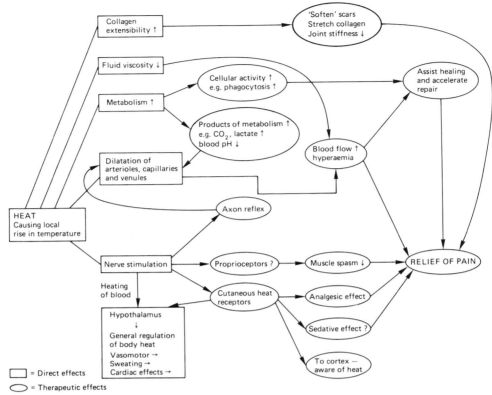

Fig. 15.6   The effects of heat.

Pain relief

Heat seems to have been used for the relief of pain throughout history and is currently used to treat many conditions, largely empirically. That heating leads to the relief of pain is well recognized but not equally well supported by research. A study of the non-analgesic methods used by cancer patients to control their pain (Barbour *et al.*, 1986) found that heat was used most frequently and helped to control pain in some degree in over two-thirds of patients. Another study (Donovan, 1985) found in a survey of patients with a wide variety of diagnoses that after medication and resting heat was the most used means to alleviate pain. The pain threshold has been shown to rise during some forms of heating (Lehmann *et al.*, 1958) and there is some evidence that patients choose intermittant heating to diminish their pain (Gammon and Starr, 1941).

The suggested reasons for pain relief are the analgesic effect and reduction of muscle spasm already noted, the raised blood flow reducing any ischaemic pain, the reduced joint stiffness, the accelerated resolution of injury and possibly the sedative effect. These responses and their interrelationships are shown in a somewhat simplified form in Figure 15.6 in which the immediate direct effects are linked to the therapeutic effects.

Clearly local effects do not occur in isolation from the general effects that maintain the constant body temperature. While local heating is taking place heat is constantly dispersed and lost from the rest of the body by vasomotor adjustment under the control of the hypothalamus.

Potential Dangers with Shortwave Diathermy

The principal danger to the patient is that of a tissue burn. This can occur if:

1. The patient is unaware of the heat either due to defective skin sensation or unconsciousness, e.g. epilepsy or fainting during treatment.

Occasionally a strong-minded or mentally unbalanced patient may stoically suffer a burn because of inadequate explanation and warning.

2. The shortwave field becomes 'concentrated' so quickly that the ensuing burn happens before the patient can react. This can occur as a consequence of many things including:

   (a) Defective positioning of electrodes.
   (b) Electrode leads too close to the patient's skin.
   (c) The presence of a low resistance pathway between the electrode and the skin, such as metal or water. All metals will act in this way even when enclosed in plastic (e.g. the metal in the plastic arms of spectacles) or metal buried in clothing like zip fasteners. What matters is the shape of the piece of metal and how it is orientated in the shortwave diathermy field. Thus if the long axis of a slender pointed metal object such as a key is parallel to the lines of the field with the point touching the skin, then current passes through the metal and will cause a burn where it touches the skin. Water droplets, such as sweat, provides a similar low resistance pathway.
   (d) Metal implanted surgically, such as a metal arthroplasty or fracture fixation by plate or wire, or metal accidentally embedded in the tissues, such as shrapnel, can provide a low resistance pathway leading to a burning at the junction of the metal and the tissues. The magnitude of this effect depends on the size and orientation of the metal. Thus small round tooth fillings embedded in dentine are insignificant, but a large long intramedullary nail is highly dangerous (Scott, 1957).

Cardiac pacemakers can be affected by the electromagnetic fields produced by various kinds of electrical equipment. The 'triggered' or demand type pacemaker is much more likely to be affected than the fixed rate type. Reported causes of pacemaker dysfunction (Jones, 1976) include a number due to shortwave diathermy as well as numerous other sources of electromagnetic energy such as electric razors. These dysfunctions, which include stopping the pacemaker and altering its rhythm, occur most frequently when the patient is within 30 cm (1 ft) of the machine but have also been reported occurring at greater distances.

It is therefore important to keep patients with

Table 15.1   Frequencies of microwave radiation

Frequency (Hz)	Approximate wavelength (cm)
2450	12.25
915	33
433.9	69

implanted pacemakers away from shortwave diathermy and microwave machines, as these effects could occur not only if the patient were being treated but also if he or she were simply close to the machine. Although there seem to be no reports of interference due to pulsed shortwave diathermy or microwave it can be inferred that this could happen.

An entirely separate danger arises by applying shortwave diathermy, microwave, or ultrasound to the region of the implanted pacemaker. As well as interfering with its function, excess local heat may be produced causing a burn in the same way as with other metal implants.

Hearing aids and other electronic devices may be affected by both pulsed and continuous shortwave diathermy. This may only cause temporary buzzing noises but could also lead to permanent damage to the hearing aid.

Microwave radiation

Microwaves are electromagnetic radiations extending from approximately 300 MHz (1 m wavelength) to 30 GHz (1 cm wavelength) found between radiowaves and infrared radiations (see figure 15.1). They are well known as radar radiations. They behave like visible or infrared radiations in that they travel in straight lines, are reflected by metal, and can be refracted.

In Europe three frequencies are available for therapeutic sources but only the first is in widespread use (Table 15.1).

The Production of Microwaves

A beam of electrons controlled by a strong magnetic field is made to pass over a number of resonant cavities causing high frequency oscillations. This device is called a **magnetron**. The principle is similar to causing sound vibrations by blowing across the top of a bottle. The oscillations are conveyed by a coaxial cable to an antenna. The output can be controlled by varying the power to the magnetron, but the frequency is fixed by its dimensions.

A reflector is mounted behind the antenna, and the whole assembly is called a **director** or **emitter**. These can be made in various shapes and sizes which usually give a diverging beam of differing intensity in its cross-section as described in the manufacturer's literature.

Effect of Microwaves on the Tissues

The high frequency electromagnetic field due to microwaves causes heating in the tissues by provoking the movement of ions, rotation of dipoles, and electron orbit distortion in the same way as described for shortwave diathermy (see Figure 15.5). In the case of microwaves the energy is 'beamed' onto the skin and passes into the body. It might be expected that heating would be greatest at the surface and diminish progressively; however, it is not quite that simple.

Microwaves are strongly absorbed by water so that highly vascular tissues such as muscle, are preferentially treated. Fat and bone on the other hand absorb less. For 2450 MHz radiation the half value depth for fat and bone is about 3.4 cm but for muscle about 0.7 cm. Thus much of the energy will pass through the superficial fat and be absorbed in the underlying muscle causing heating. What tissue is heated clearly depends on the thickness and relationship of the various tissues involved; thus joints with little overlying muscle tissue, like the knee, may be quite successfully heated but not joints such as the hip, buried beneath thick muscle. Thus microwaves will heat skin and superficial muscle especially; in practice absorption is very irregular so that 'hot spots' are likely to occur and significant amounts of radiation are reflected from the skin.

The application of microwaves

The patient should be comfortably supported so that the part to be treated can be fully and conveniently exposed. The procedure and the nature of the treatment should be explained to the patient and the patient's thermal sensation tested. The emitter to be used, determined by the size of the 'target' being treated, is adjusted to ensure that radiations strike the surface at right angles. The emitter – skin distance is important in determining both the size of the area treated and the intensity. A diverging beam leads to a large area treated with a low intensity at greater distances and *vice versa* at smaller distances. Many emitters give an appropriate heating pattern at 10 cm, approximately the width of a hand, but closer application, 2 cm, is used and recommended. The intensity control on the machine is used to adjust the heating and will thus compensate for different distances up to a point.

The required heat level, 'normal' or mild warmth, should be described to the patient who must also be warned to call out if excessive heating, pain, or any acute discomfort occur. This is essential since knowledge of heating in the tissues depends entirely on sensations felt by the patient; the output of the machine is usually shown by a meter but this gives no indication of tissue heating which varies with distance, nature of the tissues and blood flow as already noted.

Normal treatments are usually given for about 20 min to allow time for the vascular adjustments to occur (see Figure 15.11a). The deeper parts take longer than the superficial tissues to reach their maximum steady temperature; at depths greater than 2 cm the temperature is still rising after 10 min (Boyle *et al.*, 1950).

Potential dangers with microwaves

Effects of metal

Metal reflects microwaves, so any metal on the surface will shield the underlying tissues. Overheating due to reflection into the part could also occur, e.g. placing the treated part close to large metal surfaces that could turn the scattered radiation back into the tissues. Similarly metal implants can cause overheating. This is much more likely with superficial rather than deep implants.

Eyes

Microwaves are strongly absorbed by the water of the eye, as the lens does not dissipate heat easily; also cataracts have been provoked in animal experiments. It is therefore not advisable to allow microwaves to enter the eye. If the beam is to be applied close to the eye then protective goggles should be worn; these are either glass with a thin metallic film or 2 mm wire mesh, both of which are almost impervious to microwaves. (It must be clearly understood that these are *not* interchangeable with ultraviolet or laser goggles.)

Testes

Although quite small temperature increases can interfere with spermatogenesis in mammals, it is thought that very high doses would be needed to produce testicular damage in man. Nonetheless, it is sensible to avoid the testes because they are close to the surface and there is some evidence that microwaves may be more damaging than other forms of heating.

General Safety with Microwaves

Many patients, familiar with microwave ovens, may feel some alarm. It should be explained that microwaves reflected in an enclosed oven will be applied to, and absorbed by, the food from all sides. As the heat cannot be dissipated it will increase the temperature rapidly thus cooking the food. In the living body microwaves applied to one area, as in therapeutic application, cause local heating which is passed to other areas and lost to the atmosphere so that no increase in total body heat will occur. It is generally accepted that the human body could easily dissipate 10 mW/cm² of radiation which is the permitted maximum continuous exposure for general purposes (higher levels are permitted for temporary exposure). These limits do not apply to the therapeutic application of microwaves under medical supervision.

The safety of microwaves in physiotherapy has been investigated (Scowcroft *et al.*, 1977; DHSS, Medical Scientific Services, 1980) and is considered perfectly safe provided that the radiation is confined to the treatment site. Based on measurements with various emitters it was found that the physiotherapist was quite safe for short periods near the emitter and was safe for indefinite periods at 1 m from the front and 25 cm from the back of the emitter. Radiation monitors are recommended to delineate microwave patterns.

Ultrasonic therapy

Ultrasonic waves are mechanical vibrations in the form of longitudinal pressure waves. They are called ultrasonic because they lie beyond the frequencies recognized as sound by the human ear, approximately 30 Hz to 20 kHz. The commonly used therapeutic frequencies are 0.75 MHz, 0.87 MHz, 1.0 MHz, 1.5 MHz, and 3.0 MHz.

1. Infrasound or infrasonic waves, 0–30 Hz, are felt as a vibration.
2. Sound waves have a frequency of approximately 30 Hz–20 kHz.
3. Ultrasonic waves have a frequency of approximately 20 kHz–10 GHz.
4. Therapeutic ultrasonic frequencies are 0.5–3.5 MHz.
5. Commonly used therapeutic frequencies are 0.75 MHz, 0.87 MHz, 1.0 MHz, 1.5 MHz and 3.0 MHz (see Figure 15.1).

Sonic waves are distortions of the medium through which they pass. They are waves of particle compression and rarefaction moving continuously in the direction of travel. Ultrasonic waves can travel through solids, liquids, and gases. At megahertz frequencies they cannot be seen or felt. Low frequency 'standing waves' can be made visible on the surface when ultrasound is passed in water and reflected from the wall of a container. This is a useful way to demonstrate the presence of an ultrasonic output in the clinical situation. This mechanism accounts for the 'buzzing' sensation sometimes experienced by patients during ultrasound treatment.

Velocity of Sonic Waves

There is a simple relationship between the velocity, frequency and wavelength of sonic waves.

$$\text{Velocity (m/s)} = \text{Wavelength (m)} \times \text{Frequency (Hz)}$$

Since ultrasonic waves distort the medium through which they travel their velocity depends on the nature of that medium. Thus ultrasonic waves travel at different velocities in different tissues as shown in Table 15.2 below.

Table 15.2   Approximate velocities for sonic waves (m/s)

Air	343
Water	1480
Blood	1560
Muscle	1585
Fat	1450
Bone	3360

Passage of Ultrasonic Energy in the Tissues

At the interface of different types of tissue, the ultrasonic beam can be reflected or refracted. This is made use of in ultrasonic imaging for diagnosis where reflections from interfaces are picked up and displayed. Through any given volume of tissue some ultrasonic energy will be absorbed and the rest transmitted.

Heating of the tissues depends both on the rate at which energy is absorbed (see Figure 15.14) and the amount of reflection from these interfaces within the tissues. This latter depends on the difference in the nature of the tissues at the junction. Actually it is the difference in acoustic impedance of the tissues, the acoustic impedance depending on both the density and elasticity of the tissues. In the tissues differences between fat, muscle and other soft tissue are very small so little reflection occurs; however, differences between bone and soft tissues are larger.

As fat does not absorb ultrasonic energy readily, little heating occurs in subcutaneous fat and much more energy is absorbed by muscle which is therefore heated. When the ultrasonic beam impinges on bone the energy is absorbed almost at once. Additionally there will be reflection from the muscle/bone interface causing further heating. This calculated large temperature elevation in the periosteal region is believed to account for the deep 'bone' pain which is sometimes experienced when high doses of ultrasound are used. This is illustrated diagrammatically in Figure 15.7a for 1 MHz ultrasonics, and in Figure 15.7b for 3 MHz ultrasonics, which has a lower half value depth of penetration and therefore gives a different pattern of heating. However, other factors are involved, notably the rate of heating which is influenced by the blood flow. In highly vascular tissues, such as muscle, the heat would be rapidly dissipated preventing a large rise in temperature. Fat and dense connective tissue, being less vascular, become relatively more heated leading to a more even distribution of heat between the various tissues. This is suggested in the dotted line on Figure 15.7a and b. There is evidence that ultrasonic therapy preferentially heats collagenous tissues.

The wavelengths at a velocity of 1500 m/s and the approximate half value depths of penetration (the result of absorption in a mixture of tissues) are given below in Table 15.3 and depend on the frequency as shown.

Table 15.3 Frequency, wavelength and published half vale depth of penetration for ultrasonics at 1500 m/s in tissues

Frequency (MHz)	Wavelength (mm)	Half value depth (cm) (from different published sources)		
0.75	2	10		
0.87	1.724	9		
1.0	1.5	6.5	5	4
1.5	1.0	5.5		
3.0	0.5	3	1.5	2.5

The ultrasonic beam passing through the tissues diverges somewhat, more especially with lower frequencies and smaller transducer heads. Furthermore, in the area close to the transducer, the **near-field** or **Fresnel zone**, the ultrasonic beam is very irregular; in the **far-field** or **Fraunhofer zone** it becomes more uniform but this is of little consequence since in most therapeutic situations the tissues are in the Fresnel zone, the extent of which depends on

$$\frac{\text{Radius of transducer head}^2}{\text{Wavelength}}$$

The tissues that are heated by therapeutic ultrasonics cannot be determined with great precision due to this irregularity.

Effects of Ultrasound Therapy

The biological effects of ultrasonics are those due to heating and those due to the other, mainly mechanical effects.

Thermal effects

As a direct consequence of the heating and as a result of the metabolic changes there will be an increase in blood flow, dilatation of blood vessels, and more rapid exchanges across capillary walls and cell membranes. Such changes are believed to hasten the resolution of chronic inflammatory processes; this may account for the pain relief often experienced when chronic lesions are given ultrasonic treatment (see Figure 15.6).

Heating fibrous tissue structures such as tendons, ligaments or joint capsules can cause an increase in their extensibility. This also applies to scar tissue. Hence ultrasonic treatment coupled with active movement or passive stretching can lead to an increase in joint or tissue mobility in

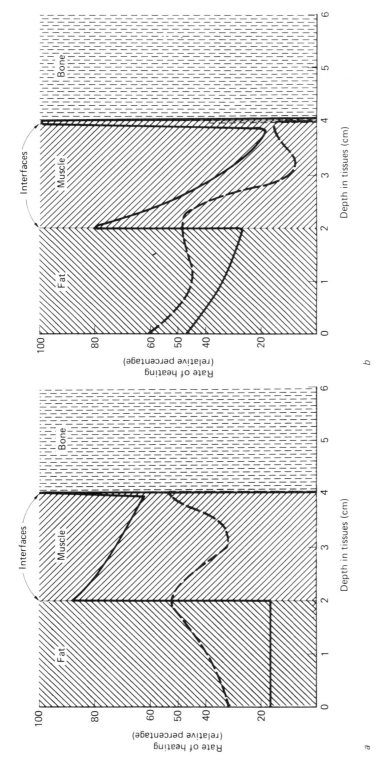

Fig. 15.7 The ultrasonic heating pattern predicted for a three-layer system of fat/muscle/bone; each layer is 2 cm thick (modified from Ward, 1980). –, Initial heating pattern . . ., Heating pattern suggested when thermal conductivity and blood flow are considered. (Note that this line only illustrates the change of pattern and is not based on any measurements.) *a*, Ultrasonic heating at 1 MHz. *b*, Ultrasonic heating at 3 MHz.

conditions such as Dupuytren's contracture or joint adhesions.

The advantages of using ultrasonics for therapeutic heating lie in the fact that it preferentially heats collagen-rich tissues as well as the periosteal region. Thus it is possible to achieve significant temperature increases in deeply placed joint capsules or intramuscular fibrosis without overheating the skin or other overlying tissues.

Non-thermal effects

Cavitation

This is due to the activity of bubbles under the influence of an acoustic field, and is of two kinds. Stable cavitation involves minute gas bubbles (a few microns) moving to and fro with the ultrasonic pressure waves and occurs during ultrasonic treatment. It is believed to contribute to changes observed in the cell membrane of nerve and muscle which could be involved in the relief of pain (Dyson, 1985). Transient cavitation, on the other hand, appears to occur only at ultrasonic intensities greater than those used therapeutically and describes rapidly growing bubbles which implode violently causing cell destruction. The essential point about cavitation is that it concentrates ultrasonic energy locally.

Acoustic streaming

The rapidly oscillating ultrasonic pressure waves cause a regular to and fro movement of particles. It also causes continuous particle motion in one direction; this latter is acoustic streaming. It occurs at boundaries such as the cell membrane.

Pulsed Ultrasonics

The principle of pulsed treatments is described on p. 166 (see Figure 15.11b). In ultrasonic therapy the pulses are described as either: (1) the **duty cycle**, which is the ratio of time *on* to total time, usually expressed as a percentage; or (2) the **mark–space ratio**, which is the ratio of **on** to **off** time. Thus if the output were **on** for 2 ms and **off** for 8 ms the duty cycle would be 20% and the mark–space ratio 1:4; the pulse frequency would be 100 Hz. The effect is to reduce the energy applied to the tissues to one-fifth. The same total energy could be applied if the pulsing treatment were given for five times the duration at the same

intensity or at five times the intensity for the same duration. However, tissue heating will depend on the rate of energy absorption not on the total energy because of heat dissipation in the tissues (see Figure 15.11b). Thus pulses will generate 'bursts' of mechanical disturbance in the tissues without significant local heating, so higher intensities can be safely used. It is reasonable to suppose that there is a threshold below which mild mechanical agitation has no effect, however long-continued, whereas short bursts of vigorous agitation can produce marked effects. It has been found that rates of ion diffusion across cell membranes are increased by ultrasonic application (Dyson, 1985). This is thought to be due to increased particle movement on either side of the membrane and perhaps to increased motion of the phospholipids and proteins which make up the membrane. The use of a flour sieve or garden riddle provides an analogy. Some particles are pushed through the sieve by gravity, but many more drop through if the sieve is gently vibrated, like the effect of continuous ultrasonics. However, there comes a time when none of the remaining particles will pass through the mesh and gentle vibration is ineffective no matter how long-continued. If the sieve is now shaken vigorously a further shower of particles is produced. So that intermittent vigorous agitation has a different effect from continuous gentle vibration.

It is also possible that the frequency of the pulsing cycle (often 100 Hz as in the example above) may have some special effect. Pain relief has been achieved in other modalities such as interferential and transcutaneous nerve stimulating currents using frequencies in the region of 100 Hz. Many studies showing increased rates of healing have used pulsed ultrasonics, (e.g. Dyson and Suckling, 1978). For a full discussion of these mechanisms see Dyson (1987).

Therapeutic Effects and Indications

After tissue injury the acute inflammatory processes are accelerated by mild doses of ultrasonics. This may be due to the gentle agitation of the tissue fluid causing increased phagocytosis or the increased motion of other particles or cells, it may also be due to increased histamine release from mast cells which has been shown to occur (Dyson, 1987). Local oedema is believed to be decreased but it is not known by what mechanism, and it may account for the reduction of pain that occurs. Very low intensity pulsed ultrasound has been shown to reduce swelling and pain after tooth extraction (Hashish *et al.*, 1986). During tissue healing the synthesis and secretion of collagen by fibroblasts is an important process that has been shown to be accelerated by ultrasonic treatment (Harvey *et al.*, 1975). It may also assist repair by increasing the blood flow (improved blood flow has been found to occur in ischaemic muscle after ultrasonic treatment). In the later stages of repair, remodelling of the scar tissue is improved by ultrasonic treatment making it somewhat stronger and more resilient.

Ultrasonic treatment has been clearly shown to increase the rates and strength of skin healing in several situations by the mechanisms described above. It seems reasonable to suppose that other soft tissues behave similarly. Experiments have indicated that the early stages of fracture healing are also accelerated (Dyson, 1985).

Thus ultrasonics can be successfully used to aid the resolution of soft tissue injuries (see, e.g., Binder *et al.*, 1985), but especially those involving collagenous tissues. As the reparative processes are increased and fibrous tissue rendered more flexible so degenerative processes, such as tendon calcification or degenerative arthrosis, will benefit. Lehmann *et al.* (1958) applied ultrasonic therapy to the region of the ulnar nerve in ten volunteers and found a statistically significant rise in pain threshold over the little finger; this suggests that ultrasonic therapy applied to the nerve had a true analgesic effect. (He also achieved similar results with infrared radiation.) Such effects on peripheral nerves could account for the benefits claimed in the treatment of neurogenic pain or phantom limb pain by ultrasound, although these have usually been achieved with much lower doses than those used by Lehmann *et al.*

Increased flexibility and extensibility of fibrous tissue results from ultrasonic application; hence it is useful in the treatment of scarring, joint contractures, adhesions, Dupuytren's contracture, scleroderma and other conditions involving inflexibility of collagenous tissues. While the mechanisms of these changes remain unclear, therapeutic levels of ultrasonics have been shown to increase protein synthesis in fibroblasts (Harvey *et al.*, 1975). For a critical evaluation of the efficacy of ultrasonic therapy see Partridge (1987).

Production of Therapeutic Ultrasonics

The high frequency mechanical vibration needed to produce ultrasonic waves is provided by the reversed piezo-electric effect exhibited by certain crystals. If an oscillating electric field is applied at a frequency which matches the natural resonant frequency of the crystal maximum amplitude is achieved. The crystal is bonded to a metal plate which therefore also vibrates and this assembly, enclosed in a metal case, forms the transducer or treatment head. Sustained electrical oscillations are produced to drive the crystal by means of an oscillator circuit.

Some therapeutic ultrasonic sources operate on one frequency only, often 1 MHz, in others different frequencies can be chosen and this may involve using a different transducer. Many allow more than one pulsing pattern, e.g. 1:1 and 1:4 mark–space ratio, and the power output is displayed in total watts (W) and W/cm² on a meter. Apart from mains and ultrasonic output indicator lights, some machines have a useful additional indicator which shows whenever the treatment head is not in full contact with the tissues.

Methods of Applying Therapeutic Ultrasonics

In order to transmit ultrasonic energy to the tissues it is necessary to provide a **couplant**. Virtually no transmission occurs through air, the treatment head simply heating up as energy is absorbed at the transducer/air interface. Ultrasonic energy is absorbed by air bubbles so degassed water is best if water is being used as the couplant.

When the treatment head is applied to the skin a couplant must be interposed. As the skin is not flat the air pockets must be filled with fluid (Figure 15.8), and this fluid has to be sufficiently viscid to stay in place. Thixotropic gels are semisolid substances that become fluid on vibration and are thus ideal for this purpose. They are available under various trade names, or may be made in a hospital pharmacy. Glycerine or various oils such as liquid paraffin or arachis oil can also be used but are less efficient transmitters than either thixotropic couplants or water. Compensation for transmission loss can be made by increasing the intensity but heating of the skin may limit the treatment when oil is used. The fluid couplant also provides lubrication for movement of the treatment head over the skin.

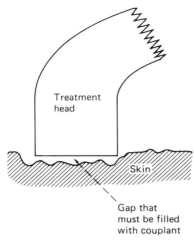

Fig. 15.8   A cross-section of a transducer on the skin surface.

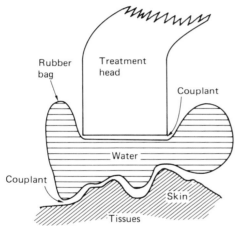

Fig. 15.9   A cross-section of a transducer and water bag on the skin surface.

A way of applying treatment to very irregular areas that cannot be submerged in water is to use a rubber or plastic bag filled with water (Figure 15.9). Couplant must be used between the bag and the skin and between the bag and the treatment head. The treatment head can be moved by either sliding over the surface of the bag or by deforming the bag so that the head moves relative to the skin. Only a minimal depth of water should separate the treatment head from the tissues.

Technique of application

The skin of the area to be treated must be examined. Inflammatory skin lesions or open wounds

are avoided. The nature of the treatment should be explained to the patient. In many ultrasonic treatments the patient will feel no sensation so that there is no check on the output. It is therefore advisable to test the machine by putting the transducer just below the surface in a bowl of water and observing the standing waves which appear. High frequency vibrations are reflected from the side of the bowl interfering with one another to produce waves of large amplitude and low frequency which are visible on the surface.

Direct contact treatment

Couplant is placed on both the area of skin to be treated and the treatment head which is then pressed upon the skin before the output is turned on. The transducer can be damaged if high intensities are applied while it is in air. The treatment head is moved over the area with a pressure sufficient to maintain even contact between the whole surface area of the head and the skin. Much skill in applying ultrasound lies in performing this movement correctly. The ultrasonic beam emitted is very irregular and is unevenly absorbed. Moving the treatment head ensures uniform treatment of the target tissue and obviates the risk of damage due to local high intensities. The speed of this movement must be slow enough to allow the skin and superficial tissues to deform and thus remain in contact with the rigid treatment head as it moves; if it is too slow the physiotherapist has difficulty maintaining an even pressure. Rates of movement of between 2 and 5 cm/s are appropriate.

The pattern of movement of the treatment head can be a series of overlapping circles, figures-of-eight or parallel overlapping strokes. This latter is likely to give less even treatment due to the longer time taken changing direction at each end of the stroke (Figure 15.10). It is essential to keep the treatment head flat on the surface and in contact at all times. Altering the angle will lead to scattering and marked energy loss and if an air gap forms transmission is completely prevented.

Supporting the part to be treated in a suitable position is obviously important in view of the need to apply even pressure during movement of the transducer. If possible the treatment head should be applied downwards and moved horizontally. This is less tiring for the physiotherapist as the weight of the treatment head contributes to the pressure and it is easier to move at a constant rate; also the couplant does not tend to flow downwards away

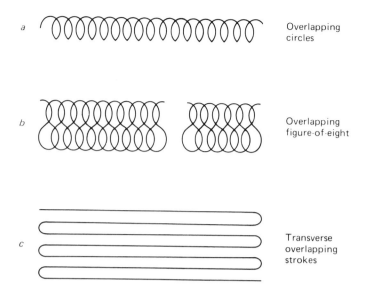

a   Overlapping circles

b   Overlapping figure-of-eight

c   Transverse overlapping strokes

Fig. 15.10   Patterns of movement of the ultrasonic transducer on the skin surface.

from the area. It is important that patients are not in such a position that they have to oppose the pressure of the ultrasonic head with their own muscular effort. Apart from the discomfort and fatigue, this is likely to lead to a less constant pressure.

Water bath technique

The water temperature should be above skin temperature and comfortable for the patient. The position of the bath and the patient should be so adjusted that the hand, forearm, ankle or foot can be rested comfortably in the bath with the patient sitting. The treatment head should be moved parallel and about 2 cm away from the surface following the surface contour as far as possible. The transducer face and the skin surface should be wiped clear of bubbles at intervals because bubbles will absorb ultrasonic energy. Using degassed water reduces bubble formation.

The main advantage of this method is that very irregular surfaces can be treated; also tender areas are not touched by the treatment head. Little additional energy is absorbed by the water.

Water bag method

Ordinary rubber balloons can be used in this method, and plastic containers have also been recommended. In each case the bag is filled with warm water, preferably degassed, and as much air as possible is excluded before the bag is sealed. Couplant is smeared onto the bag, skin and treatment head. It is often necessary to have an extra pair of hands, sometimes the patient's, to hold the bag in position. The treatment head is pressed into the bag so that an appropriate thickness of water separates it from the irregular surface. Movement of the head can be effected both by deforming the bag and sliding on its surface. Considerable energy losses are likely to occur at the various interfaces so that the intensity must be increased considerably (by about 75%) to compensate (see Figure 15.9).

Dosage

The energy absorbed in the target tissues depends on:

1. The **frequency** (Hz). As already noted, lower frequencies penetrate further, thus of the commonly used frequencies for therapeutic ultrasonics: 3 MHz penetrates least and is therefore absorbed superficially; 1.5 MHz penetrates further; 1.0 MHz penetrates further still and 0.75 MHz penetrates furthest and is thus absorbed in both superficial and deeper tissues (see Figure 15.14 and Table 15.3).

2. The **intensity** (W/cm²). Since the output is very irregular this is more correctly the space averaged, time averaged intensity. It may be shown on the meter in total W, W/cm² or both, usually to a maximum of 3 W/cm².
3. **Pulsing pattern** – duty cycle or mark – space ratio, e.g. 1:4.
4. Total **time of the treatment**.
5. The size **of the area being treated**.
6. Nature, size and position of the 'target' tissue to be treated. Since the actual intensities absorbed at any point in the tissues cannot be known dosage is, to some extent, a matter of judgement. It is first necessary to decide which is the target tissue and what effect is required, and then consider:

(a) **Depth of the target from the**
    surface   **Superficial** → **Deep**
    Frequency (see Table 15.3)   3 MHz   0.75 MHz
    Intensity   0.1 W/cm²   3 W/cm²
(b) **Size of the target area to be**
    treated   **Small**   → **Large**
    Time   3 min   15 min
(c) **Condition**   **Acute**   → **Chronic**
    Intensity   0.1 W/cm²   3 W/cm²
    Time   3 min   15 min
    Pattern   Pulsed   Continuous
(d) **Heating required**   **No heat** → **Heat**
    Intensity   0.1 W/cm²   3 W/cm²
    Time   3 min   15 min
    Pattern   Pulsed   Continuous

Each – (a), (b), (c), and (d) of the above – can vary independently so that the choice of intensity is influenced by (a), (c), and (d) and the time controlled by (b), (c), and (d). Clearly these modifications can sometimes cancel each other out. Thus a lesion may warrant a low intensity treatment because of its acute nature, but a higher intensity because it is deeply placed. It is important to remember that what matters is the ultrasonic energy delivered at the target tissue.

There seems to be little agreement on how much to vary these treatment parameters. Structures within 1 cm or so of the surface (i.e. skin, subcutaneous tendons or ligaments, etc.) are considered superficial and treated with 3 MHz ultrasound, deeper structures being treated with lower frequencies. If only one frequency is available (e.g. 1 MHz) it must be recognized that treatment will still lead to considerable energy absorption in the superficial tissues (see Figure 15.14).

Increasing the intensity to compensate for ultrasonic energy losses due to absorption and scattering at greater depth is a reasonable adjustment. Adding 0.25 W/cm² intensity for each centimetre of depth can be used as a rough guide.

The area covered by the moving treatment head must, obviously, be the main determinant of the time taken by the treatment. A useful guide is 1 min for every 10 cm² (1.5 in²), thus an area such as the palm of the hand (about 50 cm²) would be given 5 min treatment. Treatment of even the smallest target is likely to cover 20–30 cm² so that 2 or 3 min are regarded as the shortest reasonable treatment times. Usually, 15 min is considered the longest appropriate treatment time.

When using pulsed ultrasound, which, as already noted, would produce no heating (see Figure 15.11b), it is usual to compensate for the reduced energy input by increasing both the intensity and time of treatment. Intensities of 1 or 2W/cm² are often used; this is the pulse intensity, not the average intensity which would be very much lower. Increases in the time of pulsed treatments are usually not such as to completely compensate for the pulse intervals.

Potential Dangers with Ultrasonics

There seems to be no reported evidence of damage due to therapeutic ultrasonics, but reasonable presumptions and some experimental evidence to suggest the following. Ultrasonic therapy should not be applied to:

1. Neoplasms, because it may accelerate growth and cause metastases.
2. Tissues recently treated with X-ray or other ionizing radiation, because it could lead to further damage and possibly neoplastic changes.
3. Areas where haemorrhage might be provoked, e.g. an enlarging haematoma or recent haemarthrosis, or in uncontrolled haemophilia.
4. Acute infections, because the infection might spread.
5. Severely ischaemic areas, e.g. local arterial disease, because of the diminished heat transfer and possibly greater risk of arterial thrombosis.
6. Tuberculous lesions, because of the risk of reactivating encapsulated lesions.
7. The pregnant uterus; it is suggested that there might be some risk to the rapidly dividing tissues of the fetus from larger therapeutic doses. (Diagnostic ultrasonics uses very low intensities which are quite safe.)

8. Over recent venous thromboses where part of the clot might be freed causing an embolus.
9. The eye, since the fluid-filled chamber may allow good transmission damaging the retina.

There are some other circumstances where high doses should be avoided, notably anaesthetic areas because the patient may be unaware of pain and thus allow damage to occur. It must be realized that the pain commonly produced by overdosage is deep periosteal pain and that thermal sensation can only be felt on the skin. High doses have been shown to damage cells in the central nervous system, but only when applied directly. There seems to be no danger normally, and large therapeutic doses have been applied to the tissues around the spinal cord for many years without ill effects; but circumstances where the CNS is exposed, e.g. in spina bifida, should be avoided. Rapidly dividing tissues, such as the gonads and even epiphyseal plates have been considered to be at risk but without evidence. Similarly, treatment over the vagus nerve and cervical ganglia in cardiac disease is considered dangerous by some. Treatment over an implanted cardiac pacemaker should not be given as it may affect the pacemaker's stimulating frequency.

Surgical metallic implants cause reflection of the ultrasonic beam at their interface with the tissues causing increased energy absorption in this area. This does not, however, lead to a temperature rise in the implant or the surrounding tissues because the high thermal conductivity of the metal allows heat to be rapidly conducted to cooler untreated areas. Experiments have been done with implants (in pigs) without ill effects. It is therefore suggested that metal implants present no hazard when giving ultrasonic treatment (Lehmann and de Lateur, 1982). However, the effects might well be different with superficially placed and smaller implants so that cautious low doses are advisable in these circumstances.

High density polyethylene or other plastics used in replacement surgery should be avoided because their effect on ultrasonic energy absorption is, as yet, unquantified.

Theories of Therapeutic Mechanisms for Ultrasonics

There have been two schools of thought for some time. One, which might be called the American view, emphasizes the importance of heating. This approach recommends quite high intensities and sees little value in low intensity and pulsed treatments; the term **ultrasonic diathermy** is often used. The other, mainly European, is more impressed with neural and low intensity mechanical effects and uses low doses that are often pulsed. To some extent the historical development of these differing views, well described by Fyfe and Bullock (1985), has contributed to the lack of agreement over ultrasonic dosage. Other factors are the calibration inaccuracies of ultrasonic sources, uncertainty over how the energy spreads in the tissues and a lack of clinical research (Partridge, 1987).

Diathermies

It will have been noted that shortwave, microwave and ultrasound all provoke increased motion of tissue particles at a subcellular level by rapid electrical or mechanical oscillation. The atoms, molecules and macromolecules of all matter are in constant motion which increases directly with temperature. This motion is what is understood as heat. The deeper tissues of the body are at an average temperature of around 36.8 °C and the superficial tissues, especially of the extremities, usually somewhat cooler. Thus these modalities will lead to local heating (see Figure 15. 11a) which is limited by removal of the heat energy to other tissues and eventually balanced by heat loss to the environment to maintain thermal homeostasis.

Of course a temperature rise in the tissues is only recognized as heat by the patient if it is sufficient to be perceived as such. Even the most trivial absorption of energy must lead to some temporary local increase in temperature but this may not be recognized. Very low intensity treatments may not be regarded as 'heat' treatments at all. Low intensity shortwave treatments, so-called 'athermic' treatments are used and, as considered later, pulsed shortwave falls almost entirely into this category. Similarly, ultrasound and certainly pulsed ultrasound produce no detectable heating for many treatments. Some authorities on the other hand believe ultrasonic heating to be therapeutically important, as noted above.

Some of these modalities can produce significant detectable heating in the tissues, it may be asked whether there is anything to choose between them, or for that matter between them and any other form of tissue heating, such as a hot water bottle.

Skin is an organ concerned with the control of body temperature, and therefore heat applied to the surface of the skin, either as radiation or by conduction, will have only a limited effect on the deeper tissues. As the skin surface is heated vasodilatation occurs rapidly dissipating the local heat; furthermore, the subcutaneous fat acts as efficient thermal insulation preventing much heat passing to the underlying tissues by conduction. This is not to say that there will be no transfer of heat to the deeper tissues but that the skin can exert thermal control over heating methods like infrared or conduction heating due to hot water or hot air, the natural sources of heat. On the other hand, shortwave, microwave and ultrasonic diathermy are able to generate heat throughout the tissues thus, in a sense, being able to bypass the thermal barrier of the skin. Certainly, in most therapeutic situations using shortwave diathermy or microwave the skin is made hotter than the subcutaneous tissues, but deeply placed tissues are also directly heated in patterns which depend on the modality used and the structure of the tissues. Thus heating of the tissues occurs in a similar way to normal metabolic heating, heat being generated within the tissue rather than being transferred from the outside. This provides some justification for preferring these diathermic modalities.

Pulsed Diathermies

As already described, ultrasound can be applied in a pulsed form and pulsed electromagnetic energy, pulsed shortwave; microwaves can also be pulsed for therapy. The principle is the same in all; the energy is delivered in a series of discrete 'bursts' which are usually made very short compared to the intervals between pulses. The time between the pulses allows the heat generated by each pulse to be dispersed so that there is no significant overall heating (see Figure 15.11b). The effects are thus ascribed to mechanical or biological changes. The result of superimposing this low frequency cycle on the diathermy frequency is to reduce the average rate of adding energy to the tissues but allowing brief inputs which can be of high power. This concept is illustrated in Figure 15.11b but it must be recognized that this is not based on any real measurements. For many pulsing duty cycles the heat due to each pulse may well not exceed the

normal random temperature fluctuation at any point in the tissue. Thus pulsing can be seen as a means of giving a low intensity dose. There is considerable evidence to support the efficacy of pulsed ultrasound and pulsed shortwave (e.g. Bentall and Eckstein, 1975, Dyson and Suckling, 1978). There is still no certainty over whether the pulsing is the important feature or whether it is a matter of achieving a suitably low dose. This dichotomy has already been mentioned.

Pulsed electromagnetic energy (PEME) – pulsed shortwave

The output of a shortwave diathermy source can be pulsed in the same way as ultrasonics and with the same consequence, i.e. negligible heating. Although considerable interest in this therapy has developed in the past 15 years its origins can be traced to work done in the 1940s by Abraham Ginsberg which led to the Diapulse machine being developed. Many firms have since produced similar sources but most of the significant research has been done with Diapulse.

The Production of Pulsed High Frequency Radiations

High frequency oscillations at 27.12 MHz are produced in a conventional shortwave diathermy machine controlled by a timing circuit which allows the high frequency oscillations to be produced for a very short time, 65 μs in the case of Diapulse. These are repeated at intervals depending on the repetition rate. Thus at 100 pulses/s, each 65 μs pulse would be separated from the next by a gap of 9935 μs (a duty cycle of 0.654%). Each pulse is, of course, a series of high frequency oscillations, actually 1762.8 in this case. Other sources have other pulse lengths and repetition rates, some sufficient to produce mild heating (Figure 15.12a, b). Pulsed high frequency energy can be applied to the tissues by any of the conventional shortwave diathermy methods, but the Diapulse and others use a drum type electrode containing a flat spiral coil, a small 'pancake coil' (Figure 15.13).

The maximum instantaneous power, i.e. the power in watts of each pulse can be large, 975 W, but the average power is, obviously, very low – it is about 38 W at maximum in the Diapulse. However, as

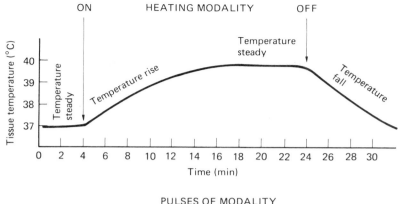

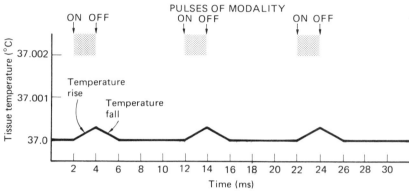

Fig. 15.11   *a*, A representation of tissue heating. As heat is added the local temperature rises, but at the same time the body's thermoregulatory system reacts removing heat until a steady state is reached at a new, higher temperature. (The temperature changes shown in these figures are not based on actual measurements.) *b*, A representation of tissue heating due to a pulsed modality. The small, negligible temperature rise due to each pulse is dissipated during the pulse intervals. Note the different time and temperature scales of part (*a*).

pointed out by Barker *et al.* (1985) this is a significant fraction of the average adult basal metabolic rate.

Pain Relief and Other Effects of Pulsed High Frequency Energy

Experimental evidence

Artificially produced haematomas in rabbits' ears have been shown to heal faster under treatment (Fenn, 1969). Experimentally induced skin wounds showed less oedema when treated (Cameron, 1961). Experiments on the median-ulnar nerve of rats indicated that those treated for 15 min/day showed more rapid and more complete regeneration than the controls (Wilson and Jagadeesh,

1976). Carefully designed experiments involving the division and suture of the common peroneal nerve of rats demonstrated statistically significant benefits with pulsed energy treatment; degeneration, regeneration and maturation of myelinated nerve fibres were accelerated and fibrosis was reduced (Raji, 1984).

Clinical investigations

In a study on children after orchidopexy, less bruising and more rapid recovery was found in those treated with pulsed electromagnetic energy (Bentall and Eckstein, 1975). A double blind study on donor site healing after split skin graft removal showed significantly greater healing at 7 days in those treated compared with the controls (Goldin

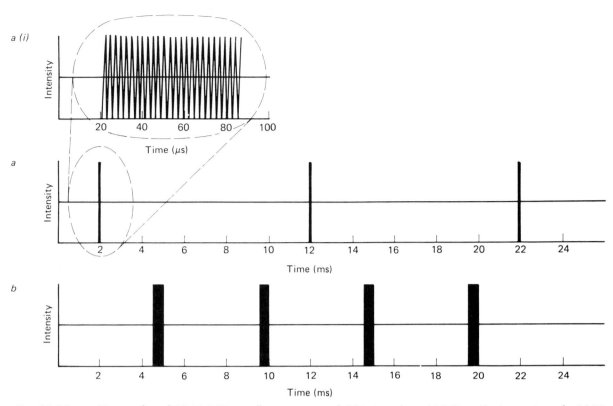

Fig. 15.12   *a*, 65 μs pulse of 27.12 MHz oscillations repeated 100 times/s at 100 Hz. *a(i)*, Approximately 1800 oscillations during a 65 μs pulse. *b*, 400 μs pulses of 27.12 MHz oscillations repeated 200 times/s at 200 Hz.

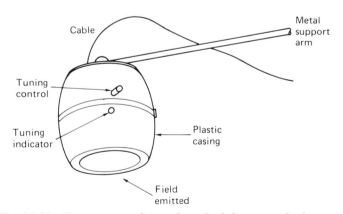

Fig. 15.13   Drum-type applicator for pulsed shortwave diathermy.

et al., 1981). Ankle injuries have been used to assess the efficacy of pulsed energy; one study showed marked reduction of pain and disability (Wilson, 1972), while another (Pasila *et al.*, 1978) resulted in a less dramatic improvement. There have been several other clinical studies published.

There is therefore good reason to expect that pulsed shortwave diathermy can accelerate the healing of soft tissue and, perhaps most important, regenerating nerve. In many of the clinical studies, comment was made on the pain relief experienced by the patients treated.

Therapeutic Uses of Pulsed High Frequency Energy

It is appropriate to treat all recent trauma both accidental and postoperative at an early stage, thus recent injuries, such as a sprained ankle, a crushed hand, muscle haematomas, local burns or acute synovitis can be treated immediately. Acute infections, such as paranasal sinusitis or pelvic inflammatory disease, may also benefit from treatment. As well as clinical impressions (Wilson, 1981), the strong experimental evidence indicates that early treatment of peripheral nerve lesions would accelerate recovery. Treatment of all these may give pain relief, especially the relief of postoperative pain, but also some more chronic conditions, such as degenerative arthritis and pelvic inflammatory disease appear to become pain free, or have their pain reduced, after treatment with pulsed high frequency energy. Neurogenic pain – as in Sudeck's atrophy, phantom limb pains and osteoporotic pain – may also be helped (Wilson, 1981).

Application of Pulsed High Frequency Energy

There is some uncertainty concerning the dosage to be given, but the following provides a rough guide:

1. For acute conditions low average energy is used, 40 or 65 μs pulses with repetition rates of 400-600 pulses/s and either three 20 min treatments each day or, if that is impossible, a 1 h treatment each day.
2. If the intensity can be altered it is sensible to use higher intensities for more deeply placed targets. Where a drum-type applicator is used it is positioned as close to the affected area as possible but not touching the skin, leaving a space of a centimetre or so.
3. Chronic lesions seem to benefit from rather more average energy so that the longer pulses are used, again at 400-600 pulses/s.
4. For the relief of pain, moderate pulse lengths of 65 or 100 μs at 100 or 200 pulses/s for 10-20 min are used.

This does not entirely conform with other published opinions; Hayne (1984) recommends 200–300 pulses/s for pain relief and lower repetition rates (100–200 pulses/s) given two or three times a day in 15 min sessions for acute lesions.

There is also a widely held opinion, not shared by the author, that short treatment times of 5–10 min are just as effective as the longer. Clearly, an open mind and more evidence on the matter are both needed. (It may be noted that the three quoted trials – Wilson, 1972; Bentall and Eckstein, 1975; Goldin *et al.*, 1981 – used 600 pulses/s for 1 h, 500 pulses/s in three 20 min periods and 400 pulses/s in four 10 min periods respectively, for each day.)

Mode of Action of Pulsed High Frequency Energy

This is not clearly understood. There is disagreement about whether the effects are specific or simply due to the mild heating. Some, e.g. Lehmann and de Lateur (1982), maintain that all the proven effects can be accounted for by mild heating and consider there is no specific therapeutic indication for pulsed output. Others, pointing to the variety of effects, suggest that electrical changes may influence cellular membrane function. Cell damage is associated with depolarization and it is suggested that recovery may be assisted by ionic movement provoked by the varying electric field. Cell division and other cellular activities may be aided by the vibrating charges. For some interesting further details see Hayne (1984). Another unresolved question concerns the pulsing parameters, pulse length, frequency and shape, and what influence they have on the effects. Almost all the research has been done with Diapulse so those parameters are often used and cited (Table 15.4).

Table 15.4 Some Pulsed High Frequency Energy Sources

	Apparatus		
Function	Diapulse	Megapulse	Curapuls and ultramed
Mode	Pulsed only	Pulsed only	Continuous and pulsed
Pulse width (μs)	65 only	Various from 20–400	400 only
Pulse repetition rates (pulses/s)	80–600	100–800 or 25–400	15–200
Intensity	6 settings	Not variable	10 settings
Maximum instantaneous power (peak power) (W)	975	approx. 500	1000
Average maximum power (W)	38	35	70

Potential Dangers with Pulsed High Frequency Energy

There have been no reported ill effects of this modality. In view of the supposed mode of action it would seem sensible to avoid rapidly dividing tissues, such as the fetus, or uncontrolled tissue growth, such as neoplasms. Similarly, tuberculous lesions should be avoided (because of the possibility of reactivating encapsulated lesions) and so should markedly hyperpyrexic patients.

Since there is no significant heating there is no risk of burns due to concentration of the field by metal on or in the tissues, or by water on the surface. However, it must be remembered that the treatment is relatively, not absolutely, athermic; the longer pulses at higher frequencies can cause heating and therefore some risk of overheating. None the less, low intensity treatments are entirely safe and have been used in the presence of metal implants.

Like other high frequency sources they could affect cardiac pacemakers causing arrhythmias; less seriously, they can also affect hearing aids and other electronic equipment, such as modern telephones.

Low Power Pulsed High Frequency Energy

Machines are available which generate pulses similar to those described above but delivering only a tiny fraction of the power, e.g. the Therafield Beta. Claims made for their efficacy were not substantiated in a controlled trial (Barker *et al.*, 1985). Other studies, however, have found that these devices can aid wound healing; for example, Nicolle and Bentall (1982) found that oedema and bruising were diminished more often on the treated side in a controlled study of bilateral blepharoplasty.

Therapeutic Radiations

It has already been noted that rapid electron oscillation leads to the production of electromagnetic radiations; microwaves have already been considered and some aspects of visible and infrared radiation will be dealt with in the next section. From the point of view of their behaviour, sonic waves are a different kind of radiation – being longitudinal mechanical rather than transverse electromagnetic waves – but follow the same principles.

When radiations travelling in one medium, such as air, meet a new medium, such as the tissues, three interactions can occur:

1. They may be reflected from the surface of the new material
2. They may be transmitted, through the new material, either in a straight line or in some other line because they have been refracted.
3. They may be absorbed.

In the last case they will give up their energy to the new material, usually heating it.

In fact all three happen in some degree; the relative amount of reflection, transmission or absorption varies with the nature of both the radiation and the new medium. For radiation of the infrared and visible spectrum most is either reflected or absorbed by the skin surface. There is a band of radiations from about 650 nm to 1500 nm, the red visible and near infrared (see Figure 15.1), in which rather more transmission (penetration) into the tissues can occur. Microwave radiations with wavelengths of several centimetres will pass through the tissues much more readily than infrared, as will an ultrasound beam, but again in both the energy will be absorbed and reflected.

Any radiation penetrating the tissues will lose energy as it travels. Some of the energy will be absorbed in the main path of the beam but some radiation will be scattered so that energy is absorbed in the region around the beam. As the amount absorbed at any point depends on the total energy at that point it follows that the decrease will be approximately exponential. The energy absorption will depend on the nature of the tissues and the wavelength of the radiation.

It is not possible to determine a point at which all the energy is absorbed, i.e. a point to which the modality penetrates, so it is usual to specify the **half value depth**. This is the depth at which half the initial energy has been absorbed. In the example in Figure 15.14, the radiations penetrate to 3 cm before losing 50% of their energy, at 6 cm 25% remains and even at 12 cm over 6% of the original energy remains. This, of course, is an idealized example; in real tissues the penetration and absorption would be much more irregular.

The same concept is sometimes expressed as the **penetration depth**, the distance travelled until the energy is reduced to 37% of the original. At twice the penetration depth the energy is reduced to 37% of 37%, i.e. 14% of the original energy and so on.

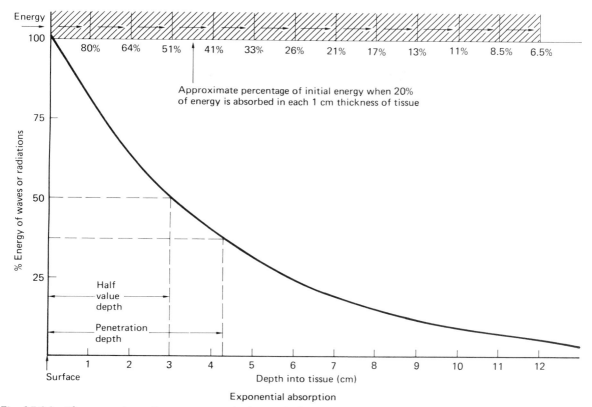

Fig. 15.14   The percentage of energy waves (radiations) absorbed by the tissues at different depths. Suppose 20% of energy is absorbed in each 1 cm of tissue, the approximate percentage of initial energy at each 1 cm layer is given.

Penetration depth = Half value depth × 1.44

and

$$\text{Half value depth} = \frac{\text{Penetration depth}}{1.44}$$

Lasers

Laser is an acronym for light amplification by the stimulated emission of radiation. It refers to a beam of radiations with the characteristics of:

1. Monochromaticity, i.e. it is of a single wavelength.
2. Coherence, the peaks and troughs of radiation are all 'in step' so that they occur at the same time and they are all travelling in the same direction. The radiations thus have both temporal and spatial coherence (see Figure 15.15).

3. Collimation, a consequence of spatial coherence as the radiations do not diverge but travel in the same narrow beam. This property allows the laser to propagate over long distances in the same narrow beam making it a valuable tool for aiming and measuring purposes.

Laser radiation can now be generated fairly easily and cheaply so that it has found many applications in recent years; at low intensities for aiming, measuring, as bar-code and compact disc readers, and at higher intensities for cutting various materials. Thus lasers have been used in surgery for some time. The tissue surrounding laser-made surgical cuts was thought to heal particularly rapidly which led to the suggestion that low intensity laser treatment may accelerate wound healing. A considerable interest developed in the use of low intensity lasers for treatment – low level laser therapy (LLLT) – of soft tissue lesions. The major

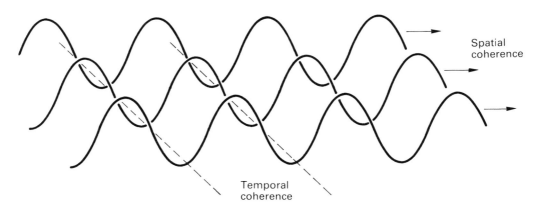

Spatial
coherence

Temporal
coherence

All three waves are travelling in the same direction – spatial coherence
in step at the same time – temporal coherence

Fig. 15.15   Coherence.

Table 15.5   Classification of lasers

No effect on eye or skin	1 2	} Low power	'cold' or 'soft'	Blackboard pointer Supermarket bar code reader
Safe on skin not on eye	3A 3B	} Mid power		Therapeutic – physiotherapy models up to 50mW mean power
Unsafe on eye and skin	4	High power		Surgical – destructive

Physiotherapy treatment = 3A + 3B also called 'low level laser therapy'.

uses are to alleviate pain and promote healing. See Table 15.5 for a classificatiion of lasers.

Principles of generating laser radiation

Electrons in orbit around the atomic nucleus occupy certain specific energy levels or 'shells' around the nucleus. When the atom gains energy, say by being heated, some electrons take up the energy by moving to higher energy levels (See Figure 15.16). This energy is given up as discrete 'packets' of radiation energy called photons; the wavelength (hence frequency) of each photon depending on the particular energy level change or transition. Under ordinary circumstances many different wavelengths are emmitted, a tungsten filament electric light bulb, for example, would emit many different wavelengths of visible and much infrared radiation. It is possible to arrange that many electrons in certain materials can be held at high energy levels so that the release of one photon can trigger the release of an identical photon from another atom which can provoke others. Thus there is a rapid build-up of identical photons which is emitted from one side of the material in a narrow beam.

Therapeutic lasers are of various types but are all classed as low or mid-power lasers. (See Table 15.5). Helium-neon lasers consist of a tube of these gases at low pressure with a means of adding energy – exciting – the atoms and reflecting ends to the tube so that the photons are reflected to and fro producing further photon emission and emerging as a narrow beam from one partially transparent end. The output, which has a wavelength of 632.8 nm, is often conveyed to the tissues by a fibreoptic cable.

Semiconductor diode lasers are of various kinds involving gallium aluminium arsenide. In these

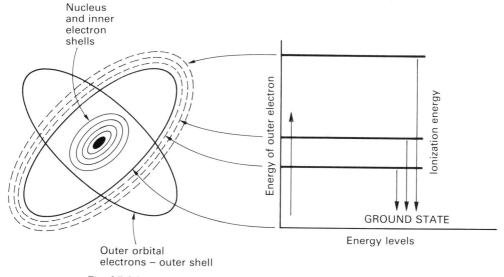

Fig. 15.16   Representation of an atom with orbiting electrons.

electrons are excited by a suitable electrical potential leads to the emission of a photon which provokes the emission of identical photons to produce laser radiation. These devices are relatively robust and cheap so that they are becoming more widely used. One very important feature is that they can be built to emit different wavelengths. This is done by varying the ratio of gallium to aluminium and building the diode in a very precise manner.

Measurements of laser energy

The rate of production of laser energy measured in watts (1 joule per second equals one watt) is usually described. Most lasers used in physiotherapy have output power in the region of a few milliwatts. However, for treatment the energy per unit area is important – called the energy density – measured in joules per cm². Many therapeutic lasers can be pulsed, which affects the amount of energy. As with other modalities pulsing allows short bursts of relatively high intensity to be applied. Pulsed injection lasers have high peak power outputs but very low average power which can be altered by changing the frequency. Thus peak values may be of several watts each lasting for a very short time, 200 nanoseconds for example, which with a pulsing frequency of several thousand Hertz would give a few milliwatts aver-

age power. The average is often deduced from the peak power, pulse length, and frequency but this is only valid if the peak power is applied for the whole of each pulse, which is not usually the case (King, 1989).

It must be clearly recognized that the energy delivered from the laser is not the same as the dosage. The dose is the energy absorbed and there are unquantified losses between the laser and the tissues; some in the fibreoptic cable, some as reflection from the skin surface and others.

The extent to which laser radiation penetrates the tissues depends, as already noted, on the wavelength and the nature of the tissues. Early suggestions that the nature of laser radiations allowed greater penetration than equivalent non-coherent radiation have been discounted as coherence is lost on entering the tissues. Confusion also arises because of the misunderstanding of terms; penetration depth refers to the distance travelled until the energy is reduced to 37% of the original, (see Figure 15.14). It has been suggested that the penetration depth of red light in soft tissue is about 1–2 mm and about twice that for 800–900 nm infrared (King, 1989). However, theoretical work leads to the belief that penetration depth is very much less so that at 3 mm only 1% of the radiation is left and the exponential absorption pattern of Figure 15.14 is too simplistic; for instance the intensity of radiation just below the skin surface may be much greater than the original beam due to backscattering (van Breugel, 1992).

Dosage

Dosage is usually expressed in J/cm² or mJ/cm², which is the energy density. If the power density in W/cm² is given it is simple to calculate the energy density from the length of time the laser is applied (W = J/s). If the total output power is given then the power density is found by dividing by the area of the beam.

There is very little agreement on the dosage required for various conditions and recommendations range from 0.5 J/cm² to 20 J/cm², doses between 4 and 10 J/cm² are most widely applied.

Application of lasers

Many therapeutic laser sources are hand-held and applied in contact with the skin, while some are mounted on a stand. In both cases the laser can be applied at a distance from the tissues; this may be useful for treating open areas or very tender points. A single laser provides a very narrow beam so that it is a 'spot' treatment. The laser must be applied successively to several points to cover a larger area. Some types of therapeutic laser use a collection of laser diodes giving different wavelengths, called cluster diodes; others deliberately allow the beam to spread out before it strikes the skin thus enabling a larger area to be treated.

The position of the patient must be chosen so that the area to be treated is accessible and supported, the skin surface should be clean (grease or dirt will obviously tend to obstruct the radiations) and the patient given an explanation of the nature of the treatment. If there is any risk of the radiations entering the eye, either directly or by reflection, the patient should wear goggles of an appropriate construction. The laser is applied to the skin or positioned so that it is at right angles to achieve maximum penetration and is switched on for the appropriate length of time, often a matter of a minute or so. If several spots are to be treated the laser is reapplied in a new place. For safety and accuracy of dosage it is recommended that the machine be switched off while the position is changed. Some machines are operated with a key to ensure that use is restricted to authorized therapists.

Therapeutic applications of low intensity laser

The two areas that have found most favour for the use of lasers are the relief of pain and soft tissue healing. The use of laser therapy for the control of pain seems to be quite extensive, being principally used for musculoskeletal pain syndromes and neurogenic pain (Baxter et al., 1991). However, a wide variety of actute and chronic conditions are also treated, including rheumatoid arthritis, osteoarthritis, various types of back pain and other conditions (England, 1988; Seitz and Kleinkort 1986). Neurogenic pain, notably post-herpetic neuralgia, has been treated very successfully (Walker, 1983; Moore, 1992). The laser is also widely used on trigger or acupuncture points (Ong, 1986).

The use of laser therapy in tissue healing and skin disease is also widespread and is supported by a considerable body of *in vitro* experimental evidence indicating effects at a cellular level.

There is considerable doubt concerning the efficacy of laser treatment. This is due to the absence of any satisfactory theoretical basis for its action and the difficulty of interpreting the often contradictory results of clinical trials. A recent meta-analysis of randomized clinical trials (Beckerman et al., 1992) concluded that many of the trials were flawed but there was some suggestion that laser therapy may have a specific effect, particularly for post-traumatic joint disorders, myofascial pain and rheumatoid arthritis; but the degree of certainty concerning laser efficacy was rather weak. (Also see Kitchen and Partridge (1991) for a review of laser therapy.)

References

Barbour, L.A., McGuire, D.B. and Kirchoff, K.T. (1986) Nonanalgesic methods of pain control used by cancer outpatients. *Oncology Nursing Forum*, **13**(6), 56–60

Barker, A.T. et al. (1985) A double-blind clinical trial of low power pulsed shortwave therapy in treatment of a soft tissue injury. *Physiotherapy*, 71(12), 500–4

Baxter, G.D., Bell, A.J., Allen, J.M. and Ravey, J. (1991) Low level laser therapy: current clinical practice in Northern Ireland. *Physiotherapy*, **77**(3), 171–8

Beckerman, H., de Bie, R.A., Bouter, L.M. et al. (1992) The efficacy of laser therapy for musculoskeletal and skin disorders: a criteria-based meta-analysis of randomized clinical trials. *Physical Thera.*, **72**(7), 483–91

Becker, R.O. and Marino, A.A. (1982) *Electromagnetism and Life*, State University of New York Press, New York

Belcher, J.F. (1974) Interferential therapy. *NZ. J. Physiother.*, November, pp. 29–34

Bentall, R.H.C. and Eckstein, H.B. (1975) A trial involving the use of pulsed electromagnetic therapy on children undergoing orchidopexy. *Kinderchirurgie*, **17**(4), 380–2

Binder, A., Hodge, G., Greenwood, A.M. *et al.* (1985) Is therapeutic ultrasound effective in treating soft tissue lesions? *Br. Med. J.*, **290**, 512–14

Boone, C. (1981) Applications of iontophoresis In *Electrotherapy* (ed. S.L. Wolfe), Churchill Livingstone, New York, pp. 99–121

Boyle, A.C., Cook, H.F. and Buchanan, T.J. (1950) The effects of microwaves: a preliminary investigation. *Br. J. Phys. Med.*, **13**, 2–8

Brighton, C.T. *et al.* (1981) A multicentre study of the treatment of non-union with constant direct current. *J. Bone. Joint. Surg.*, **163**A(1), 2–13

Cameron, B. (1961) Experimental acceleration of wound healing. *Am. J. Orthopaed.*, **53**, 336–43

Csillik, B., Knyhàr-Csillik, E. and Szücs, A. (1982) Treatment of chronic pain syndromes with iontophoresis of vinea alkaloids to the skin of patients. *Neurosci. Letts*, **31**, 87–90

De Domenico, G. (1982) Pain relief with interferential therapy. *Aust. J. Physiother.*, **28**(3), 14–18

DHSS Medical Scientific Services (1980) *Health Equipment Information*, No. 88. HMSO, London

Donovan, M.I. (1985) Nursing assessment of cancer pain. *Semin. Oncol. Nursing*, **1**(2), 109–15

Dyson, M. (1985) Therapeutic applications of ultrasound. In *Clinics in Diagnostic Ultrasound*, vol. 16 (*Biological Effects of Ultrasound*) (eds W.L. Nyborg and M.C. Ziskin), Churchill Livingstone, New York

Dyson, M. (1987) Mechanisms involved in therapeutic ultrasound. *Physiotherapy*, **73**(3), 116–20

Dyson, M. and Suckling, J. (1978) Stimulation of tissue repair by ultrasound: a survey of the mechanism involved. *Physiotherapy*, **64**(4), 105–8

England, S. (1988) Introduction to mid laser therapy. *Physiotherapy*, **74**, 100–2

Evans, P. (1980) The healing process at cellular level: a review. *Physiotherapy*, **66**(8), 256–9

Fenn, J.E. (1969) Effect of pulsed electromagnetic energy (Diapulse) on experimental haematomas. *Canad. Med. Assoc. J.*, **100**, 251–4

Forster, A. and Palastanga, N. (1985) *Clayton's Electrotherapy, Theory and Practice*, 9th edn, Bailliere Tindall, London

Fyfe, M.C. and Bullock, M.I. (1985) Therapeutic ultrasound: some historical background and development in knowledge of its effects on healing. *Aust. J. Physiother.*, **31**(6), 220–4

Gammon, G.D. Starr, I. (1941) Studies on the relief of pain by counterirritation. *J. Clin. Invest.*, **20**, 13–20

Goldin, J.H., Broadbent, N.R.T., Nancarrow, J.D. and Marshall, T. (1981) The effects of Diapulse on the healing of wounds: a double-blind randomized controlled trial in man. *Br. J. Plast. Surg.*, **14**, 267–70

Haag, W. (1979) Practical experience with interferential current therapy in gynaecology. *Der Frauenarzl*, **1**(20), 44–8

Harris, R. (1963) The effect of various forms of physical therapy on radio sodium clearance. *Ann. Phys. Med.*, **7**, 1–10

Harvey, W., Dyson, M., Pond, J.B. *et al.* (1975) The stimulation of protein synthesis in human fibroblasts by therapeutic ultrasound. *Rheumatol. Rehabil.*, **14**, 237

Hashish, I., Harvey, W. and Harris, H. (1986) Anti-inflammatory effects of ultrasound therapy: evidence for a major placebo effect. *Brit. J. Rheumatol*, **251**, 77–81

Hayne, C.R. (1984) Pulsed high frequency energy – its place in physiotherapy. *Physiotherapy*, **70**(12), 459–66

Jones, S.L. (1976) Electromagnetic field interference and cardiac pacemakers. *Phys. Ther.*, **56**(9), 1013–18

Kanui, T.L. (1985) Thermal inhibition of nociceptor-driven spinal cord nerves in rats. *Pain*, **21**, 231–40

King, P.R. (1989) Low level laser therapy: a review. *Lasers Medi. Sci.*, **4**, 141–50

Kitchen, S.S. and Partridge, C.J. (1991) A review of low level laser therapy. *Physiotherapy*, **77**(3), 161–7

Layman, P.R., Argyras, E. and Glyn, C.J. (1986) Iontophoresis of vincristine versus saline in post-herpetic neuralgia: A controlled trial. *Pain*, **25**, 165–70

Lehmann, J.F. and de Lateur, B.J. (1982) Therapeutic heat. In *Therapeutic Heat and Cold*, 3rd edn (ed. J.F. Lehmann), Williams and Wilkins, Baltimore, Md

Lehmann, J.F., Brunner G. D. and Stow R.W. (1958) Pain threshold measurements after therapeutic application of ultrasound, microwaves and infrared. *Arch. Phys. Med. Rehabil.*, **39**, 560–5

Lehmann, J.F., Masock, A.J., Warren, C.G. *et al.* (1970) Effect of therapeutic temperatures on tendon extensibility. *Arch. Phys. Med. Rehabil*, **51**, 481–7

Low, J. and Reed, A. (1990) *Electrotherapy Explained. Principles and Practice.* Butterworth-Heinemann, Oxford

Low, J. and Reed, A. (1994) *Physical Principles Explained.* Butterworth-Heinemann, Oxford

McQuire, W.A. (1975) Electrotherapy and exercises for stress incontinence and urinary frequency. *Physiotherapy*, **61**(10), 305–7

Millard, J.B. (1961) Effect of high frequency current and

infra-red rays on the circulation of the lower limb in man. *Ann. Phys. Med.*, **6**, 45–66

Moore, K.C. (1992) Clinical patterns of symptom relief during laser therapy for ophthalmic post-herpetic neuralgia. Second Meeting of the International Laser Therapy Association, London, UK, 18–20 September 1992

Nicolle, F.V. and Bentall, R.H.C. (1982) Use of radio-frequency pulsed energy in the control of post-operative reaction in blepharoplasty. *Aesthet. Plast. Surg.*, **61**, 169–71

Nikolova-Troeva, L. (1967a) Interference-current therapy in distortions, confusions and luxations of the joints. *Münch Med. Wochensch.*, **109**(11), 579–82

Nikolova-Troeva, L. (1967b) Comparative studies on therapeutic results obtained by means of interference therapy and other methods in arthrosis deformans. *Phys. Med. Rehabil.* **8**(3) 239–61

Ong, K.L.T. (1986) Handling the patient in pain *Physiotherapy*, **72**, 184–8.

Pärtan, J., Schmid, J. and Warum, F. (1953) The treatment of inflammatory and degenerative joint conditions with interferential alternating currents of medium frequency. *Wiener Klin. Wochensch.* **31**, 624–8

Partridge, C.J. (1987) Evaluation of the efficacy of ultrasound. *Physiotherapy*, **73**(4), 166–8

Pasila, M., Visuri, T. and Sundholm, A. (1978) Pulsating shortwave diathermy: value in treatment of recent ankle and foot sprains. *Arch. Phys. Med. Rehabil.* **59**, 383–6

Presman, A.S. (1970) *Electromagnetic Fields and Life*, Plenum Press, New York

Raji, A.M. (1984) An experimental study of the effects of pulsed electromagnetic field (Diapulse) on nerve repair. *J. Hand Surg.* **9B**(2), 105–11

Rennie, S. (1988) Diadynamic current therapy. In *Current Physical Therapy* (ed M. Peat), B.C. Decker, Toronto pp. 207–11

Savage, B. (1984) *Interferential Therapy*, Faber and Faber, London

Scott, B.O. (1957) *The Principles and Practice of Diathermy*, William Heinemann Medical Books, London

Scott, S.M. and Purves, C.E. (1991) The effect of interferential therapy in the relief of experimentally induced pain; a pilot study. Proceedings of 11th International Congress of World Conferderation of Physical Therapy, Book II, p. 743.

Scowcroft, A.T., Mason, A.H.L. and Hayne, C.R. (1977) Safety with microwave diathermy. *Physiotherapy*, **63**(11), 359–61

Seitz, L.M. and Kleinkort, J.A. (1986) Low power laser: its application in physical therapy. In *Thermal Agents in Rehabilitation* (ed. S.L. Michlovitz), S.A. Davies, Philadelphia, pp. 217–37.

Taylor, K., Newton, R., Personius, W. and Bush, F. (1987) Effect of interferential current stimulation for treatment of subjects with recurrent jaw pain. *Phys. Ther*, **67**(3), 346–50

Van Breugel, H.F.I. (1992) A Monte Carlo model for laser light distribution in tissue: effects of intensity profile and divergence of the laser beam. Second Meeting of the International Laser Therapy Association, London, UK, 18–20 September 1992

Wadsworth, H. and Chanmugan, A.P.P. (1980) *Electrophysical Agents in Physiotherapy*, Science Press, Marrickville, NSW Australia.

Walker, J. (1983) Relief from chronic pain by low power laser irradiation. *Neurosci. Lett.*, **43**, 339–44

Ward, A.R. (1980) *Electricity Fields and Waves in Therapy*, Science Press, Marrickville, NSW Australia

Wilson, D.H. (1972) Treatment of soft tissue injuries by pulsed electrical energy. *Br. Med. J.* **2**, 269

Wilson, D.H. (1981) PEME, the new beam for fractures. *World Med.*, November, pp. 97–8

Wilson, D.H. and Jagadeesh, P. (1976) Experimental regeneration in peripheral nerves and the spinal cord in laboratory animals exposed to a pulsed electromagnetic field. Proceedings of the Annual Scientific Meeting of the International Medical Society of Paraplegia 1975, Part III. *Paraplegia*; **14**, 12–20

Wright, V. and Johns, R.J. (1961) Quantitative and qualitative analysis of joint stiffness in normal subjects and in patients with connective tissue diseases. *Ann. Rheumatol. Dis.* **20**, 36–46

Wright, V. (1973) Stiffness: a review of its measurement and physiological importance. *Physiotherapy*, **59**(4), 107–11

16 *Heat and cold*

NIGEL P. PALASTANGA

Introduction

The use of various forms of heat and cold continues to be one of the cornerstones of physiotherapy practice. Arguments concerning the relative merits of one versus the other in the management of pain have been long and protracted and have as yet only been superseded by arguments about the mechanism by which heat or cold can be applied. Each of these modalities has its advocates who extol the virtues of a particular favourite, often with little or no evidence to support their assertions. The situation where therapists are faced with a mass of conflicting opinion and data has, if anything, become worse in recent years as month by month new and more sophisticated apparatus appears on the market. Research into the effects of some of these modalities is beginning to take place as the culture of physiotherapy education has changed world wide and graduate physiotherapists are equipped to evaluate the effects of their treatments using scientific method.

In this chapter an attempt will be made to rationalize the use of heat and cold in the treatment of pain. In the first part, various forms of therapeutic heat will be discussed, followed by a similar discussion on cold. As in the previous edition of this book, details of technique will not be included in this chapter and the reader is referred to texts on electrotherapy and cold therapy (Forster and Palastanga, 1985; Low and Reed, 1990) for this information.

Heat

The history of the use of heat to relieve pain is as old as medicine itself. Therapeutic heat has been applied to the human body by conduction from heated stones, sand, oils and water, or by radiant heat from the sun or fires (Licht, 1984). Historically heat has proved itself to be a very useful method of reducing pain, and although much of the supporting evidence is empirical it cannot be ignored as a form of treatment. Even when used today some of the techniques of conductive heating or immersion in heated fluids must be very similar to those used by the Ancient Greeks and Romans. However, the advent of a more precise scientific and technological society has allowed the development of many different sources of therapeutic heat, the application of which can be accurately monitored in terms of depth of penetration and temperature rise achieved (Lehmann and de Lateur, 1984). The net effect of applying heat is, however, a local or general rise in temperature, and it is this which is considered to produce the physiological effects responsible for a reduction in perceived pain.

Physiological Effects of Heat

The primary aim of this short chapter is to consider the modulation of pain utilizing the effects of either heat or cold. In other sections of this book authors will have described in detail how pain is perceived, transmitted and modulated. In this part only the mechanisms involved when heat is applied will be discussed, followed later by a similar discussion of the mechanisms involved when cold is utilized.

To some extent the physiological effects produced by heat will depend upon the depth of penetration and the level of temperature increase developed within the body tissues. Human beings are homeothermic with the core temperature of deeply placed organs and structures remaining fairly constant while the skin temperature is much more variable. This variation of skin temperature is accounted for by the fact that the skin, as the largest organ in the body, has an important role in temperature regulation. This regulation is achieved by the skin preserving or losing heat depending upon the differential between body and the surrounding temperature. The difference in temperature between the body's core and its surface is because of the insulating nature of subcutaneous tissue, principally fat. The flow of heat from the deeper tissues across this barrier is achieved by blood flow in order to cool the body. The converse situation also operates where cold skin is isolated from the warmer core tissues by this fat and a vasoconstriction preserves heat.

The receptors in the skin which are stimulated by an increase in temperature have in the past been identified anatomically as Ruffini end organs and those stimulated by a decrease in temperature as Krause's end bulbs. This distinction is now much less certain and thermal perception is much more likely to be the result of central interpretation of impulses from free nerve endings in the basal layer of the epidermis (Low, 1990). Thermal sensations become merged with and are then superseded by pain at an upper temperature of 45°C, and a lower temperature of 15°C. Hence the range of comfortable thermal sensations is fairly narrow.

Excessive heating of the tissues is dangerous and the signalling of excess heat as a noxious stimulus is a warning of impending tissue damage. If the tissue temperature rises above 50°C (only 5°C above the level of noxious stimulation) then collagen will start to shrink and melt (Mason and Rigby, 1963). This signalling mechanism has formed the basis of the safe application of heat to patients for many years, whereby the patient perceives the heat and is asked to report if it becomes uncomfortable. It is essential therefore that any patient being treated with therapeutic heat has an intact thermal sensory mechanism and understands the level of heat to be experienced. For medico-legal and patient safety reasons it is therefore essential that prior to the first heat treatment patients:

1. have their thermal sensation tested (and will only be given heat if it is normal);
2. understand the level of heat they are expected to experience (and know what to do if it becomes excessive).

Even though the technology used to produce therapeutic heat may be highly sophisticated, it is interesting that the basis upon which the degree of heating produced in the patients is assessed still relies upon the patients reporting their subjective feelings of warmth.

Increased Circulation

As described above, heat is known to increase the circulation to superficial tissues and this is visible as an erythema. Some modalities produce deeper heating, for example microwave produces measurable levels of heating in muscles (Low, 1990). This increase in circulation is usually attributed to a local vasodilatation of the capillaries and arterioles produced by the direct effect of heat on their walls. Local axon reflexes may also operate, whereby sensory neurons have sensory collaterals connected to blood vessels, which again produce vasodilatation. The heat itself will produce an acceleration of metabolic rate (van't Hoff's rule) with a subsequent rise in metabolites in the area. These metabolites can cause a vasodilatation of the blood vessels by a direct action on their walls.

Overall, this increase in local circulation could well be responsible for reducing the level of nociceptive stimulation in a number of circumstances.

1. Pain associated with secondary muscle spasm or tension syndromes is attributed to local ischaemia resulting from partial occlusion of blood vessels within the muscle. Heat produces a hyperaemia within the muscle which resolves the ischaemia and reduces pain.
2. Where pain is the result of nociceptor stimulation by the chemicals produced or released as the result of trauma or inflammation, a local increase in circulation could remove these chemicals and therefore reduce pain.
3. Where local swelling is placing pressure on nociceptive endings and causing pain, local gentle heat could reduce the swelling via its circulatory effect and thus reduce pain. Cold therapy is probably more effective in this situation, however, as heat could exaggerate the swelling and make the situation worse in the acute stage.

Increased extensibility of collagen

Following injury there is a cascade of events which leads to bleeding, inflammation, swelling and pain (Halvorson, 1990). Unless normal function of the soft tissues is restored within a reasonable amount of time then collagen in soft tissues will shorten into the position in which it is being maintained. This loss of extensibility in collagen-rich structures such as ligaments and capsules associated with joints will lead to a loss of range of movement. Associated with this shortening of collagen fibres is the fact that they contain sensory endings which act as mechanoreceptors (type I, II and III) and nociceptors (type IV) (Wyke, 1967, 1972). The function of these receptors in ligaments and capsules will be affected adversely by this shortening. Mechanoreceptors will give an altered pattern of kinaesthetic information, and the nociceptors in capsules and ligaments will be stimulated earlier in their range of movement by tension. The overall effect of this shortening of collagen will be a loss of normal function, the only solution to which is to stretch the offending tissue to its normal length, without damaging it.

Heat has been shown to increase the extensibility of collagen (Gersten, 1955) and so it follows that the application of heat at therapeutic levels to shortened collagen would be useful prior to the application of manual or other techniques designed to stretch it. The increased extensibility of collagen would mean that the point at which nociceptive stimulation resulting from the stretch was reached would be further into range. Hence the increase in range before pain signalling was produced would be a useful effect of heat. This heat could be produced by a modality such as ultrasound which can have useful direct effects on scar tissue (Dyson and Suckling, 1978).

Pain Modulation

The Gate Control Theory

The gate control theory (see Chapter 9) of pain modulation was first proposed by Melzack and Wall (1965) and has been subject to revision by them (1982). There have been critics of the theory (Nathan. P. 1972) but the basis of the theory in pain modulation is still widely accepted. A detailed explanation of the theory has been given earlier in this book (see Chapter 9), consequently only its relevance to heat (and later cold) will be addressed here. If it is accepted that the thermal sensation produced by local heat is carried to the posterior horn of the spinal cord in large diameter myelinated nerves, then it fulfils the criteria for 'closing' the gate to predominantly small diameter nociceptive impulses. The synapses within the substantia gelatinosa and nucleus proprius will transmit the thermal sensation through to consciousness in preference to nociceptive (pain) impulses.

Descending Pain Suppression Systems

This system involves areas of the brainstem releasing endogenous opiates within the central nervous system (Basbaum and Fields, 1976) resulting in a reduction of the levels of pain perceived (see Chapter 9). For this system to be operative, the level of heat applied has to be sufficiently powerful to produce strong (almost noxious) afferent stimulation. Although this might be possible with water at a sufficiently high temperature, the levels of heating required are at a level close to those at which thermal injury could be produced (a burn) and so is not used in practice. However, it is likely that endogenous opiates are produced as the result of a strong placebo effect which operates when any form of physical therapy is applied to the patient, especially if the technology involved is impressive.

Methods of Heating Tissues

The distribution of heat within the tissues depends upon a number of factors, for example:

1. The amount of energy which is absorbed and converted to heat.
2. The specific heat of the tissues as this will affect its thermal properties.
3. Other biological systems such as blood flow, sweating etc., which have a marked effect upon the heat developed in the tissues.

Heat has to be transferred to the tissues by some mechanism and this could be by conduction or some other form of energy being absorbed and converted to heat by the body. A range of methods can be utilized to achieve this, and some will be described in the following pages.

Conductive Heating

Conductive heating as therapy involves the transfer of thermal energy from a heated substance to the body tissues by conduction. The thermal energy will move from the body containing the greatest thermal energy to the one with least. This transfer will continue until the thermal condition of both bodies is the same. Commonly a number of conductive methods of heating are used to modulate pain; some of which will now be described.

Immersion

Immersion of the whole body or body parts has been a popular method of treatment of joint pains for thousands of years. Today, patients are treated in hydrotherapy pools heated to around 37°C for a range of painful conditions ranging from rheumatoid arthritis and ankylosing spondylitis, to fractures and low back pain. This form of treatment has the added advantage that the physical forces which exist in the water can be used to assist or resist movements of patients as they exercise. Consequently pain can be reduced by the direct effect of heat, and also by the fact that exercises which are difficult on land can be used to produce mechanoreceptor stimulation in order to close the pain gate. Local immersion can be used when treating small parts of the body such as the hands and feet. This makes it a manageable form of therapeutic heat for patients to use at home.

Hot Packs

These 'hydrocollator' packs are made from cotton fabric cases which contain a silicate gel. The gel has the capacity to absorb large quantities of water. The packs are immersed in hot water at a temperature of around 80°C, and when some of this hot water is absorbed by the gel it contains a considerable amount of thermal energy. The pack is wrapped in dry terry towelling and applied directly to the part being treated. Heat is conducted to the body tissues from the hot pack, but some authorities feel that there is some electromagnetic radiation in the infrared spectrum radiated to the tissues by the pack (Low and Reed, 1990). The temperature rise developed by the hot pack after 20 minutes is approximately 2°C at a depth of 1 cm and 1°C at a depth of 2 cm in underlying muscle (Halvorson, 1990).

Electrically Heated Pads

These pads resemble small electric blankets and utilize the thermal effect of an electric current to produce heat in the wires they contain. The whole pad is wrapped in terry towelling and the heat is conducted to the tissues, plus possibly some radiated infrared. Generally these pads are applied to flat areas of the body such as the back or neck prior to some form of manual therapy.

Paraffin wax

Paraffin wax with some mineral oil added is kept in its molten state in a thermostatically heated bath at a temperature of around 44°C. The patient applies (by dipping) or has the molten wax applied to the part to be treated – usually the hands or feet. On contact with the patient the wax solidifies to form a thick coating of wax over the part. As the wax changes state from liquid to solid, kinetic energy is released in the form of latent heat, and this combined with the heat from conduction of the wax to the tissues forms the basis of the heating. Consequently a very pleasant, all-enveloping form of heat is developed which is very useful in managing the pain in conditions such as rheumatoid arthritis.

Absorption of electromagnetic rays

Infrared

Infrared electromagnetic radiation lies in a band between 750 and 4 000 000 nm in the electromagnetic spectrum. In the past infrared was described as Near (770–1400 nm) and Far (1400–3000 nm), both of which were used therapeutically. This has, however, been superseded by a classification of infrared A, B and C, with A equating to Near and B to Far, with C being the long infrared (Low and Reed, 1990).

Any heated body emits infrared radiations, but for therapeutic purposes specific generators have been developed to produce wavelengths which are most likely to be absorbed by the patient. True infrared treatment is carried out without contact between the patient and the generator and the thermal effect is achieved when the electromagnetic radiation is converted to thermal energy within the patient's tissues when it is absorbed. In physiotherapy practice two types of generator are available for the production of infrared.

1. Non-luminous generators. These utilize the principle of heating some material (e.g. fireclay or metal) via a wire carrying an electric current. Once heated, this material starts to emit electromagnetic radiation in the infrared range, with a peak emission of around the 4000 nm wavelength. Most of this infrared is absorbed and converted to heat in the epidermis which must then be conducted to deeper tissues in order to have a useful effect.

2. Luminous generators. Infrared is invisible to the human eye as its wavelengths do not stimulate the receptors in the retina. This generator is named because of the visible light which it also produces. The electromagnetic radiation is produced from a bulb which in terms of its infrared spectrum has a peak emission at a wavelength of around 1000 nm. This wavelength is absorbed and converted to thermal energy in the dermis, and so has a deeper penetration than the non-luminous generator. However, this is still relatively superficial and would have to be conducted to deeper tissues to have a useful effect.

In terms of pain relief, infrared is a very superficial form of heat and the only advantage enjoyed over conductive heating is its non-contact application. The treatment of deep painful structures depends upon the conduction of this superficial heat down to them, or for some of the mechanisms previously described (e.g. stimulation of superficial thermoreceptors connected to large diameter afferent nerve fibres closing the pain gate) to operate. In practice the application of gentle infrared has proved to be a very useful method of reducing pain prior to the application of other physiotherapeutic measures such as manipulative procedures or exercise.

Microwave

Microwaves are also a form of electromagnetic radiation which when absorbed by the patient's tissues are converted to heat. In Europe three wavelengths are commonly used, these being approximately 12, 32 and 69 cm. Of these, the most commonly used is the 12 cm wavelength, but this is considered by some authorities not to be the best wavelength for heating purposes (Low and Reed, 1990). The microwaves are produced by a specialized valve called a magnetron and conveyed via a coaxial cable to an antenna housed in an emitter. From here they are projected to the patient through an air space.

Microwaves penetrate the patient's tissues to a depth of up to 3 cm. They are absorbed most effectively by tissues with a high water content such as muscle, where they produce electron orbit distortion, dipole rotation and ionic movement, all of which produce heat. Consequently microwaves are useful when heat needs to be produced in deeper soft tissues, and as such can be of value in the management of soft tissue pain.

Shortwave diathermy

Shortwave diathermy is used to produce heat deep within the tissues. The technique of application is such that the patient's tissues are influenced predominantly by either an electrostatic or electromagnetic field. Shortwave diathermy operates at a wavelength of 11 m with a frequency of 27.12 MHz (see Chapter 15).

Capacitor heating is a method in which the patient's tissues are placed between two capacitor plates attached to the machine. A high frequency current oscillates between these two plates and the patient's tissues are subjected to a strong electrostatic charge first in one direction and then in the other. Overall this high frequency alternating electric current will exert an influence on charged particles within the field in such a way that heat is generated. The particles influenced are found in fluids (dipoles and ions) and in insulators (cell membranes and fat). Considerable heat is developed by the capacitor field method of application of shortwave diathermy. This is produced by the oscillation of these charged particles, but unfortunately the greatest levels of heating are produced in fat, and this limits the amount of energy that can be applied during the treatment.

In terms of its depth of penetration shortwave diathermy should, in theory, produce heating right the way through the tissues, as its name implies. In practice, however, this is not the case. The distribution of the field within the tissues and consequently the amount of heat developed will depend very much upon the arrangement of the tissues and positioning of the electrodes. Provided that an appropriate technique is chosen (Forster and Palastanga, 1985; Low and Reed, 1990), shortwave diathermy can form a useful method of applying heat to deep painful joints such as the hip. A number of important points of technique of application need to be observed in order to avoid potentially hazardous concentration of the field which could result in thermal damage to the patient's tissues (Forster and Palastanga, 1985; Low, 1990). The mechanisms involved in pain relief have been described earlier, but the effects of shortwave diathermy as a form of deep heat have made it a very popular method of managing painful joints associated with degenerative conditions such as arthritis. In some cases, however, for example osteoarthritis of the hip, the application of shortwave diathermy has produced an increase in pain, probably associated with vascular engorgement in the area.

Inductive heating utilizes the strong electromagnetic field which is generated around the middle section of an inductothermy cable carrying a high frequency current. The inductothermy cable is wound in such a way that the magnetic field passes through the target tissues. Eddy currents are produced around these magnetic lines of force in the patient's tissues of low impedence, e.g. muscle. The eddy currents themselves will generate a thermal effect within the tissues, and as such form a very useful method of fairly superficial heating. An advantage of inductothermy is that the cable can be wound totally around a limb or placed as a flat coil on a surface such as the back. The mechanism by which heat is generated, and the technique of application, makes inductothermy a useful form of heat in the treatment of musculoskeletal pain.

Pulsed electromagnetic energy is a form of treatment where the danger of thermal damage which exists with continuous shortwave diathermy has been reduced by breaking up the applied energy into very short pulses (e.g. 65 μs) of very high energy (e.g. 975 W). Thus the term 'pulsed shortwave' has been used to describe this form of treatment (Low and Reed 1990). The pulsed nature of the application means there is no appreciation of heat by the patient, but some authorities claim that there is still an imperceptible thermal effect taking place within the tissues (Lehmann and de Lateur, 1984). It has been speculated that the strong electromagnetic effect which is applied to injured tissues could have an effect on electrical potential of damaged cells (Hayne, 1984). The removal of the danger of thermal damage to the patient's tissues has made this a popular method of treatment. In the management of recent injuries the effect of pulsed electromagnetic energy to the tissues has been shown to accelerate repair and reduce pain (Bentall and Eckstein, 1975; Wilson, 1982; Barclay et al., 1983). In the management of painful conditions it has also been shown to be effective (Wagstaff et al., 1986).

Ultrasound

Therapeutic ultrasound is produced by the high frequency oscillation of a piece of piezoelectric material. The oscillation is the same as the frequency of the electric current producing it, and can be set at 0.75, 1, 1.5, or 3 MHz for treatment purposes. In the early days of its use ultrasound was applied as a method of producing heat. This was the result of the acoustic energy being absorbed and converted to heat at that point. Although the thermal effect is still recognized, other therapeutic effects have been identified which are useful in tissue repair (Dyson and Suckling, 1978; Dyson, 1987). Even when ultrasound is used in a pulsed mode, where short periods of ultrasound are interspersed with silences, a slight thermal effect is still produced.

The thermal effect of ultrasound, if sufficiently strong, could reduce pain perception by the mechanisms attributed to heat described earlier. In addition, it is probable that the mechanical stimulation of mechanoreceptors by ultrasound could have an effect on the transmission of nociceptive impulses at a spinal level (i.e. the pain gate).

The technique of application for ultrasound requires the patient's tissues to be linked to the applicator by a medium which can transmit the ultrasonic energy. This 'couplant' can be water or a special gel; air will not transmit ultrasound. As the ultrasonic beam is transmitted through the patient's tissues it undergoes marked attenuation as a result of: diffraction at tissue interfaces, scatter of the beam and absorption. The ultimate result of this attenuation is that at useful depths of penetration the beam has been reduced considerably in power. Consequently ultrasound is most useful when treating fairly superficial musculoskeletal conditions. For more detailed explanations of the effects, methods of application, dangers and contraindications the reader is referred to more specific electrotherapy texts (Forster and Palastanga, 1985; Low and Reed, 1990).

Ultrasound has proved to be useful in the treatment of sports injuries because of its effect on reduction of pain and acceleration of repair.

Cold

Cold has a long history of medical use and has been applied to patients to relieve pain for thousands of years (Licht 1984). Originally snow and ice was used for treatment and this had to be transported from mountainous regions, or stored in deep vaults after the winter. The result of this was to make 'ice' something of an expensive treatment, available only to those who could afford it. Once ice could be produced commercially in large quantities in the nineteenth century it became widely available and much cheaper. This led to a reduction in its appeal as a form of treatment.

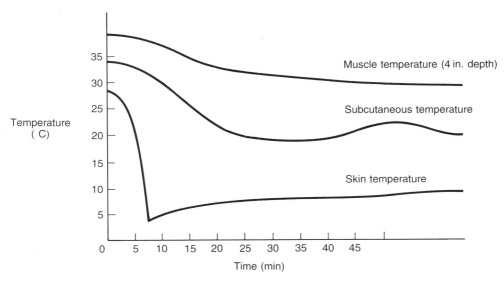

Fig. 16.1 The approximate temperature changes experienced in the tissues when an ice pack has been applied to the skin. (After Low and Reed, 1990.)

A reduction in the temperature of the tissues can also be achieved by spraying liquid spirits such as ether onto the skin where they change state into a gas, a process which requires large amounts of energy (latent heat). Plastic packs filled with gel can be cooled to very low temperatures and then be wrapped in towelling and applied to the patient. Heat is transferred from the patient to the pack by the process of conduction, the net result of which is a cooling of the tissues and warming of the pack. Cold compresses have always been used to reduce pain, and the 'cold sponge' still plays an important part in the management of painful sports injuries.

Today, ice forms the most common method of application of cold to the body. When ice is placed on the patient's skin, heat is conducted from the patient's body to the ice which then changes its state from solid to liquid – it melts. This simple process requires a considerable amount of energy. For example, 1 g of ice at 0°C requires 491 J of energy to form water at body temperature = 37°C, whereas 1 g of water at 0°C requires only 155 J to be raised to 37°C. This is an important fact in therapy and reinforces the need to use ice rather than just ice cold water for treatment purposes.

When ice is placed on the patient's skin dramatic and immediate cooling occurs in the superficial tissues which experience a temperature drop of 15°C (30–15°C) within 2–5 minutes. Deeper tissues are not cooled as much and usually only experience a temperature drop of about 5°C (35–30°C) and this can take up to 20 minutes to occur, longer if there is a thick layer of subcutaneous fat. In a normal, intact physiological system by far the greatest amount of cooling has occurred in the subcutaneous tissues, with only a small temperature reduction at a depth of 2.5 cm. Many of the effects of cooling are therefore achieved by the effect on skin and other superficial tissues. This suggests that the physiological finding of a reduced velocity of conduction when axons are cooled has little significance for all but the most superficial nerves. Many of the older theories for reduction of pain and spasticity cite reduced (or stopped) rates of conduction as the mechanism involved (Douglas and Malcomb, 1955), but the results of laboratory investigations on exposed nerves do not necessarily transfer to the intact physiological situation (see Figure 16.1).

Physiological effects of cold

The two physiological effects which are most likely to produce a reduction of pain are that on the local circulation and the effect on the nervous system.

Circulatory effects

The initial response of the skin to the application of cold is an attempt to preserve heat by producing a local vasoconstriction. The overall effect of this is for the skin to become very cold. At this stage the skin attempts to restore its normal temperature by producing a local vasodilatation to allow more warmed blood through the area. There then follow short periods of alternating vasoconstriction and vasodilatation as the circulation 'hunts' for its normal level in order to prevent tissue damage. This is called 'Lewis's hunting reaction' (Keatinge, 1961) where the circulation goes through periods of stasis and flushing as illustrated in Figure 16.2.

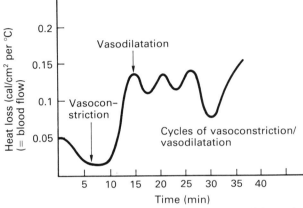

Fig. 16.2 A diagrammatic representation of 'Lewis's hunting reaction' to show the effect of prolonged ice application on the circulation through the tissues of the hand, as shown by measurement of heat loss from the skin, which equates to circulation. (After Keatinge, 1961.)

In the management of recent injuries, use is made of the initial vasoconstriction which can last for up to 10 minutes. The cold should be applied immediately to the injured area in an attempt to limit the extravasation of blood from damaged vessels into the tissues. This vasoconstriction is attributed to reflex activity via sympathetic fibres and the direct effect of cooled blood on the vessel walls. Pain may be reduced, or prevented, by a reduction of swelling (and therefore pressure) which itself stimulates nociceptors. In practice the cold application is usually followed by some form of compressive bandage.

The vasodilatation which occurs later, and then the alternate flushing effect, could usefully help reduce pain by removing substances produced as the result of trauma or inflammation which stimulate nociceptors. This effect is frequently utilized in the management of the more chronic conditions where established swelling contributes considerably

to the pain experienced. The circulatory effect of cold also has a benefical effect on the rate of repair.

Neural Effects

When ice is applied to normally innervated skin it acts as an extremely powerful sensory stimulus. This sensory experience can be used in the treatment of hypertonic muscle states and pain.

When muscles are in spasm (the reversible condition of hypertonic muscles following injury) or are spastic (as the result of an upper motor neuron lesion), pain is often a consequence because of the accumulation of metabolites within the muscle. Ice applied to these hypertonic muscles has been shown to have a dramatic effect in reducing their tone, which will allow the previously compressed vessels within to carry blood through the muscle and remove these metabolites. Frequently the secondary pain produced by spasm is greater than that from the injured tissue, and once the spasm has been reduced normal movement of the part can be encouraged. In cases of spasticity, ice can reduce tone sufficiently for a similar effect on pain, but is far more important for its role in allowing the application of techniques to remedy the spastic patterns of movement.

In terms of pain modulation via its sensory effect, the sensation of cold would be carried to the posterior horn by large diameter myelinated fibres and would thus have a marked effect on the perception of pain. As described elsewhere (see Chapter 9), the pain gate would be closed to nociceptive impulses.

The application of ice in itself to the tissues can be considered a noxious stimulus, and as such the afferent (noxious) stimuli generated could cause centres in the brainstem (notably the periaqueductal grey and raphe nucleus) to release endorphins at a spinal level and thus reduce pain. In clinical practice these theories are borne out, and ice can often produce a dramatic reduction in the level of pain patients perceive. Frequently the severe pain of acute joint inflammation experienced by patients with rheumatoid arthritis can be successfully reduced. Even the pain emanating from relatively deep structures responds well to cold application, and will allow other procedures to be implemented. Cold can in fact be considered as a treatment in its own right, but is frequently used as part of a comprehensive treatment programme. Cold can be applied in a number of ways to the body and the choice of packs, towels, immersion or ice massage depends upon the area to be treated, patient condition and facilities available to the therapist. Even the simplest method of application, ice cube massage, has been shown to be effective in reducing low back pain (Melzack *et al.*, 1980). The same technique is utilized in 'Cryokinetics', where ice is massaged over painful tissues, e.g. patellar tendon, in an attempt to remove inhibition of muscles due to pain. In this pain-reduced condition the quadriceps could be exercised more effectively (Halvorson, 1990).

Cooled gel packs can be applied to the patient, but it has been found that melting ice on the skin has a much greater cooling effect (McMaster *et al.*, 1978). Further details on methods of application, contraindications and other effects can be obtained from basic texts on the subject (Forster and Palastanga, 1985; Low and Reed, 1990).

Alternate application of heat and cold

It has been shown in the preceding pages that the process of adding energy to the tissues (heating) and removing heat (cooling) both have beneficial effects on pain. Contrast baths utilize a technique whereby the tissues are first placed in hot water (40–50°C) and then into iced water (10–15°C). The immersion time can be set at 4 minutes hot to 1 minute cold, or the part is left in the heated or cooled water until the patient gets used to the sensation when it is switched to the other bath. The total treatment time is usually around 30 minutes. Contrast baths are claimed to have a marked effect on the circulation, a claim supported by the vivid erythema produced. The circulatory effect would modulate pain, and the strong alternate sensory stimulus would affect the transmission of nociceptive traffic – both by the mechanisms already described.

Heat versus cold

In clinical practice there are circumstances when heat is preferable to cold and vice versa. For example, in the management of acute sports injuries cold is preferred by the therapist as it limits the local extravasation of blood into the tissues and therefore limits the pain produced by swelling. It could be the case that the application of heat in this acute situation might make matters worse as the vasodilatation produced could increase bleed-

ing and therefore pain. It has been claimed that athletes tolerate cold application badly (Halvorson, 1990), but it is undoubtedly the treatment of choice in the acute stage. Cold application is usually followed by the application of compressive bandaging which should help maintain the restriction in bleeding. Cold would be the method of choice for the first few days, but as the lesion becomes more chronic, then the application of some form of therapeutic heat might be considered. If the problem were to be fibrosis of the lesion which also involved the surrounding tissues, then ultrasound, microwave or shortwave diathermy could be applied in an attempt to increase extensibility, and allow the application of more vigorous stretching techniques.

Cold has been shown to have a dramatic effect on muscle spasm, but occasionally the application of cold can make the spasm worse. If the patient problem being managed is spasm of muscles surrounding an acute neck or back pain, the irritative effect of ice combined with the weight of the pack, which for safety reasons has to be placed on top of the part, could increase the tone of surrounding muscles. In this situation the application of some form of gentle heat to the area in the form of non-contact infrared, microwave or shortwave diathermy might be used. As an alternative, conductive heating applied as heated hot packs or electrically heated pads with the patient lying on top of them might be used. Once the desired effect on muscle tone has been achieved using either heat or cold, other manual techniques can be applied.

Occasionally the determined preference of the patient may have to influence the choice of therapeutic modality used by the therapist. The elderly do not usually tolerate cold well and frequently associate the level of pain and stiffness of their condition to the cold weather. If, in the therapist's opinion, the idea of the application of cold so terrifies the patient that the benefits anticipated are outweighed by the psychological stress, then some form of therapeutic heat would seem to be a reasonable alternative. If, however, the therapist can persuade the patient to have a short trial treatment, then frequently the benefits experienced, especially on their pain, can be so great that they will tolerate the discomfort and allow cold to be used.

Anatomical considerations might also affect selection of the treatment modality. The hip for example is such a deep joint that the only effective form of heat therapy is shortwave diathermy. It is highly doubtful whether the application of cold would penetrate as deeply as the hip joint, even if it were practical to apply ice in this region. The same arguments apply to the sacroiliac joint, but here ice can have a useful effect on pain via its effect on the soft tissues behind the joint.

The eventual decision as to which modality should be applied rests with the physiotherapist who, as a result of their patient assessment, will formulate a clinical diagnosis and patient problem list. At this stage of problem solution the advantages, disadvantages and anticipated effects of each modality will be considered in order to choose the most effective treatment. Once a course of treatment has been implemented, the results of every treatment session are reassessed and appropriate changes made to the programme.

References

Barclay, V., Collier, R. and Jones, A. (1983) Treatment of various hand injuries by pulsed electromagnetic energy. *Physiotherapy*, **69**, 186–8

Bentall, R. and Eckstein, H. (1975) A trial involving pulsed electromagnetic energy on children undergoing orchidopexy. *Kinderchirurgie*, **17**, 380–2

Douglas, W. and Malcomb, J. (1955) The effect of localized cooling on conduction in cat nerves. *J. Physiol.*, **130**, 53–71

Dyson, M. and Suckling, J. (1978) Stimulation of tissue repair by ultrasound. *Physiotherapy*, **64** (4), 105–8

Dyson, M. (1987) Mechanisms involved in therapeutic ultrasound. *Physiotherapy*, **73**(3), 116–20

Forster, A. and Palastanga, N. (1985) *Clayton's Electrotherapy, Theory and Practice*, 9th edn, Bailliere Tindall London

Gersten, J. (1955) Effect of ultrasound upon tendon extensibility. *Am. J. Phys. Med.*, **34**, 362–9

Halvorson, G. (1990) Therapeutic heat and cold for athletic injuries. *Physician Sportsmed.*, **18** (5), 87–94

Keatinge, W. (1961) Cold vasodilatation after adrenalin. *J. Physiol.*, **159**, 101–10

Lehmann, J. and de Lateur, B. (1984) Therapeutic heat. In Lehmann, J. (ed.), *Therapeutic Heat and Cold*, 3rd edn, Williams and Wilkins, Baltimore, Md

Licht, S. (1984) History of therapeutic heat and cold. In Lehmann, J. (ed.), *Therapeutic Heat and Cold*, 3rd edn, Williams and Wilkins, Baltimore, Md

Low, J. and Reed, M. (1990) *Electrotherapy Explained: Principles and Practice*, Butterworth Heinemann, Oxford

McMaster, W., Liddle, S. and Waugh, T. (1978) Laboratory evaluation of various cold therapy modalities. *Am. J. Sports Med.*, **6** 291–4

Melzack, R. and Wall, P. (1965) Pain mechanisms: a new theory. *Science*, **150**, 971–9

Melzack, R. and Wall, P. (1982) *The Challenge of Pain*, Harmondsworth, Penguin

Melzack, R., Jeans, M., Stratford, J. and Monks, R. (1980) Ice massage and transcutaneous electrical stimulation: comparison of treatment for low back pain. *Pain*, **9**, 209–17

Nathan, P. (1976) The gate control theory of pain: a critical review. *Pain*, **99**, 123–58

Wagstaff, P., Wagstaff, S. and Downey, M. (1986) A pilot study to compare the efficacy of continuous and pulsed magnetic energy (shortwave diathermy) on the relief of low back pain. *Physiotherapy*, **72**, 563–6

Wilson, D. (1974) Comparison of shortwave diathermy and pulsed electromagnetic energy in the treatment of soft tissue injuries. *Physiotherapy*, **60**, 309–10

Wyke, B. (1967) The neurology of joints. *Anns. R. Coll. Surg. Engl.*, **41**,: 25–50

Wyke, B. (1972) Articular neurology – a review. *Physiotherapy*, **58**, 94–9

17   Manipulative procedures

PETER E. WELLS

Introduction

The use of the hands for skilful and dextrous treatment is central to the practice of physiotherapy. Direct intervention by physiotherapists to alleviate pain is most clearly illustrated by those aspects of professional practice which involve various forms of handling and manipulative therapy. As the surgeon is typified by the cutting, repairing and replacing of tissues so is the physiotherapist by therapeutic handling and the various types of passive movement.

From the earliest part of their training physiotherapists begin to acquire the refined manual skills which make up the various manipulative procedures including massage and passive joint mobilization. However, the so-called 'art' of manipulation is less a matter of acquiring ever more techniques, but more the skilful assessment of when and how they should be used. In this respect the selection, application and assessment of manipulative procedures for the treatment of pain is arguably the most 'skilful' aspect of manipulation.

Whatever the emphasis given in any particular case to the use of manipulative procedures, these are always considered alongside such things as the need for muscle re-education, relaxation, postural realignment and careful education of the patient. There is evidence that a combination of such treatment is more effective than the use of any one of them alone (Coxhead *et al.*, 1981).

General indications

Manipulative procedures are applied to treating parts of the musculoskeletal system when pain and restricted movement, or occasionally excessive movement, have resulted from trauma, degenerative change and long-term postural stress. A large and varied range of ailments, the origins of which lie in some dysfunction or malfunction of neuromusculoskeletal structures, respond to carefully selected and suitably modified manipulative treatment. The tissues of the spine, trunk, head and limbs are equally amenable to treatment by these methods.

The neuromusculoskeletal structures include the joints with their ligaments and joint capsules, muscles and tendons including the tenoperiosteal junctions, the cartilaginous junctions between the vertebral bodies referred to as discs and the fascia which commonly exists in dense sheets which envelop the muscular compartments of the body and forms the subcutaneous connective tissues (see also Chapter 18) and neural tissues.

Classification of manipulative procedures

Since the subject of manipulation is bedevilled by semantics, it has come to mean different things to different people. For example, many of the general public and even the medically qualified associate manipulation with high velocity thrust techniques and little else, and many seem to believe that it involves very forceful and even aggressive procedures.

To those who regularly employ manual therapy in their day-to-day clinical work it covers a wide range of procedures from the very gentle to the more firm or vigorous.

Clearly there must be a framework within which can be defined the many procedures which are commonly employed across the wide spectrum known as manipulative therapy. Such a framework, now used by most physiotherapists, is as follows:

1. Soft tissue techniques (massage).
2. Regional mobilization.
3. Localized mobilization.

4. Regional manipulation.
5. Localized manipulation.

It should be made clear what is meant by each of these categories. First what is the difference between **mobilization** and **manipulation**?

Mobilization consists of passive movement techniques usually employing repetitive movement, which is under the patient's control. This means that if the patient for any reason communicates to the operator that he wishes the technique to be stopped then it can be. The patient is, of course, relaxed throughout and does not control the procedure by any active movement on his part. Repetitive oscillatory movements to relax muscles, relieve pain or carefully elongate tight structures come under the grouping of **mobilization**.

A **manipulation**, on the other hand, consists of a single, high velocity thrust applied to a joint or series of joints and soft tissues. This procedure gaps or moves the joint very quickly and is carried out to create extra freedom of movement and to relieve pain. Because of its speed and the fact that it is only ever attempted while the patient is relaxed, the technique is not under the patient's control. It is over almost before he knows it has been done.

The categories that have been set down may now be defined and discussed.

Soft Tissue Techniques (Massage)

Whereas this range of procedures is sometimes grouped together as 'massage' the tendency now is to use the expression 'soft tissue techniques', since the word massage has acquired a very general and non-medical connotation. This is unfortunate since skilled massage administered by the medically trained and experienced physiotherapist can give very beneficial effects in a number of conditions, especially orthopaedic and rheumatological ones.

The growth in the popularity of generalized and non-specific massage, administered by an assortment of non-medical masseuses and aimed at helping the individual relax, has been accompanied by a decline in the widespread use of massage by physiotherapists. One reason for the more restricted use of massage within physiotherapy is that recent decades have seen the growth in our knowledge of neuromusculoskeletal biomechanics and neurology. As a result it is becoming clear that many problems previously thought to arise principally within soft tissues, such as muscles, do in fact owe more of their cause to joint disturbances and disturbances of nervous system mobility and sensitivity. These problems then manifest themselves secondarily in muscles, fascia and so forth, e.g. fibrositis. In situations where patients complain of pain, tenderness and 'stiffness' of muscles, e.g. those of the neck and scapular area, more attention is now placed upon analysing very specifically the joint and movement abnormalities underlying the problem and less emphasis given to treating purely the soft tissue disturbances accompanying it.

Nevertheless, massage or soft tissue techniques maintain a rightful place in the field of natural medical alternatives to drug therapy and surgery. Their use is now restricted to very specific instances when they are judged to be particularly beneficial. In the treatment of painful musculoskeletal conditions and impaired function, massage is usually used in conjunction with other passive joint mobilizing procedures. Where this is so, it goes without saying that each procedure is assessed independently, both for its inclusion in treatment and also its effects.

It is interesting to note the results of an investigation by Danneskiold-Samsøe *et al.* (1986) into the effects of massage. The reporting, by 21 patients out of 26 with myofascial pain, of a steady improvement in their symptoms during a course of ten massage treatments (each of 30–45 min) was accompanied by a gradual decline in the increase (following each massage session) of plasma myoglobin concentration. A parallel gradual decline in muscle tension was also reported. It is clear from this investigation that the effects of massage are not all in the mind (important though that is) but that measurable biochemical changes may be observed as a result, and that these changes accompany the subjective reporting of improvement by patients with what is termed in this investigation '**myofascial pain syndrome**'.

While it is known that massage often produces a sense of well-being and may gain the confidence of the patient, its use by physiotherapists is perhaps best confined to those patients whose pain or other symptoms can be shown to arise from their muscles or other soft tissues. Those physiotherapists working in the field of psychiatry may take exception to this rule.

The principal massage techniques used for the relief of pain are:

1. Effleurage.
2. Stroking.
3. Kneading (petrissage).
4. Vibration.
5. Frictions.

Different techniques clearly have different effects and therefore reduction in pain during and following their use may be achieved by different mechanisms. It is easy to speculate upon some of these mechanisms but clearly it is not known for certain how the results observed are mediated. The selection of techniques will depend upon the cause as well as the intensity and reactivity (irritability) of the pain and other symptoms.

Effleurage

This technique consists of a stroking movement in the direction of the flow in the veins and lymphatics. The essential aspects of technique which will ensure the maximal effect are:

1. The relaxation of the hands which must mould to the shape of the part being treated.
2. The use of even pressure, the degree and rate of which must vary in order to be maximally effective but not aggravate the patient's symptoms. This pressure must be maintained throughout the movement.
3. Each stroke must be carried to the nearest group of superficial lymphatic nodes. When small irregular areas are treated the technique is carried out using the fingers or thumb.

The effects of effleurage may be summarized as:

1. The hastening of the flow of blood towards the heart by mechanical pressure upon the superficial veins.
2. The acceleration of lymph flow in a similar manner.
3. The stretching of subcutaneous soft tissues.
4. The increase of circulation in the skin.
5. The stimulation of pressure and touch receptors in the skin.

The use of effleurage for the relief of pain is particularly justified when soft tissue oedema (especially that causing very high tissue pressure) and the resultant high concentration of metabolic by products such as histamine bradykinin etc., appear to be contributing to the patient's discomfort or frank pain.

Part of the effect in modulating pain may occur as a result of alterations in somatosensory biasing in the central nervous system by the considerable sensory stimulation resulting from the technique.

Stroking

This technique is similar to effleurage but exerts less pressure and is performed in any direction on the body surface. When employed in the presence of pain, it is always slow, light and rhythmical. The whole palmar surface of the relaxed hand is used with even pressure, and care must be taken not to tickle or irritate the patient when lifting off the hands at the end of each stroke.

The effect of stroking is purely sensory. When carried out in a careful, rhythmical manner for a period of time its effect in calming and relaxing the tense and anxious patient may be considerable. Conversely, if there is any sign that the patient does not like being handled in this way and cannot accept the technique then it is, of course, abandoned. Any decrease in pain which results is probably due to sedative sensory effects and the effect upon the reduction of tension and the 'holding' effect of muscles.

Kneading (petrissage)

The various techniques of kneading are primarily directed at muscles and the connective tissue coverings which surround and divide them. The subcutaneous tissues are also affected. The tissues are either:

1. Compressed and then released, as with circular kneading, a circular movement is carried out with one or both hands with pressure exerted inwards and upwards. Small areas are treated with the fingertips or thumbs.
2. Grasped, lifted up, squeezed and then relaxed as with the technique of picking-up. Alternatively, the muscles may be grasped with both hands and lifted up, the hands then moving alternately backwards across the direction of the muscle fibres, as with wringing (Figure 17.1).
3. Rolled between the fingers and thumb with the hands lying flat on the surface, as with the technique of skin rolling. The tissues are rolled

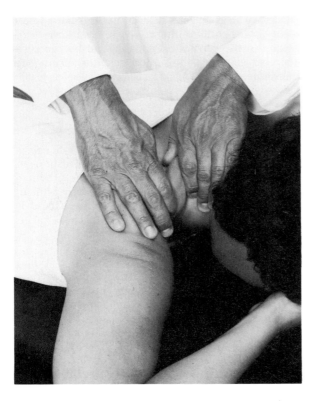

Fig. 17.1   Wringing. An example of a soft tissue technique to stretch and relax sore, tense muscles often found accompanying a chronic joint problem.

forwards by the thumbs and backwards by the fingers.

The effect of the kneading techniques are similar to those of effleurage as far as the circulation of the tissues being manipulated is concerned. In addition, muscle tissues are stretched by the slow deep technique and a mobilizing effect may be achieved. The same occurs with the skin as a result of skin rolling. Slow, rhythmic kneading may also have a general sedative effect.

The use of kneading techniques for pain relief is mainly indicated in the more chronic situations where sore, tender, aching muscles frequently accompany underlying joint problems, e.g. in the paraspinal muscles and the other large muscles of the neck and trunk, particularly in the case of chronic recurrent cervical and lumbar spinal problems. In these situations, it is clearly vital to assess and treat any underlying joint problems as the

first priority, thereafter employing soft tissue techniques, such as kneading when indicated. The same, of course, applies to muscle pain and tenderness in the upper and lower limbs and its relation to spinal or peripheral joint problems and neural mobility.

Where pain of a more severe nature and possibly a more recent onset is being treated, kneading techniques must be used with great care since any severe or irritable symptoms will be easily stirred, e.g. when treating a haematoma in a recently traumatized muscle. Both the rhythm and depth of the techniques must be adapted to the patient's response guided by a continuous assessment of the symptoms throughout the treatment session. Another example of this situation would be the early treatment of a cervical whiplash injury (i.e. within the first few weeks).

Vibration

This technique is a fine form of tremor conveyed through the hands or fingertips. It is a difficult technique to achieve. It is used in order to induce relaxation in muscles where soft tissue trauma, such as tears and haematomas are accompanied by severe muscle spasm. It is often the earliest and safest technique which may be given directly over a muscle haematoma for example.

The rationale for using vibrations in the treatment of acute soft tissue pain is two-fold: first, fine vibration appears to have a sedative effect. In situations where pressure and stretching of the soft tissues is not tolerated, vibrations may be the first step in establishing a manual approach and gaining some muscle relaxation. Secondly, the fine mechanical effect in and around the centre of the lesion may assist in hastening the resolution of inflammation.

It is interesting that many who suffer from chronic, recurrent muscular aches and pains find the use of a battery or electrically operated vibrator, directly applied to the affected muscles, gives considerable relief of their symptoms (see Chapter 9).

Frictions

These are small penetrating movements, performed by the thumb or fingertips, in which the superficial tissues are moved on the deeper ones (Figure 17.2). They may be done in a circular or transverse

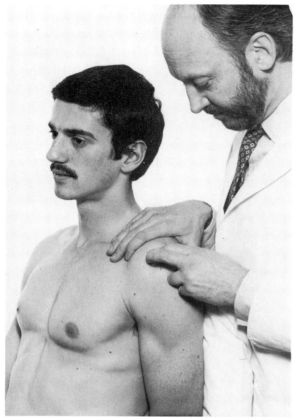

Fig. 17.2 Friction. Deep transverse frictions to the supraspinatus tendon. An unresolving tendinitis can be treated with this deep, localized stretching technique across the direction of the fibres of the tendon.

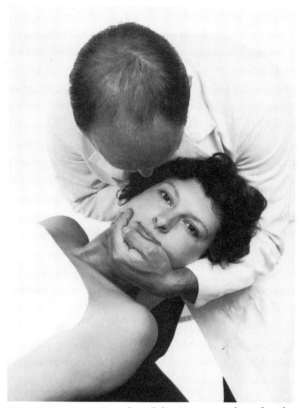

Fig. 17.3 A rotational mobilization procedure for the cervical spine. By positioning the appropriate level of the neck midway between flexion and extension, this generalized technique can emphasize motion at that level. The movement is a repetitive oscillatory one, carried out through a prescribed arc of the available range of cervical rotation, invariably away from the painful side.

direction. The painful structure being treated must be located very accurately and deep friction transmitted by a gradually increasing pressure. Transverse frictions are the most commonly used, particularly with ligamentous injuries and tendon and tendon sheath disorders. Initially, full pressure and friction cannot be given because of the local pain response, but gradually as the friction continues a deeper penetration can be achieved as the tissues appear to become numbed. Cyriax (1984) emphasizes that in order to be maximally effective, frictions must be very accurately localized, of sufficient depth and carried out for a sufficient length of time (up to approximately 20 min).

Frictions have a number of effects which may explain their usefulness in the treatment of certain types of painful soft tissue disorders such as muscular lesions, lesions of tendons (both with and without a sheath), ligamentous lesions and traumatic and other causes of pain and restriction in the capsule of the small joints such as the interphalangeal joints.

The effects of frictions are as follows:

1. They cause a local hyperaemia.
2. They aid in restoring mobility in various structures which, from their nature or position, tend to develop adhesions after injury or strain, e.g. in sprains of the medial collateral ligament of

the knee and tears within muscles such as the hamstrings.

3. They assist in restoring the natural smooth gliding between a tendon and its sheath in tenosynovitis.

There are clear indications and contraindications for these important techniques (Cyriax, 1984). Using them in order to decrease pain and avoid the formation of dense scar tissue will facilitate the restoration of more normal movement. In doing so the natural repeated stretch of the soft tissues, without which scar tissue will always shorten (Evans, 1980), will be quickly restored.

Regional Mobilization

Whereas trauma and degenerative changes frequently give rise to localized musculoskeletal disorders, in the spine it is common to find regional disturbances in movement and function associated with generalized stiffness and accompanied by varying degrees of pain.

It is in such situations that regional mobilization techniques, which affect a group of joints and their soft tissues, are used. At the same time, by careful positioning, it is possible to direct the effects of regional mobilization to a particular spinal level if this is considered necessary. As an example. regional rotation techniques are frequently employed for the cervical and lumbar spine to treat signs and symptoms arising from one vertebral level (Figure 17.3). Similarly, with some peripheral joint complexes, e.g. the elbow and wrist, a technique may affect a group of articulations while aimed at the treatment of pain arising from one of them (Figures 17.4 and 17.9).

Included in this category of regional mobilization is traction, a stretching force which is applied in general along the longitudinal axis of the tissues. The precise magnitude of the traction force, the position in which it is given and the time for which it is carried out may all bear upon its effect, and so it is important to administer traction in a very accurate and predetermined way.

This is best carried out with specialized apparatus devised to do just that (Figures 17.5, 17.6). However, this 'mechanical' traction is still clearly within the field of manipulation since the body tissues are passively moved, albeit in this case by a machine rather than by the operator's hands.

Spinal traction may also, of course, be adminis-

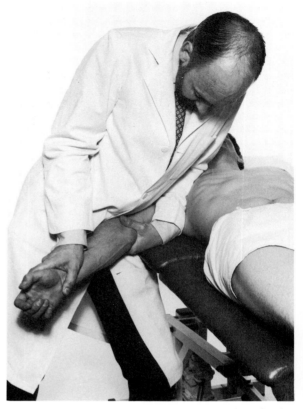

Fig. 17.4 A generalized mobilization procedure for the elbow complex exploring both the pain response and movement characteristics towards the end of the extension range while an adduction stress is applied. Useful both as an examination technique, where necessary, and a treatment for certain types of elbow problem, this procedure does not determine which specific part of the elbow joint complex is at fault.

tered by the hands, but it has the disadvantage that the physiotherapist can only sustain it for a short period of time.

Localized Mobilization

In order to direct treatment in a specific way and assess it accurately, it is important to be able to locate the source of a pain precisely to a particular joint. For example, at the elbow differentiation must be made between the humeroradial, humeroulnar, superior radioulnar and even 'radioannular' articulations. In the same way, where a vertebral cause is giving rise to local or referred pain, it is

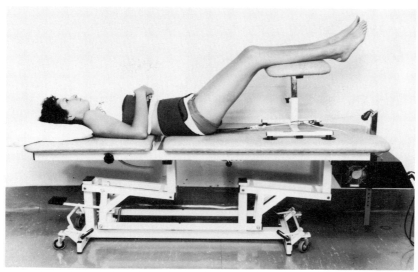

Fig. 17.5 Lumbar traction. An extremely effective passive technique for the relief of many types of lumbar pain and sciatic symptoms. The degree of hip flexion is used to determine the mid position of the relevant lumbar vertebral level being treated, and the legs are supported accordingly. Sustained or intermittent traction can be given as with the cervical spine. The lower thoracic levels can be treated with some modifications in positioning of the patient and the harness.

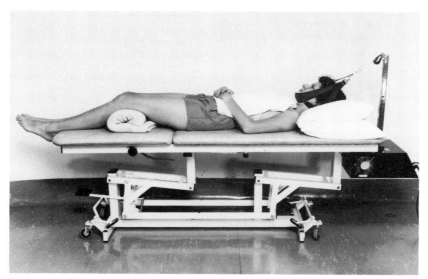

Fig. 17.6 Cervical traction. The level to which the tractive force is directed is determined by the degree of flexion of the head-upon-neck or neck-upon-trunk. In this instance, the cervicothoracic junctional region is being treated. Motorized traction such as this may be used to apply a sustained (not the same as constant) or intermittent force to take into account the degree of pain or stiffness to be treated. The upper thoracic levels can be treated with a similar arrangement.

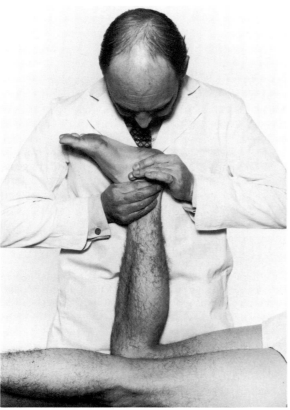

Fig. 17.7 A localized mobilization technique for the subtalar joint, utilizing the small degree of accessory rotational movement (rotational 'joint play') normally present.

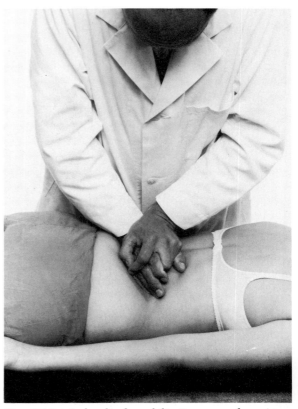

Fig. 17.8 A localized mobilization procedure in a posteroanterior direction being performed at the 4th lumbar level. A small but definite range of accessory movement can be obtained, localized by a small area of the hypothenar eminence of the underneath hand. The movement may be a sustained or an oscillatory one.

important to be able to locate precisely the level of the spine from which the symptoms are arising. When this has been done, localized mobilization procedures (Figures 17.7, 17.8) consisting of passive accessory or physiological movements are employed to move the joint or mobility segment at fault in a carefully controlled way (a mobility segment of the spine can be defined as the movable junction between two adjacent vertebrae, e.g. L5 and S1 including their associated joints and soft tissues).

While every attempt is made to localize forces with great care to the joint or the spinal level being treated, no manipulative procedure can ever be entirely localized since, especially in the vertebral column, the adjacent levels are bound to move somewhat also. Even so, it comes as a surprise to many observers to see how accurate such

techniques can be in the hands of an experienced manipulative physiotherapist.

Regional Manipulation

The majority of joint problems resolve with the use of regional or localized mobilizations and do not need a manipulative thrust technique. In the case of spinal dysfunction, a number of patients generally require one or more 'manipulations' to clear their symptoms and restore good functional movement.

If the restriction of movement affects a number of adjacent segments in the spine then a regional manipulation may be used (Figure 17.10). By care-

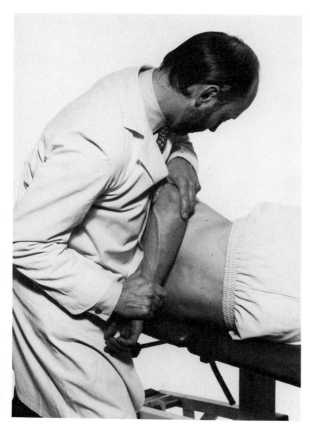

Fig. 17.9 A generalized mobilization procedure to the glenohumeral joint to improve the 'hand behind back' movement. The three components of this physiological movement – extension, adduction and internal rotation – can be mobilized separately in this position.

ful positioning and control fundamental to all manipulative procedures, these high velocity techniques of controlled amplitude can effectively regain movement simultaneously at a number of adjacent levels. However, such regional procedures are employed on far fewer occasions than the carefully localized ones.

Localized Manipulation

When mobilization has failed to gain completely the degree of joint mobility reasonably expected it may be necessary to carry out a localized manipulation (Figure 17.11). By careful positioning and a very precise application of the force used, either with short or long leverage, a degree of movement

can be obtained suddenly at a joint previously abnormally tight and restricted. The speed employed is crucial in most cases for a successful manipulation, both in the application of the force and in its release. The amplitude of the movement used is always small and very controlled, as part of the built-in safety of each manoeuvre. Considerable skill is required to carry out localized manipulation successfully and such skill takes much time and practice to acquire.

It is doubtful whether any localized manipulation is ever as entirely localized as the title suggests. Even with the most careful positioning and force application adjacent joints and tissues invariably receive some of the stress imparted by the technique. The point is that this is minimal when expertly carried out and, of course, far more localized than a generalized manipulation seeks to be.

Localized manipulation is mainly used in the treatment of spinal problems. However, it is occasionally used in the treatment of peripheral joints, e.g. the glenohumeral joint, sacroiliac joint and the small joints of the hand or foot.

Manipulation under anaesthetic (MUA)

There may come a point in treatment when mobilization and manipulation cease to improve the situation further, or progress is exceedingly slow. At this stage, the surgeon or physician in overall charge of the patient may decide that a manipulation of the spinal level or peripheral joint concerned should be carried out under an anaesthetic. While that decision is the doctor's alone, it will usually be made after consultation with the physiotherapist who has been carrying out the treatment. Obviously a procedure that can be achieved while the patient is conscious and able to respond is preferable to that performed while the individual is anaesthetized and cannot react. The subjective and physical responses to any manoeuvre are what guides treatment and the degree of gentleness or vigour used. The conscious subject can report changes in their symptoms immediately and physical testing likewise will give essential information quickly. However, if fibrosis in the soft tissues of the joint is so dense that a firm manoeuvre is required which would be too uncomfortable for the unanaesthetized patient, or if they are unable to relax or are of a body build which prevents the procedure from being carried out,

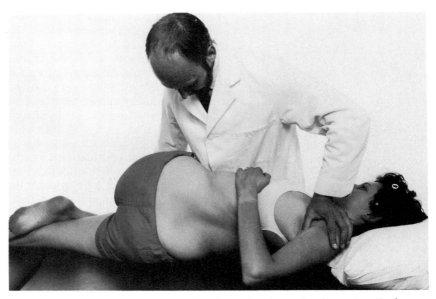

Fig. 17.10 A generalized rotational manipulation for the mid to lower lumbar spine. Such a procedure is usually performed to improve the local signs and symptoms arising from regional stiffness in the low back. Even though the force and amplitude are carefully controlled, such a procedure would not be used in the presence of segmental hypermobility within the area.

then the use of an anaesthetic may provide a way forward.

The use of this technique has been criticized on the grounds that it is like taking a sledgehammer to crack a nut. However, when used sparingly and for specific indications the results may be seen to justify the means.

Maitland (1986) has pointed out that 'follow-up' physiotherapy is only indicated if the symptoms have not responded sufficiently to MUA. If complete relief of symptoms is gained then follow-up treatment is unnecessary. He also makes the following important observation:

> Where manipulation of the conscious patient has failed, MUA may be successful. The converse is also true. Sometimes . . . patients may require a balance of both.

The treatment of pain and abnormal tension in the nervous system by manipulative procedures

Abnormal mechanics in the nervous system has long been recognized as a source of signs and symptoms, especially of pain. The passive straight leg raising test (SLR), passive neck flexion test (PNF), and the prone knee bending test (PKB) are used routinely to detect abnormal or adverse tension in the nervous system. Many orthopaedic and neurosurgeons include early and regular passive straight leg raising in the postoperative management of those who have undergone spinal surgery, in order to prevent fibrotic restriction of the sciatic nerve and nerve roots. Conversely some cases of successful disc surgery fail to gain total relief of their symptoms or suffer a recurrence of symptoms in spite of evidence that no further disc prolapse has occurred. Why is this so?

The nervous system, both central and peripheral, including the sympathetic system, is a dynamic, mobile entity, with its own mechanics. It adapts to body movement by virtue of being free to move in relation to its surrounding tissues, the interface, and also by the development of tension within itself as its 'relaxed' (and somewhat folded) state is stretched.

The nervous system must continue to conduct impulses during a remarkable range and variety of body movements. The protective coverings and connective tissues of the system must adapt mechanically to even the extreme ranges of body movement without abnormal and harmful forces developing within the system.

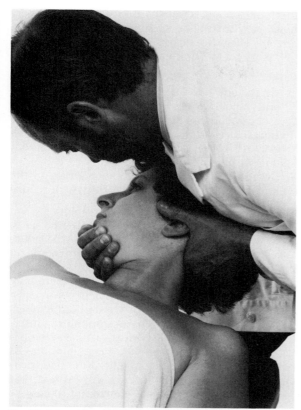

Fig. 17.11 A localized posteroanterior thrust technique to mobilize the left atlanto-occipital joint. The cervical spine is well short of full rotation and a small direct thrust with the left hand directed through the plane of the joint achieves the movement.

Physiotherapists define abnormal neural tension (ANT) as **the abnormal mechanical or physiological response produced from the nervous system when the normal movement and stretch capabilities are tested.** Muscles protect nerves, a function clearly demonstrated by a limitation of the range of passive straight leg raise in an individual suffering from sciatica, where hamstring spasm prevents the disturbance of hyperalgesic (pathologically sensitive) nerve tissue. Abnormally raised muscle tone (spasm) and pain are the major sign and symptom of abnormal neural tension, as demonstrated in the aforementioned test. Such states are extremely common in the field of musculoskeletal pain and dysfunction, to the point where it is perhaps more correct to talk in terms of the *neuro* musculo skeletal system.

To summarize then, the subject of the examina-

tion and treatment of abnormal neural tension has developed and extended in recent years based upon the hypothesis that numerous common musculo-skeletal complaints appear as a result of an interference with the, normally, painless mobility of the neural structures. Furthermore, that the main pathological changes, both pathophysiological (inflammation) and, later pathomechanical (fibrosis and restricted movement) occur principally in the connective tissues of the nervous system.

Sir Sidney Sunderland, the great neurologist, summarized it so:

> From these considerations it emerges that the role of the connective tissue components is to preserve the structural integrity of the nerve trunk and in doing so it also protects the contained nerve fibres. Should anything happen to damage and threaten the integrity of the nerve trunk, fibroblasts will react in a way calculated to restore the tensile strength of the nerve. This they do by depositing collagen and forming scar tissue. However, though this reaction is responsible for restoring the tensile strength of the nerve, the elasticity of the nerve is sacrificed and the formation of adhesions attaching the nerve to its bed costs the nerve its mobility. (Sunderland, 1989)

Numerous soft tissue afflictions are found with careful differentiating tests to have an ANT component, sometimes a major one. Examples are:

- Upper limb disorder ('repetitive strain injury').
- Chronic post-whiplash syndrome.
- Achilles tendonitis.
- Tension headaches.
- Tennis and golfer's elbow.
- Groin strain.
- Shin splints (tibialis anterior syndrome).
- Chronic sciatica.
- Acute and chronic anterior knee pain and hip pain syndromes.
- Chronic facial pain.
- Shoulder 'capsulitis'.
- Pulled calf, pulled hamstrings.
- Chronic sprained ankle pain.
- Low back pain, neck pain, thoracic pain

All these painful conditions and more are seen and treated by physiotherapists and physiotherapists have *uniquely* developed an array of tests to identify when an alteration in nervous system mobility is contributing to an individual's pain and other symptoms and to an alteration in function.

Maitland in 1978 published his first account of the Slump Test, Elvey in 1979 described the Brachial Plexus Tension Test (or Upper Limb Tension

Test), and in recent years Butler and Gifford have described further methods of testing (1989) and physiotherapists continue to investigate the scientific as well as the clinical validity of these tests.

The basis of all these procedures to detect altered neural tension is to differentiate between joints, muscles and nerves as the source of symptoms and signs. As an example, we know that the pain of an ankle inversion injury, particularly following repeated sprains, may become persistently troublesome. Nitz, Dobner and Kersey (1985) describe how grade II and III ankle sprains produce a high percentage of peroneal and tibial nerve injuries and that, particularly with grade III ankle sprains, this peripheral nerve injury contributes to the clinical disability including a weakness of gastrocnemius muscle. With this observation in mind it is interesting to test the passive straight leg raise (SLR) in such cases, but with the foot held in plantar flexion and inversion. Held thus the familiar pain over the lateral ligament and lateral border of the foot is seen to increase markedly with raising the leg (hip flexion with knee maintained in extension) and diminish with the lowering of the leg (foot maintained throughout in the same degree of plantar flexion and inversion). The rise and fall of the pain intensity with raising and lowering of the leg indicates neural mobility/tension/hyperalgesia as the underlying mechanism for the prolongation of the symptoms, in addition to any local ligamentous or other effects. The test may then be employed as treatment with the effect of relieving pain and tenderness and usually reversing the chronic progression of the condition.

Investigating a neural tissue mechanical basis of an individual's problem is a **concept** of testing and any condition or area of the body may be so examined. ANT tests are not 'positive' or 'negative' but 'comparable' or 'not comparable' with the patient's complaints, in the same way that joint problems detected with movement testing and palpation are denoted as comparable joint signs or are not comparable.

The treatment of adverse neural tension

Treatment follows upon a detailed skilled examination of the neuromusculoskeletal system. Specific techniques targeted to affect the mobility of neural structures may of course influence many other aspects of neural tissue physiology such as circulation, tissue fluid pressure gradients, local pain mechanisms and so on. We do not know, as yet, how our treatment techniques bring the undoubted effects we observe and patients report.

It is useful to think in terms of affecting nervous tissue mobility and other effects:

1. At the **interface** between the nervous system and other tissues (muscles, bones, ligaments and osseofibrous tunnels for example).
2. **Intraneurally**, that is within the nerve itself and its connective tissues (perineurium, endoneurium and epineurium).
3. By **postural** and **ergonomic** adaptations to the individual and their environment which reduce abnormal body stresses.

Details relating to these approaches as well as to the whole subject of ANT may be found in *Mobilization of the Nervous System*, the standard work on the subject by David Butler (Butler, 1991).

We realize and accept the limitations there may be with this approach to treatment in specific cases, as in all other areas of physiotherapy intervention. If, owing perhaps to an unremitting interface problem (irreversible bony/scar tissue changes with severe nerve entrapment), a condition and its symptoms is reversible by only 20–30% then treatment is not prolonged unnecessarily. When that point has been reached is of course not so easy to determine and there is no substitute for hard experience to know it. However a simple routine for the patient to maintain and even, over a long period of time, further improve the status quo, is essential.

It is important that the sufferer is taught such a routine by the physiotherapist and is given an appointment perhaps at 4-monthly or so intervals to assess any change in the condition and modify the patient's self-treatment as necessary.

Also, in treating ANT problems it is necessary to be aware of any latent or delayed responses such as may happen especially when dealing with a highly reactive or irritable condition.

The aim of treatment is to improve movement and extensibility of the pain-sensitive neural and other associated structures without causing harm. It is kept constantly in mind that it is neural tissue that is being manipulated and the safety of its impulse-conducting function is paramount. Therefore mobilization is within normal physiological limits, always bearing in mind the resting tension of the nervous system and how abnormal that may be in any given instance. We aim to mobilize at various interfaces, we do not force.

These adverse neural tension tests devised by physiotherapists, such as the brachial plexus tension test of Elvey, have begun to enter the medical literature. The *British Journal of Rheumatology* in 1989 (Quinter, 1989) published a study of upper limb pain and paraesthesia following neck injury in motor vehicle accidents which refers to the use of the brachial plexus tension test in the assessment of whiplash victims. This supports the use of the test 'in a clinical setting where arm pain and/or paraesthesia could reasonably be expected to arise from hyperalgesic cervical or brachial plexus neural tissues'.

In a further clinical research trial 60 patients diagnosed as having repetitive strain injury ('upper limb disorder') were assessed by a full examination carried out by a consultant rheumatologist. They were additionally each assessed using the BPTT of Elvey. No signs were found of any known rheumatological disorder; however in 59 of the 60 cases in the study the BPTT was found to be 'positive' (comparable!) thus supporting the concept that repetitive strain injury is manifestly a disorder of neural irritation and neural mechanics. This concept has been put to work by physiotherapists with considerable success in the treatment of this highly painful and seriously disabling disorder.

The concept and the clinical use of adverse neural tension assessment and treatment will revolutionize much physiotherapy practice over the coming years.

The effects of manipulative procedures

When the effects upon the body of various passive movement procedures are discussed, there is a danger of confusing observations of what results with how results are thought to be achieved. To guide thoughts on this matter Maitland (1986) has proposed a 'two-compartment' approach to rationalize the information obtained. First, there is the compartment in which information concerning anatomy, biomechanics, pathology and diagnosis is accumulated. The second compartment contains the history, signs and symptoms of any particular patient that has been examined.

It is natural when discussing manipulative procedures to want to rationalize what happens during and after treatment by relating any changes in the second compartment directly to alterations in the first. However, while the effects of manipulation upon the patient's symptoms and signs can be observed and can be reported by the patient, it is speculative to attempt to describe how exactly those effects have been achieved. In other words, it cannot be said precisely in any given case how improvement in the signs and symptoms has been achieved but only that it has.

Therefore, the short answer to the question: 'How and why does manipulation work?' must, in all honesty, be that it is not known for certain. However, it is possible to hypothesize mechanisms using the considerable volume of information now available and growing steadily relating to joint and soft tissue neurology, pathology, biomechanics and pain studies. The effects and uses of soft tissue or massage techniques have been discussed earlier in this chapter. Manipulative procedures directed primarily to the spinal or peripheral joints require some further consideration. First, it should be stated that the basic effects we wish to achieve in terms of the signs and symptoms are as follows:

1. To decrease pain and other symptoms.
2. To decrease muscle spasm.
3. To improve mobility of the joints and soft tissues.

The mechanism whereby these effects are achieved by treatment would probably be by one or more of the following:

1. An alteration in the bias of sensory input from the joints and soft tissues by an increase in the stimulation of the mechanoreceptors located within them.
2. Reflex effects upon spasm.
3. The prevention or limitation of the formation of inelastic scar tissue and the restoration of extensibility to the soft tissues.
4. The improvement of tissue–fluid exchange.
5. Improvement in the mobility of the nervous system and alteration in the state of neural hyperalgesia.
6. The psychological effects of being carefully assessed and treated sympathetically.

These two lists summarize the two-compartment way of thinking mentioned earlier.

It is useful when discussing the possible ways that manipulation achieves its effects to keep in mind the cycle of events, aptly named a 'vicious circle', invariably encountered when the patient is taken for treatment (Figure 17.12).

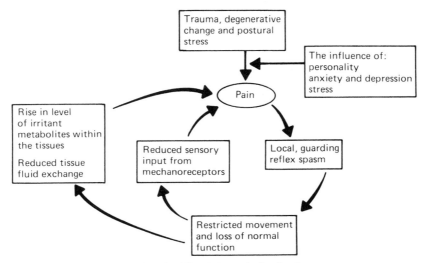

Fig. 17.12　The vicious circle of pain.

Stimulation of articular mechanoreceptors and its effects upon pain

It is only since the mid 1960s, that details of the morphology and precise function of the articular receptors have been known (Wyke, 1967). It represented an exciting breakthrough in knowledge for those concerned with the treatment of musculo-skeletal pain and dysfunction, and in particular for physiotherapists, since it provided evidence to demonstrate conclusively the mode of response of specific receptors (types I, II, III and IV) in joint structures to a wide spectrum of mechanical and nociceptive stimuli.

Types I, II and III are mechanoreceptors. Type III receptors are absent from the spinal joints (Wyke, 1981) but are present in the ligaments of peripheral joints. Type I articular receptors are located in the fibrous capsules of the spinal apophyseal joints, whereas type II receptors can be found in the deeper layers of the capsules and in the articular fat pads. Type IV are nociceptive receptors found in the ligaments and fibrous capsules of the spinal joints, in the walls of articular blood vessels and in articular fat pads. Unlike the mechanoreceptor system, the articular nociceptive system is, under normal circumstances, completely inactive, and only becomes active when levels of mechanical stress become excessive or when chemical irritants accumulate in the tissues.

Coincidentally, there was about the same time that these receptors were described the publication of a new theory on pain mechanisms by Melzack and Wall (1965). It took as one of its central themes the modulation of nociceptive afferent input in the spinal cord by continual afferent barrage from mechanoreceptors. In spite of the criticism of the theory (Nathan, 1976) and its modification over the past two decades, this central idea held firm and is of fundamental importance in any account seeking to show how manipulation achieves its effect. Stated briefly, one function of the mechanoreceptor system is pain suppression. When the nociceptive system is activated for any reason, the transmission of these impulses through the central nervous system will vary according to the degree of mechanoreceptor stimulation and impulse transmission occurring at the same time. The greater the level of mechanoreceptor activity, the greater the effect of pain suppression.

Consequently, as suggested by Wyke (1979, 1985), the passive manipulation of, or the application of traction through, limb and spinal joints has many reflex and perceptual consequences. These include the relief of pain as a result of the presynaptic inhibition of pain impulses through the synapses in the basal spinal nucleus via the mechanoreceptor stimulation that is inevitably associated with all manipulative procedures. The well-trained manipulative physiotherapist can influence this neurological mechanism with a high degree of refinement.

In other words, a large part of the total effect of manipulation is probably achieved by modulating nociceptive and sensory input from the periphery by gaining maximal inhibitory effects from the stimulation of the mechanoreceptors located in skin fascia, muscle, tendons, ligaments, joint capsules etc. By this mechanism it is possible to break into, and thereby begin to break down, the 'vicious circle' of pain and restricted movement.

Other complex effects must operate in the relief of pain and spasm and other observed responses to the techniques directed at mobilizing neural tissue (see ANT section above).

Reflex effects upon spasm

The local reflex protective spasm, which accompanies so many painful musculoskeletal conditions, often diminishes progressively as pain relief is gained. On the other hand, such spasm, as the clinician knows well, may persist and become a major obstacle 'protecting' the damaged structures well beyond the point in time where the restoration of movement is desirable. The judicious use of suitable manipulative procedures can reduce this persistent and counterproductive spasm. This in itself will hasten the return of normal movement and thus enhance a more 'normal' sensory barrage from the periphery into the central nervous system. Movement, then, begets movement provided that excessive pain is not produced.

Prevention of the formation of disorganized and inelastic scar tissue and the loss of extensibility in the soft tissues

It is a fact of pathology that either by a slow process of degenerative change or as a result of sudden or repeated trauma, fibrous scar tissue is laid down within the neuromusculoskeletal tissues. While little can be done in practice to prevent this natural healing reaction from occurring, a knowledge of the events and their time-scale helps prevent or minimize the less desirable effects of the process. The major undesirable effect of scarring within the soft tissues, including those of the joints, is that if it is not subjected to repeated stress at the right time, the fibres which give it strength will organize themselves haphazardly into a disorganized meshwork (Evans, 1980). Such an arrangement produces a weak and inextensible scar which, in turn, produces pain when stretched. In contrast, scar tissue which is stressed to an appropriate degree at the right stage will form fibres running parallel to the normal stress lines of the tissue and, with repeated movement, a mobile scar will be formed which does not restrict movement. One way of achieving some of the healthy stress upon such tissue is by manipulative techniques which utilize repeated careful stretching movements (Mealy et al., 1986), though, of course, such procedures will only achieve maximal benefit if followed up by appropriate and repeated movement by the patient. There are exceptions to this rule, such as the early treatment of a tenosynovitis arising from overuse of the affected part. In this case, rest is more appropriate between treatments.

The same rationale applies to the use of stretch in the case of a spinal nerve root which is in the process of becoming adherent to the surrounding tissues within or beyond the intervertebral foramen. Inflammation and degenerative change occurring in these tissues diminish the mobility of the nerve, which normally moves to a limited but appreciable extent during trunk and limb movements (Breig and Marions, 1963). A traumatized nerve which has become adherent in this way may be the source of chronic referred limb pain (Fahrni, 1966), and quite apart from joint manipulation, there remains the effect (Figure 17.13) in such cases of 'mobilizing' the nerve and its coverings within the intervertebral foramen. Particular techniques are used to achieve this effect and can be applied in treating the cervical as well as the lumbar spine. (See Section above on the treatment of pain and abnormal tension in the Nervous System.)

Improvement of tissue–fluid exchange

The repeated functional movement of joints and their associated tissues and the contraction and relaxation of the muscles which move them during everyday activities promote the normal flow of blood and lymph by a pumping and 'milking' effect. The normal nutrition and health of tissues, such as cartilage and muscle as well as collagenous structures are probably, in part, due to such regular movements (Lowther, 1985). The action of stretching, which occurs naturally throughout the spine and the peripheral joints as part of the individual's normal activities maintains the extensibility of the musculoskeletal structures, especially the collagenous tissues.

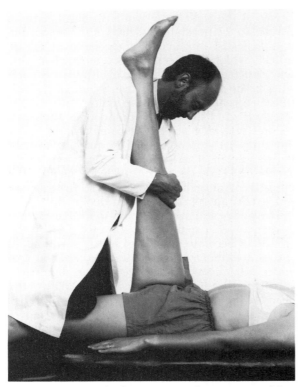

Fig. 17.13 Straight leg raising technique to mobilize the pain-sensitive structures in the intervertebral canal. This procedure is carefully graded and only ever used in the presence of chronic non-irritable symptoms when it has been estimated that some or all of the symptoms are arising from a lack of mobility between the nerve root and surrounding structures.

When pain and joint restriction reduce such movement, often in a very masked way and for a considerable period of time, normal healthy tissue–fluid interchange is impaired (Grieve, 1981). Muscles maintained in a state of chronic guarding spasm become weak from disuse. The regular rhythmic pumping action around the affected joints is lost. The normal sensory barrage from the joint and its soft tissues is depleted. This will be the case whether it is spinal or peripheral joints or soft tissues which are affected. Manipulative techniques, by helping to restore movement, restore normal biomechanical forces to the muscles, collagenous tissues and local blood vessels and the lymphatics and neural structures. By these measures some part of the effects upon pain and mobility may be mediated.

Psychological effects

All manipulative therapy by definition involves close physical contact between the patient and operator, and the skilful and sympathetic handling of tense, painful and aching tissues. Apart from the neurophysiological effects related to manipulative therapy, the psychological benefit which may be derived from this form of treatment may be considerable. The value of 'therapeutic handling' is demonstrated every day by patients who register enormous relief when the source of their problem is found, discussed and handled very specifically and with due care. The remark 'I've longed for someone to find that spot and do something about it', is satisfying to both patient and manipulator alike and when it is followed up with a demonstrable change in the patient's signs and symptoms, it helps establish a bond of trust and a spur to recovery.

How much of this effect can be ascribed to a 'placebo response' is not possible to say. It is generally believed that some 20–30% of the improvement noted in any trial is due to the Placebo effect (see Chapter 4) and presumably manipulation is no exception. It is still not known what the mechanisms are which underlie this aspect of the total response to treatment.

On occasions, a patient may appear to be developing a psychological dependence upon being manipulated. If treatment is merely reinforcing ideas of physical dysfunction when the valid testing of signs and symptoms does not bear this out, then such treatment should be reconsidered and the patient referred back to his doctor. It should always be borne in mind that what a patient's pain and disability means to him may differ greatly from what it means to the physiotherapist. However, the limitations of manipulative procedures must be acknowledged.

Diagnosis, pathology and manipulative procedures

Dr James Cyriax and Mr Geoffrey Maitland, two great pioneers in the development of the treatment of musculoskeletal disorders, emphasize the paramount importance of a comprehensive and systematic examination and assessment of the moving parts of the body in order to make a precise diagnosis. Diagnosis is the *sine qua non* of manipulation (Cyriax, 1984; Maitland, 1986).

However, the exact cause may be unclear even

though it is recognized as a benign, mechanical one. In these cases the referral may simply state for example 'low back pain', 'backache and sciatica', 'painful, stiff shoulder' or 'retropatellar pain' and so on. It may be that the diagnosis and the pathology implied by it come within the category which requires extra care and caution, and this will be observed in these cases. Certain diagnoses, as seen, contraindicate the use of high velocity thrust techniques but do not preclude the use of carefully controlled mobilization techniques or certain soft tissue techniques. A few diagnoses actually dictate precisely what specific techniques should be used. As an example, nerve root irritation or compression arising from the cervical spine and giving severe and highly reactive symptoms into the upper limb should only ever be treated initially by gentle sustained cervical traction. Similarly, the patient suffering from a locking incident of the knee due to a meniscal tear will sometimes require a very specific manipulative procedure to free the mechanical block to movement arising from this internal derangement. The number of such instances when the diagnosis and pathology specifically dictate what technique must be used initially is small, however, when considered alongside the majority of musculoskeletal problems where the precise mechanisms causing the signs and symptoms may not be absolutely clear.

The case of the painful stiff neck is a good example. Many such patients are X-rayed and seen to have cervical spondylosis (i.e. cervical disc degeneration), a condition which is, of course, frequently asymptomatic. They may also have cervical osteoarthritis affecting the synovial apophyseal joints and the upper cervical articulations, particularly between the axis and the atlas. Disc degeneration is a normal process of ageing and one that eventually overtakes everybody's spine to some extent. That is not so in the case of apophyseal osteoarthritis which seems to occur less commonly. However, the fact remains that the ubiquitous cervical spondylosis or spondylarthritis may clinically present in a whole variety of ways ranging from a patient with a mildly aching and slightly stiff neck to someone with a truly agonizing and unpleasant pain radiating from the neck to the shoulders, arm and hand, accompanied by pins and needles, numbness and other neurological signs. Both may be diagnosed as due to 'cervical spondylosis'. The treatment approach in these two cases is entirely different. The diagnosis as such gives no indication of the precise treatment techniques to be used. It is

the particular combination of signs and symptoms, in addition to certain other factors, that guides the treatment in such situations and not the diagnosis. Obviously an understanding of the nature of the problem conveyed by the diagnostic label 'spondylosis' is essential but this more clearly defines certain boundaries within which the manipulator works rather than indicating precisely what must be done. It is certainly feasible that a number of different manipulators employing differing techniques may each provide relief to the patient with a particular type of painful stiff neck. They each achieve this in their own way for a variety of reasons obviously, but the principal one is likely to be that they understand how to handle joint problems with the appropriate degree and type of movement. Each manipulator skilfully does what is required to restore function to the painful stiff joints so that they move painlessly, even though they achieve this employing differing techniques.

Localization of the Sources of Symptoms

The most common fault in using manipulative procedures is in not directing the treatment specifically to the source of the problem, be it a specific structure or tissue, a specific joint or a specific level of the spine. Cases may be quoted where treatment by physical means has failed to achieve the relief of symptoms which is sought because it has not been directed accurately to the source of the symptoms. Obviously examples can be drawn from those cases where pain and other symptoms arise from the spinal structures, but closely resemble the clinical presentation of local disorders. Even some localized soft tissue tests such as palpation, stretch and, on occasions, isometric muscle contraction may give rise to pain where a longstanding spinal disorder is eventually implicated as the source of the symptoms. Some commonly encountered situations are quoted below as examples.

Tennis elbow

Frequently the 'classic' signs and symptoms in a patient with this condition may be altered by treatment directed to their cervical spine. Alternatively, or in addition, definite joint signs may be elicited by localized accessory movement testing directed to the humeroradial or superior radioulnar joints. It is not to deny that the soft tissue changes associated with this condition do exist and even on occasions require surgical intervention. But in at least some cases, the tennis elbow results from complex cervicobrachial mechanisms (Gunn and Milbrandt, 1976) and does not respond to techniques directed solely to the soft tissues of the extensor region of the forearm. If the condition does respond to local techniques, such as frictions and injection, but arises from an underlying joint problem or a spinal disorder it is likely to recur.

Shoulder pain

Conditions as classic as supraspinatus tendinitis and capsulitis, frequently have their origin totally or in part in the cervical or uppermost thoracic spine. A specific shoulder action or activity may be the precipitating or triggering factor and not the causative factor in the onset of symptoms in these cases.

Anterior knee pain

This commonly arises from the vertebral region somewhere between the thoracolumbar and 3rd lumbar levels (Chadwick, personal communication, CSP Congress Lecture, 1986). Much valuable time may be wasted applying a variety of locally directed treatments if the true source of the patient's pain is not revealed by careful spinal testing, especially palpation. Again, this does not deny the fact that anterior knee pain may be related to a purely local cause and respond to specific methods directed to the knee. Furthermore such pain often can be shown to be due, at least in part, to adverse neural tension (see above).

Hand symptoms

Not uncommonly the symptoms usually associated with **carpal tunnel syndrome** may be linked with vertebral dysfunction, in particular stiffness and pain elicited with passive accessory and physiological movement testing at the 4th thoracic vertebral level. Pins and needles, puffiness and dusky bluish discoloration of the hands may accompany this condition, and these may all be relieved by mobilization or manipulation directed to the relevant vertebral level. This condition may coexist with carpal tunnel syndrome and should particularly be suspected where local measures to relieve the patient's symptoms and signs have had limited effect. Commonly the mobility of cervical and thoracic neural tissues may also be shown to be involved (see section on ANT above).

In any situation such as these, where the physiotherapist suspects a source other than that quoted by the referring doctor, the doctor should be con-

sulted and the findings discussed prior to any course of treatment being undertaken. It is unacceptable that where a local cause was suspected at initial examination a different source, if suspected by the physiotherapist, is treated without discussion with the referring medical practitioner.

A rather different situation exists where the source of a patient's problem does lie within a local structure, e.g. a muscle, tendon, ligament or joint. Again a common fault in treatment when using manipulative procedures is a failure to be sufficiently specific. For example, a patient who has sustained an inversion sprain of the ankle frequently suffers from symptoms (and has signs) which have arisen from trauma sustained by the calcaneocuboid joint. If treatment is directed only to the lateral ligament of the ankle in this situation then symptoms in the region of the sprain may well persist. Similarly, e.g., a pain at the point of the shoulder may lead to treatment being directed to the glenohumeral joint or the acromiohumeral soft tissues when, by careful differential testing, the acromioclavicular joint may be found to be at fault.

The pitfalls of attempting to relate treatment by manipulative procedures or other physical measures to a 'diagnostic label' without the essential tools of meticulous differential testing are clear. Precise diagnosis should implicate the structures which are the primary source of the patient's problem.

Examination and assessment

No treatment, and particularly that in which manipulative techniques are to be included, should ever be commenced without an appropriate and sufficient examination having first been carried out by the person undertaking that treatment. Such an examination can never supplant that of the referring doctor, but is meant to supplement it. Indeed no logical treatment can ever be planned nor the response to it assessed until a thorough picture of the presenting signs and symptoms has been elicited, following the familiar format of 'listening', 'looking', 'testing' and 'feeling'.

One expert, writing of the examination preceding spinal manipulation, made the following point (Grieve, 1975):

> ... the vitally important therapist's examination is less of a diagnostic sorting procedure than an 'indications' examination concerned solely with the manner

in which a joint problem is manifesting itself, and with localization of the vertebral segment(s) involved.

Exactly the same could, of course, be said of the examination of the non-spinal joints and soft tissues. But since manipulative procedures are associated in many people's minds with spinal problems and must take into account particular considerations of the vascularity and neurology of those regions, the points made will relate in the main to examination and assessment of the cervical, thoracic or lumbar spine. The relevance of most of the points to other musculoskeletal problems should be clear.

The **subjective section** of the examination will elicit the following:

1. The problem complained of, i.e. pain, stiffness, locking, giving way, weakness and unable to work, unable to play sport, etc.
2. The precise areas and depth of the pain and its severity, any paraesthesia and any reduced or absent sensation.
3. The type of pain, e.g. burning, throbbing, shooting, stabbing.
4. The behaviour of the different areas of pain over a 24 h period related to activities, e.g. walking, running, lifting, carrying, and postures, e.g. sitting, lying, standing; particular attention must be paid to severe night pain.
5. The history of the onset, e.g. related to a particular trauma or slow and insidious.
6. The past history, to elicit previous episodes, any pattern of development and previous treatments and their effect.
7. Points which alert the physiotherapist to the possibility of a condition having developed for which the patient should be referred back to the doctor. For example, with lumbar problems the development of retention and/or 'saddle' anaesthesia as a result of involvement of the cauda equina or the presence of symptoms of spinal cord involvement at the cervical or thoracic levels or sudden unexplained weight loss.
8. Details of relevant medical history and medication, e.g. diabetes, anticoagulant therapy, steroid therapy.

Before the physical part of the examination is undertaken, literally before one places hands on the patient, it is vital to pause and consider the information elicited so far. This process of assessment, trying to resolve the meaning of information gathered, will direct the remainder of the examination. While examination and assessment are two

words often used interchangeably, they do not mean the same thing. It is one thing to be able to examine well, but another to interpret what all the information means. As already stated, the physiotherapist's examination is not the primary diagnostic sorting procedure but more an 'indications' examination and, therefore, it is the following aspects which need particularly to be decided at this point:

1. Which structures must be tested as possibly contributing to the problem? For example, a patient sent with a diagnosis of 'cervical spondylosis' may simply have localized unilateral neck pain with a slight restriction of movement and little else. On the other hand, the patient may present with more severe pain, a gross restriction of movement, weakness of the muscles of the shoulder or arm, neurological deficit from nerve root irritation or compression and a tight sore shoulder joint, apparently related to their chronic cervical problem. Tests which will incriminate or exclude structures over which the symptoms spread will need to be used. If muscle weakness and shoulder joint restriction are found to be contributing to the problem they will need to be included for treatment at some point.
2. Are the symptoms severe? Severity is conveyed by the degree to which the problem restricts the individual's activities. For example, a severely stiff and painful lumbar spine may seriously affect the ability to continue with a particular occupation or may interfere markedly with sleep. Likewise, a severely sprained ankle may markedly limit walking. Severe symptoms will need to be examined with great care, particularly when dealing with a stoical patient.
3. Is the condition irritable? Irritability is defined by three factors: the ease with which symptoms are provoked, the intensity of those symptoms, and the time taken for them to settle following the provoking activity. Irritability must be determined before any active or passive procedures or treatments are undertaken, lest the patient's pain is unnecessarily stirred.
4. What is the nature of the problem? The nature of the problem has a number of aspects upon which not only the detail of the objective examination will depend, but also to some extent the treatment. Two aspects may be mentioned:

   (a) **Serious pathology.** While it is assumed that the serious disease processes which are referred to under contraindications.

have been excluded at the time of the doctor's examination, the possibility that such pathology may begin to manifest itself during the time the patient is seen by the physiotherapist is always kept in mind.

(b) **The source of symptoms**. Special consideration needs to be given to whether, for example, a spinal problem is primarily arising from the disc or the apophyseal structures and whether the nerve root or a more widespread mobility problem of the nervous system is involved and how. The latter may manifest itself as a chronic nerve root ache or alternatively an acute and highly irritable pain. The handling of the patient's tissues and the extent to which they are encouraged, for example to move further during movement testing will pay due regard to all these factors. As another example, if dizziness is complained of, then the objective examination must explore this symptom in some detail, so that its source (particularly if seeming to come from vertebral artery problems) can be clarified with the doctor.

The **physical section** of the examination will elicit the following:

1. The presence of factors which may possibly be contributing to the present problem. Examples in the case of spinal problems include a short leg, poor posture, weakness of the abdominal muscles.
2. The movements that are limited and by how much and what limits them – pain, spasm or resistance.
3. Details of postural deformities and whether they relate to the present episode. An example might be a lumbar scoliosis shifting the upper trunk away from or towards the painful side. Alternatively a joint such as the elbow or the knee may be seen to be held in a degree of flexion, e.g. when compared with the other side. An attempt must always be made carefully to reduce such a deformity, noting its relation to pain and range of movement in order to determine whether or not it is related to the present problem.
4. The presence of neurological deficit. Power, sensation and reflexes will all be tested as a routine part of a spinal examination particularly where pain radiates beyond the proximal joint, i.e. shoulder or hip.

5. Involvement of the pain-sensitive structures of the spinal and intervertebral canal or of neural tissue in the periphery. For example, the straight leg raising, prone knee flexion and slump test (Maitland, 1986) will demonstrate abnormalities of the sensitivity and mobility of the pain-sensitive structures of the spinal and intervertebral canals (including the dura mater and other neural coverings) or of peripheral nerve tissue. These will influence treatment and may be used to assess the efficacy of that treatment.
6. Factors which aggravate dizziness (if this is complained of by the patient with a cervical problem).
7. Palpable differences in the texture of soft tissues and in passive physiological and passive accessory intervertebral movements. This last section of the examination, palpation, is arguably the most informative. Provided no other part of the examination is omitted, skilful and meticulous palpation will help tie together all the other examination findings.

The overall aim of the physical examination is to reproduce the patient's symptoms or to aggravate them provided the severity, irritability and the nature of the problem permit this to be done. The specific tests and palpation details which do this are highlighted in the examination by an asterisk (*) so that significant physical as well as subjective findings are assessed continuously to guide the treatment. When symptoms are severe, and particularly if irritable, all testing thought likely to exacerbate them is avoided, in exactly the same way as manipulative techniques judged likely to aggravate the signs and symptoms are not used.

Contraindications

Disease processes and injuries which affect bone and joint structures as well as other soft tissues and weaken them, making them especially vulnerable to stress, are contraindications to all forceful manipulative procedures. In addition, the use of certain drugs such as steroids and anticoagulants precludes any vigorous passive treatment.

The well-trained manipulative physiotherapist who works with the full knowledge of the patient's medical condition knows clearly those situations in which, for example, manipulative thrust techniques are absolutely contraindicated and those where even mobilization is barred. The physiotherapist is also aware of conditions in which care must be exercised regarding the choice of specific techniques used and the degree of vigour which may or may not be employed. The first rule of manipulative treatment (as with all therapy) is **do no harm** and the responsible operator always errs on the side of caution. When there is any doubt regarding the suitability of any procedure in a given situation it is not employed.

It is the responsibility solely of the patient's doctor to diagnose his medical condition referring the patient, as seen fit, for assessment and treatment by another properly trained professional. The referring doctor will have identified any pathology which is an absolute bar to manipulative treatment and any which requires caution. Such absolute contraindications are more usually related to certain vertebral or spinal conditions.

The cases in which spinal manipulation (i.e. the techniques using rapid, short amplitude thrust) is completely contraindicated are as follows:

1. Malignant disease of the bone or soft tissues.
2. Bone disease such as osteomyelitis, osteoporosis, (of whatever cause), and tuberculosis.
3. Spinal cord compression.
4. Cauda equina compression.
5. Recent fractures.
6. Vertebrobasilar insufficiency.
7. Inflammatory arthritis such as rheumatoid arthritis and ankylosing spondylitis.
8. Bony or ligamentous instability of whatever cause, e.g. spondylolisthesis, fractures, craniocervical and lumbosacral anomalies.
9. Severe degenerative changes and longstanding spinal deformity.
10. Severe nerve root irritation or compression.
11. Pregnancy; generally all vigorous procedures to the lower thoracic and lumbar spine are to be avoided after the 3rd month.
12. Pain of unknown origin.
13. Recent whiplash trauma to the neck.
14. Anticoagulant therapy and current or recent steroid therapy.
15. Certain psychological states where there is clear evidence that the patient has developed an obsessional dependence on 'having his spine clicked back'.

A number of these conditions also preclude the use of mobilization techniques.

Furthermore there are situations in which particular care needs to be exercised, as with the following:

1. Severe pain, particularly if it is easily stirred and takes some time to settle.
2. Acute nerve root pain.
3. If spinal movements and/or palpation reproduces distally referred symptoms.
4. Worsening signs and symptoms, such as those due to increasing nerve root compression.

Of the conditions listed as contraindications to manipulation, a number may safely be treated with mobilization techniques and soft tissue procedures provided that specific safeguards are observed. For example, the patient with known vertebral artery disease may gain great relief from pain arising from coexistent cervical problems if treated by carefully graded mobilization techniques and soft tissue procedures. Obviously rotational movements and others which reproduce their dizziness will be totally avoided. But gentle traction, localized accessory movements and attention to the cervical soft tissues are usually safe and acceptable provided they do not aggravate the dizziness.

Treatment

The use of manipulative techniques is related directly to the examination findings and the assessment of those findings. Moreover, mobilization, manipulation and soft tissue techniques are chosen from a variety of different treatment modalities which the physiotherapist may choose to employ. Eventually, following due assessment, they may be used in combination with: corrective exercise to enhance mobility or restore good muscle tone; postural correction and advice; or temporary splinting and supports such as a cervical collar, a lumbar corset, a sacroiliac belt or a wrist splint.

Manipulative therapy is not a panacea for every mechanical musculoskeletal ailment. Skilfully used, however, it may play a valuable part and is often most important in the overall management of the condition. Sometimes manipulative therapy has quite a dramatic effect, as with certain spinal problems. It is the communication of these sudden 'cures' by one patient to another or to their doctor or by one physiotherapist to another which has generated the myth that a certain type of manipulation is a 'hole in one' curative procedure. Like most myths it is powerful and, in this instance, may do considerable harm in misleading patients and doctors as to what they should expect, and in making the less experienced practitioners of the art feel a failure if they do not regularly come up with such rapid successes. Every able manipulative physiotherapist has these successes but invariably they can be predicted. Most spinal and peripheral joint problems can be divided into those which will give a quick response and those which will take longer, and even perhaps require protracted treatment. This will apply irrespective of how good the physiotherapist is. It is related to the nature of the problem and that involves the type, extent and the stage of the pathology at the time the patient is seen.

Treatment is also related not only to the relief of symptoms and signs but advising the patient how best he may avoid further episodes of pain and disablement. A knowledge of the prognosis related to various syndromes is essential therefore in order that the manipulative physiotherapist can give the patient realistic advice. For example, lumbar discogenic problems are prone to recur if the patient does not regain and maintain a good painless range of lumbar extension and flexion, habitually sits in chairs and cars with a sagging flexed posture of the lumbar spine, spends prolonged periods in sustained flexion either while seated (as when driving) or standing, and lifts incorrectly.

In the case of treatment of a joint and its immediate supporting structures one of the principal guiding factors is whether that treatment is initially to be for pain or for inert tissue resistance and stiffness. Passive mobilization procedures to treat pain which is severe and limits movement are carefully controlled so that they are carried out without provoking symptoms. They therefore are applied in the early part of the available range of movement whether it be accessory or passive physiological movement. With peripheral joint problems, pain which is severe and limits movement early in range is treated with small amplitude accessory movements. The use of movements of too great an amplitude or the employment of passive physiological movements at this stage would provoke and aggravate the symptoms rather than settle them. When pain is not severe nor irritable and does not limit movement markedly the techniques used may be applied further into the range. Eventually it may be necessary to work into the pain, when this is permissible, to clear the symptoms and signs. If, on the other hand, restriction of movement is due to the resistance imposed by changes in the various inert soft tissues then the techniques used will generally be applied up to and at the point of restriction, assuming that pain and muscle spasm are minimal.

A number of other factors guide the choice of technique and how it is performed. For example, in the cervical spine, if rotation is to be used it is carried out towards the painless direction. If an acute joint-locking is manipulated, a procedure is used which safely and painlessly opens the joint with great speed.

Where a manipulative thrust technique is judged necessary, it is because it has been preceded by gentler techniques which have failed to achieve the degree of progress expected. In spite of having been applied with suitable vigour at the limit of the reduced range of joint movement, mobilizations in this case will cease to have further effect; a manipulation may achieve the final improvement. On the other hand, mobilization procedures may be continued after manipulation and frequently in these circumstances then achieve further improvement and progress. The same is true of the use of various soft tissue techniques.

A manipulative thrust technique is used when the pain felt by the patient is a local one and only spreads locally. This is invariably related to an abnormally tight vertebral mobility segment which has been localized by passive testing. A hypermobile joint or a case of spinal instability is never manipulated nor does a manipulation ever push through spasm.

There are then factors which guide the manipulative physiotherapist in selecting techniques and there is an order of efficacy to further guide the order in which they are employed. One important guiding principle is that the force used is the minimal possible to achieve a reasonable result. That force is carefully controlled and graded at all times, irrespective of what type of manipulative technique is being used.

It is the ability to monitor and interpret changes (sometimes subtle) in the many aspects of the signs and symptoms that make up one particular patient's problem, which is the key to successful treatment by manipulative therapy. Finely tuned assessment is the secret of the effective manipulator, and not an ever increasing store of techniques. The precise level of the spine or the specific joint to be treated, the type of technique used and its gentleness or vigour, the modifications, additions and subtractions to what is done are all aspects of assessment upon which the degree of success will depend. In turn, all of these aspects hinge upon

Table 17.1 The Features of Spondylosis and Osteoarthritis Compared

Spondylosis	Osteoarthritis
Common	Less common
Acute episodes; may be complete freedom between bouts of symptoms; may be asymptomatic and not need treatment	Never completely free of symptoms, which should be treated
Nerve root pressure common; spinal cord pressure may occur	Nerve root pressure is uncommon, but root irritation may occur on certain movements
Stiffness in acute episodes spread over weeks or months	Daily variability of stiffness, easing with movement
Commonly affects: lower cervical mid thoracic lower lumbar	Commonly affects: upper cervical upper and lowest thoractic lower lumbar
Routine X-rays commonly show changes	Routine X-rays frequently reported as normal
Pain aggravated by some positions, eased by others	Posture or position makes little difference in general

Source: Stoddard, 1969.

the abilities of the physiotherapist as a communicator. Details of the subtle and involved process that goes to make up that skill would require another chapter!

The Use of Orthoses

The management of a painful musculoskeletal problem may involve the use of an orthotic device to support and rest the part. The prescription for a permanent support, such as a rigid collar for a patient with a painful and unstable rheumatoid neck, is clearly the responsibility of the doctor. Many orthotic devices, however, are used as a temporary measure to protect the part and control pain, mainly between physiotherapy treatments, especially when the patient is required to carry out activities or take up postures which are known to exacerbate their symptoms.

Examples of orthoses include the following:

1. Lumbar support (belt or 'corset').
2. Sacroiliac belt, especially for painful, hypermobile joints.
3. Lumbar–sacroiliac support for pregnancy.
4. Cervical collar.
5. Wrist splint.
6. Elbow splint (for tennis elbow).
7. Thumb splint (carpometacarpal or metacarpophalangeal).
8. Sorbo rubber insoles/shock pads for various ankle and foot problems, osteoarthritis of the hip.

The following points should be considered prior to providing a patient with any orthosis:

1. Do not provide any orthotic device unless it is *specifically* indicated, i.e. it can be shown to be advantageous to the patient and fulfils a specific aim. For example, of the large number of patients with painful neck problems referred for physiotherapy, only some benefit from the use of a cervical collar. Those who may do fall, in the main, into the spondylotic as opposed to the arthritic group (Table 17.1).

   Providing a collar for a patient with predominantly arthritic cervical problems may well worsen his symptoms, since the 'stiffness' associated with such degenerative change is usually in great need of graduated mobilization and frequent specific exercise by the patients themselves. Furthermore only *certain* spondylotic problems benefit significantly from a cervical support. This would be firstly when the symptoms are severe, particularly those referred into the upper limb; secondly when cervical movement is markedly restricted by pain and spasm, and thirdly when sleep is interrupted because of pain. The symptoms must be shown to be improved in these aspects by the use of the collar.

2. Fit the orthosis *personally* (i.e. do not hand over the task to a colleague to do if you are busy), making sure it is the correct size and shape, comfortable and supports, stabilizes or immobilizes as required. Make certain the patient or his helper can apply the device correctly and knows how to remove it if it becomes uncomfortable.

3. Explain when it is given that it is a *temporary measure* and will soon be discarded as treatment settles the symptoms and painless movement is regained. Start to decrease the amount of time that the patient wears the device as soon as possible. For the patient who complains of night pain, which is relieved by use of a soft collar, the abandonment of its use at night should

only be advised once the daytime pain is under control without the use of the collar. There is some evidence (Mealy *et al.*, 1986) that initial immobilization (for 2 weeks in this study) with rest in a soft collar following whiplash injury gives rise to prolonged symptoms compared with early active management.

4. Where the patient's history is of a chronic, recurring problem and his work or hobbies include activities which may provoke the pain, advice to wear the support while undertaking these activities may help prevent an attack.

An example is the wearing of a lumbar support during prolonged periods of gardening for an individual with a degenerative low back problem. It should be stressed, in such cases, that the wearing of the support or splint is only necessary as a temporary measure and a period of regular specific movements to maintain the ranges of movement of the affected area should always be undertaken daily as a priority, while the orthosis should for most of the time be kept stored away.

Recurrence of symptoms

The nature of many joint problems, particularly those of the spine, is that they are liable to recur and even grow worse. If patients are not careful about their lifestyles, they will continue, perhaps unwittingly, to predispose themselves to further painful episodes.

Manipulative treatment aids recovery, but the maintenance of the improvement gained is the responsibility of the individual patient himself. The most important points of prophylaxis are the maintenance of a full range of movement in all directions for the joint, and the avoidance of postures and activities which give rise to symptoms. Every patient should expect and receive careful instruction as how best to avoid further problems and how to maintain full range painless movement. Manipulation may be an important factor in the patient's recovery but it is never the only one. It is often the case, e.g. with low back pain, that the eventual answer to a particular patient's problem in the long term is a regular regime of specific mobility exercises and meticulous attention to seated posture. The manipulative physiotherapist is failing in her duty if this is not made very clear to the patient and pursued with sufficient emphasis.

Research

The effectiveness of manipulative techniques is not an easy aspect to research, particularly in the case of spinal pain. Many investigations have been undertaken, particularly with regard to low back pain, to compare manipulation with other forms of treatment, but a large proportion of these trials have proved very unsatisfactory for various reasons. The main reasons are outlined below.

The Selection of Patients

For example, in the case of low back pain a variety of mechanical causes are included. So far there is no universally accepted categorization of the causes and mechanisms of low back pain and therefore a heterogeneous mix of pathologies and syndromes are invariably admitted into a trial. It may be that it will eventually be shown that manipulative therapy is highly effective for some conditions, less so for others or, more likely, that it achieves rapid results in certain clinical situations and slower results in others.

A useful analogy can be drawn from the use of ergotamine for migraine where it has been stated that if this drug were used in a trial for headaches of a wide variety of causes it should be shown to be ineffective. However, it is, as we know, a highly effective treatment for migraine headache.

Measures for Improvement

The criteria chosen to assess progress during a trial of manipulative techniques ultimately depend upon the patient's interpretation of pain, a subjective and highly personal experience. Even the attempts to make objective observations, such as measuring movements and the straight leg raising test used in the assessment of certain lumbar problems, rely to a great extent on the way that pain affects the individual. The criteria of when a patient returns to work is again not a very reliable measure of real progress because individuals may or may not return to work for a variety of reasons. Often these reasons are not known to those treating them. Financial and social pressures may persuade some patients to return to work even though they still have considerable pain, while others may not return to work even though their symptoms appear minimal.

One experienced researcher in the field stated:

More sensitive measures of progress need to be established along with the criteria which would allow the early identification of those patients who are likely to respond to manipulation. (O'Donaghue, 1983)

Personal Skills of the Manipulator

If it is believed that skills of assessment and of the choice of techniques and the way in which they are carried out have a bearing upon the outcome of treatment, then the danger of measuring the individual skills of the operator and not 'manipulation' *per se* becomes obvious. In a trial which uses many manipulators (and it must to obtain sufficient patient numbers in the specified time), great attempts need to be made to describe exactly what is being done under the umbrella of 'manipulation'. This is not easy and when the choice is made too constricting, e.g. with 'one rotational manipulation each week for 3 weeks', the criticism is immediately advanced that it is not a treatment that any other manipulator would have chosen to do anyway and if it was to fail nobody would be surprised.

The Double Blind and Single Blind Trial

The classic double blind trial, devised to test the efficacy of drugs, requires that both the patient and the doctor assessing him are unaware which treatment has been received. Clearly the patients are always aware whether they have or have not received 'manipulation'.

The single blind trial, when only the assessing doctor is unaware of the treatment, is possible but it is not easy to always guarantee that the doctor remains unaware of the type of treatment given.

A more comprehensive discussion of manipulation trials can be found in Grieve (1986).

References

Breig, A. and Marions, D. (1963) Biomechanics of the lumbo-sacral nerve roots. *Acta Radiol. (Diagn.)*, **1**, 1141–60

Butler, D. and Gifford, L. (1989) Concept of adverse mechanical tension in the nervous system. *Physiotherapy*, **75**(11), 622–36

Butler, D. (1991) *Mobilisation of the Nervous System*, Churchill Livingstone, London/Edinburgh

Coxhead, C.E., Inskip, H., Meade, T.W. *et al.* (1981) Multicentre trial of physiotherapy in the management of sciatic symptoms. *Lancet*, **1**, 1065–8

Cyriax, J. (1984) *Textbook of Orthopaedic Medicine*, vol. 2, 11th edn, Bailliere Tindall, London

Danneskiold-Samsøe, B., Christiansen, E. and Andersen, R.B. (1986) Myofascial pain and the role of myoglobin. *Scand. J. Rheumatol*, **15**, 174–8

Elvey, R.L. (1979) Brachial plexus tension and the pathoanatomical origin of arm pain, In: *Aspects of Manipulative Therapy* (eds E.F. Glasgow and L. Twomey), Lincoln Institute of Health Sciences, Melbourne, pp. 105–10

Elvey, R.L., Quinter, J.L. and Thomas, A.N. (1986) A clinical study of R.S.I. *Aust. Family Phys.*, **15**(10), 1314–22

Evans, P. (1980) The healing process at cellular level: a review. *Physiotherapy*, **66**(8), 256–9

Fahrni, W.H. (1966) Observations on straight leg raising with special reference to nerve root adhesions. *Canad. J. Surg.*, **9**, 44–8

Grieve, G. (1975) Manipulation. *Physiotherapy*, **61**(1), 11–18

Grieve, G. (1981) *Common Vertebral Joint Problems*, Churchill Livingstone, Edinburgh

Grieve, G. (1986) *Modern Manual Therapy of the Vertebral Column*, Churchill Livingstone, Edinburgh

Gunn, C.C. and Milbrandt, W.E. (1976) Tennis elbow and the cervical spine. *Canad. Med. Assoc. J.*, **114**, 803–7

Lowther, D.A. (1985) The effects of compression and tension on the behaviour of connective tissues. In *Aspects of Manipulative Therapy, 2nd edn* (eds E.F. Glasgow, L.T. Twomey, E.R. Scull and A.M. Kleynhans), Churchill Livingstone, Edinburgh, pp. 16–22

Maitland, G.D. (1978) Movement of pain sensitive structures in the vertebral canal in a group of physiotherapy students. Proceedings of the Inaugural Congress of the Manipulative Therapists Association of Australia, Sydney.

Maitland, G.D. (1986) *Vertebral Manipulation*, 5th edn, Butterworths, London

Mealy, K., Brennan, H. and Fenelon, G.C. (1986) Early mobilisation of acute whiplash injuries. *Br. Med. J.*, **292**, 656–7

Melzack, R. and Wall, P.D. (1965) Pain mechanisms: a new theory. *Science*, **150**, 971–9

Nathan, P. (1976) The gate-control theory of pain: a critical review. *Brain*, **99**, 123–58

Nitz, A.J., Dobner, J.J. and Kersey, D. (1985) Nerve injury and grades II and III ankle sprains. *Am. J. Sports Med.*, **13**(3), 177–82

O'Donaghue, C.E. (1983) Controlled trials of manipulation. *Manipulation Association of Chartered Physiotherapists Newsletter*, **14**, 1–6

Quinter, J.L. (1989) A study of upper limb pain and paraesthesiae following neck injury in motor vehicle accidents: assessment of the brachial plexus tension test of Elvey. *Br. J. Rheumatol.*, **28**, 528–33

Stoddard, A. (1969) *Manual of Osteopathic Practice*, Hutchinson, London

Sunderland, Sir S. (1989) The mischievous fibroblast: friction trauma, fibrosis and adhesions. In Proceedings of the Manipulative Therapists Association of Australia, Adelaide, Australia

Wyke, B.D. (1967) The neurology of joints. *Ann. R. Coll. Surg.*, **41**, 25–50

Wyke, B.D. (1979) Neurology of the cervical spinal joints. *Physiotherapy*, **65**(3), 72–6

Wyke, B.D. (1981) The neurology of joints: a review of general principles. In *Biology of the Joint. Clin. Rheumat. Dis*, **7**(1), 223–9

Wyke, B.D. (1985) Articular neurology and manipulative therapy. In *Aspects of Manipulative Therapy*, 2nd edn (eds E.F. Glasgow, L.T. Twomey, E.R. Scull and A.M. Kleynhans), Churchill Livingstone, Edinburgh, pp. 72–7

18 Connective tissue massage

JEAN and LOUIS GIFFORD

Introduction

The discovery and development of connective tissue massage (CTM) can largely be attributed to the observations and insight of Elizabeth Dicke, a German physiotherapist, who in 1929 suffered a severe postinfection circulatory disturbance in her right lower limb. The severity of the condition was such that amputation of her lower leg was advised. While bedridden during the illness, she experienced severe back pain, and her leg, as well as being painful, was cold, bluish and the dorsalis pedis pulse was absent to palpation. She attempted to relieve the back pain by applying pulling strokes on the skin over the painful areas of the back and sacrum. She discovered that the inelastic, hypersensitive and fixed tissues on the painful side were loosened by these strokes, and the tension of the skin was lowered to the level of the uninvolved side. Simultaneously, the pain in the back eased and an acceptable sensation of warmth took its place.

While persisting on successive days with the stroking, pins and needles were gradually felt in the affected leg, followed by an agreeable sensation of warmth. In further treatments, she incorporated areas around the greater trochanter and along the iliotibial tract. Gradually the superficial venous circulation reappeared in the thigh and leg, and within 3 months a satisfactory reduction in her symptoms was established.

After recovering she systematically observed her patients, and was soon able to pinpoint areas of tension consistently related to known pathological states in the viscera and extremities. She found the regions of increased tension or resistance, generally visible as retracted areas (Figure 18.1), by stroking the patient's back with her finger.

Unknown to Elizabeth Dicke, Head (1893) and Mackenzie (1909) had previously published works relating surface changes to internal disorders.

Henry Head, an English neurologist, was the first to show that in diseases of the internal organs, certain skin areas innervated by the same cord segments became hypersensitive to touch, pressure and temperature. These areas, which appear during the acute phase of disease and disappear with its recovery, are commonly known as **Head's zones**. For example, in pathology of the gallbladder, hyperalgesia is found in the segments T6 to T10.

Later, Mackenzie (1909) observed hypertonic alterations and hypersensitivity in muscles belonging to the same segment as diseased organs. Dicke had independently stumbled upon and described visible and palpable changes in the tension of the skin, subcutaneous and other connective tissues that were segmentally related to visceral pathology in a similar way to the observations of Head and Mackenzie.

It seems likely (Ebner, 1972) and reasonable to assume that all tissues of the same segment, including the circulation, are subject to changes in the presence of organ pathology. The connective tissue areas observed by Dicke have remained relatively unchanged over the years, and are referred to as **connective tissue zones** or **reflex zones** in more recent literature (Luedecke, 1969; Ebner, 1975). They are generally located homolaterally in the segment of the affected organ, and, as a rule, do not occupy the segment uniformly. Thus certain *maximal points* of tension within the reflex zones are especially noticeable. An example is the zone affected by liver and gallbladder malfunction (Figure 18.2). Tension is particularly increased between the right scapula and the vertebral column at the level of T4 to T6 and over the inferior angle of the right scapula. The inferior costal margin on the right frequently appears to be drawn in, and there is increased tension over the lateral margin of the right latissimus dorsi. Maximal points also occur in the liver and gallbladder

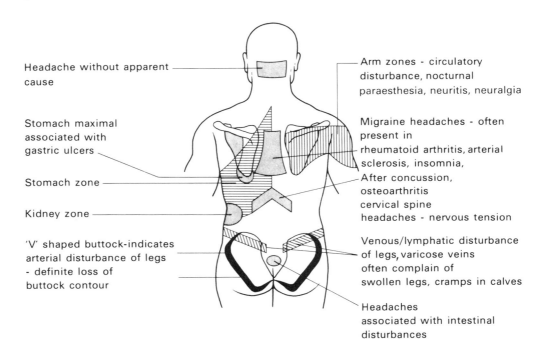

Headache without apparent cause

Stomach maximal associated with gastric ulcers

Stomach zone

Kidney zone

'V' shaped buttock-indicates arterial disturbance of legs - definite loss of buttock contour

Arm zones - circulatory disturbance, nocturnal paraesthesia, neuritis, neuralgia

Migraine headaches - often present in rheumatoid arthritis, arterial sclerosis, insomnia, After concussion, osteoarthritis cervical spine headaches - nervous tension

Venous/lymphatic disturbance of legs, varicose veins often complain of swollen legs, cramps in calves

Headaches associated with intestinal disturbances

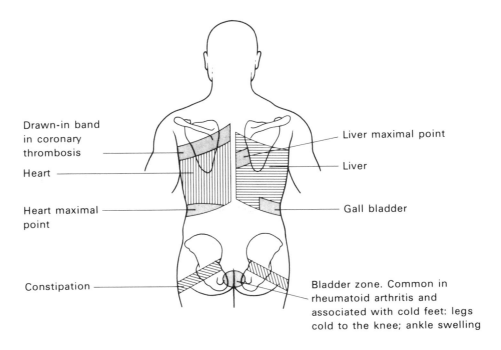

Drawn-in band in coronary thrombosis

Heart

Heart maximal point

Constipation

Liver maximal point

Liver

Gall bladder

Bladder zone. Common in rheumatoid arthritis and associated with cold feet: legs cold to the knee; ankle swelling

Fig. 18.1   The connective tissue zones – with some practical notes. (After Ebner, 1975)

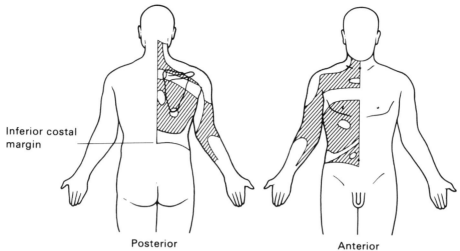

Inferior costal margin

Posterior   Anterior

Fig. 18.2   Liver and gallbladder connective tissue zones. The shaded area represents maximal points. (After Ebner, 1975.)

zones anteriorly on the chest and laterally over the right shoulder (Figure 18.2).

Head's zones of hypersensitivity (Figure 18.3*b*) and Mackenzie's zones of increased muscle tone (Figure 18.3*a*) are commonly viewed as being mediated via the viscerocutaneous reflex mechanism (Luedecke, 1969; Hall, 1979).

The development of the connective tissue zones are also considered to be via similar pathways (Bischof and Elmiger, 1963), although the more widespread and sometimes remote zones are yet to be convincingly explained. Ebner (personal communication) views the expansive and interconnecting nature of the body's connective tissue as a possible mediator of tension to regions beyond those embryologically related to the diseased organ. Her theory is simply explained if one imagines a tight cotton sheet being pinched between finger and thumb at any chosen point. Widespread folds of tension are seen to radiate surprisingly far from the small area held by the fingers (Figure 18.4). Ebner (1975) further emphasizes that since all structures function *inter*dependently, a disorder in any one part of the body can have far reaching effects, even to the extent that it may interfere with the function of the whole organism.

Both Mackenzie and Head limited the use of their observations purely to diagnosis. Kohlrausch in 1937 (Kohlrausch and Leube, 1953) was the first to try to influence internal organs through treatment of the body surface using 'fine vibra-

tions' and 'loosening frictions'. In the following year he began his collaboration with Elizabeth Dicke, and together with Leube (Luedecke, 1969), they defined CTM as it is practised today. They discovered that the application of CTM led to the reappearance of normal tension in the connective tissue zones and the simultaneous recovery of the internal complaint.

For many years man has tried empirically to influence morbidity in organs by treatment of the body surface. Nearly everyone has at some stage experienced the soothing warmth of a simple hot water bottle when suffering from some minor disturbance. It is impossible that heat reaches the internal organ, yet comforting responses are received. It is well known that segmental irritation of the skin can produce impulses which are received by the organ of the same segmental innervation level (Sato *et al.*, 1975). The responsible neural pathway is known as the **cutaneovisceral reflex**, knowledge of which has helped explain and lead to the development of many successful therapeutic procedures directed at apparent deeper tissue dysfunction (Travell and Rinzler, 1946; Stoddard, 1962, 1969).

The mechanism of the effectiveness of CTM has not been explored or clarified completely. Bischof and Elmiger (1963) take the view that the specific stimulation of the 'pull' on connective tissue provides sufficient stimulus to elicit the cutaneovisceral reflex, and that this is solely responsible for

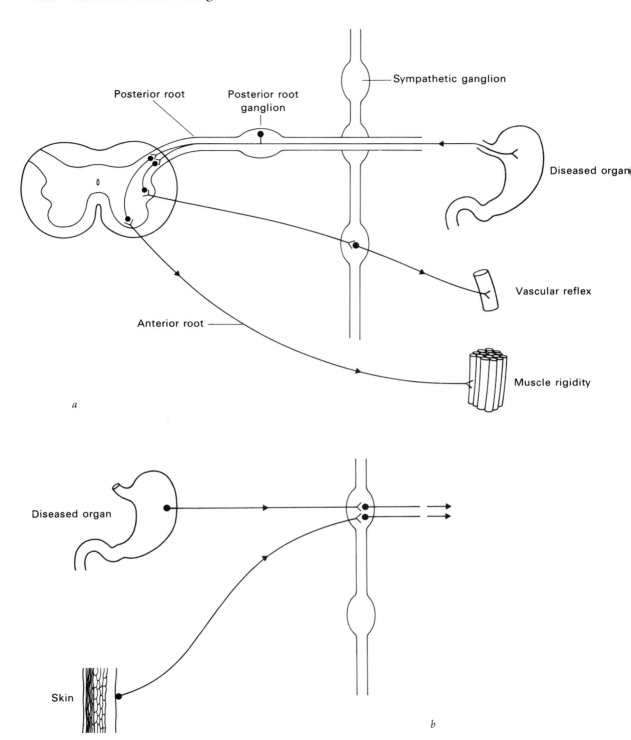

Fig. 18.3   *a*, Reflex arc at the spinal level. The impulse from a diseased organ is referred to muscle and blood vessels. *b*, impulses arising from the diseased organ associated with cutaneous hyperalgesia.

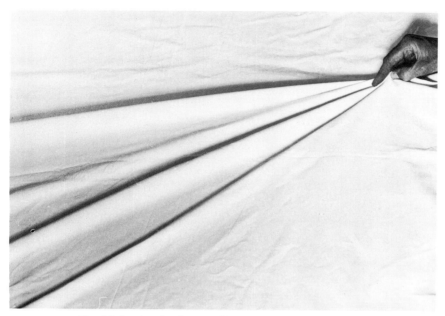

Fig. 18.4   A tight sheet to illustrate tension radiation.

the effects of the massage. Luedecke (1969) more openly felt that its mode of action could not be explained purely as a result of this reflex, as the treatment often influences tissues not segmentally related to the regions treated. Most authors (Luedecke, 1969; Ebner, 1978) are of the opinion that autonomic reflex pathways, widespread circulatory changes and endocrine release are involved in the production of the frequently powerful reactions to CTM.

The stroke

CTM involves the special stroking manoeuvre first described by Dicke (1954). The stroke consists of a tangential pull on the skin and subcutaneous tissues away from the underlying fascia. The deft, deceptively easy manipulation is carried out by the middle finger assisted and supported by the ring finger. The proper stroke of CTM is *always* a pull on the tissue, *never* a push or a pressure. Three stages are recognized that may help in understanding the procedure (Figures 18.5 and 18.6). These are:

1. Touch firmly, with distal interphalangeal joints flexed slightly.

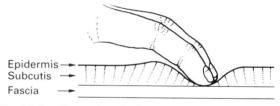

Fig. 18.5   The stroke – 'Take up the slack'.

2. 'Take up the slack'.
3. 'Pull' from the shoulder and the body.

Stage (2) is produced by the long finger flexor muscles, and stage (3) by flexion of the elbow which makes it incumbent so that the **radial aspect of the wrist** always leads the stroke (see Figure 18.6).

Two types of stroke are performed:

1. The short stroke just described, where no movement of the fingers on the skin occurs.
2. The long stroke, in which the fingers, maintaining tension from stages (1) and (2), are allowed to run through the tissues. With this stroke, healthy tissue passes as a fluent fold in front of the moving finger. When resistance is encountered in faulty connective tissues, the stroke must never be forced through them. The

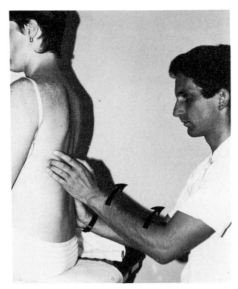

Fig. 18.6 Stage 3 of the stroke showing elbow flexion and radial aspect of the wrist 'leading the stroke'.

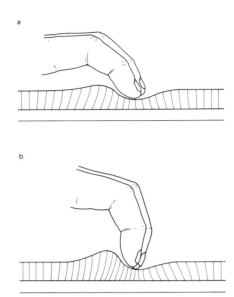

Fig. 18.7 Diagram to show how the strength of the stroke can be altered by changing the angle of the terminal phalanx to the skin.

physiotherapist should then alter her technique and may choose either to (a) substitute the long with short strokes; (b) to slow the stroke, or (c) to reduce the strength of the stroke by slightly extending the distal interphalangeal joints of the manipulating fingers (Figure 18.7).

Responses to CTM

Subjective

Normal sensation

When the fingers stroke normal tissues, relatively little resistance is felt and the patient reports only a mild scratching sensation, which is indicative of correct application of the technique. If more tense tissues are stroked, the patient may feel a sensation resembling cutting or scratching, as if the pull were with the finger nails instead of the finger tips. Leube and Dicke (1944) consider the cutting sensation as pathognomonic for recognising the proper nervous reflex. As tension decreases with use of the technique, so the intensity of the cutting sensation also decreases. The cutting sensation should cease simultaneously with the end of the stroke, and it should not persist after treatment ends.

Abnormal responses and undesirable reactions

Feelings of diffuse, dull pressure locally or in remote regions; cardiac oppression; shortness of breath; abdominal discomfort; dull pressure in the bladder; signs suggestive of shock and itching are all undesirable reactions that may be encountered. These are indicative of poorly executed and sometimes excessive use of the technique, or that CTM was an inappropriate treatment. Bischof and Elmiger (1963) view these reactions as being 'expressions of increased disturbance of the autonomic nervous system'. They are generally seen during the early use of CTM in automatically labile patients, and imply initial caution and strict attention to technique.

Objective

When the strokes are performed in abnormally tense connective tissue zones, or even normal tissues if the technique is executed vigorously, the three stages of the triple response occur. First a red line confined to the area of the stroke appears; this is later followed by a 'flush' of spreading redness and finally, if the tissues are particularly tense or the stroke vigorous, an area of superficial swelling emerges. The strength and duration of the skin reaction is directly proportional to the tension of the surface connective tissues. In some conditions, where chronically tense tissues are encountered, the skin reaction may still be visible for up to 36 h. Again, as tension is relieved, so the intensity of the reaction subsides.

In contrast, in most peripheral vascular conditions such as Raynaud's disease, the expected cutting sensation and skin reactions can only be obtained very faintly, if at all, even though tension in appropriate zones is found to be very high. In a similar, but reciprocal way to most other conditions, as tension is relieved, so normal sensory and skin responses concomitantly *increase* to normal in parallel with the improvement of the condition.

Profuse sweating is frequently seen following or during CTM, even in those who do not usually visibly perspire, suggesting parasympathetic stimulation (Ebner, 1968). If CTM is performed on one side only, it is possible to observe homolateral perspiration. Other 'autonomic' reactions that are frequently encountered include the appearance of gooseflesh and the enlargement of the pupils, both of which may present when only the caudal portion of the sacrum is treated.

Ebner (1975) reports that Volker and Rostovsky (1949) measured skin temperature of the foot in patients with circulatory disturbances of the leg and showed that dilatation occurred following CTM administered to the sacral and lumbar areas. Hall (1979) noted a 6.5°C increase in the temperature of the big toe of a normal subject following similar proximal treatment. It appears that CTM has a powerful effect on the vascular system. Bischof and Elmiger (1963) have pointed out that the vasodilatory effect of CTM was greater than that obtained with pharmacological agents, and as good as that seen following a sympathetic block. It is also noteworthy that dilatation of upper extremity vessels has been shown to occur when the pelvis is treated (Ebner, 1975), and that maximum skin temperature increase occurs 30 min after CTM, and can persist for up to 1 h. These observations tend to deny the role of the segmental reflex mechanism, and it has been suggested that humoral mechanisms are more likely to account for these effects (Ebner, 1975). However, some autonomic nervous system reactions are seen from 1 to 2 h following CTM in the form of fatigue, a pleasant desire to sleep, bowel movement and diuresis. It is probably upon these findings that Terich-Leube (1957) bases his postulation that the massage slightly emphasizes the general state of the auto-nomic nervous system on the parasympathetic side.

The following is a summary of the effects of CTM outlined by Ebner (1975):

1. CTM helps harmonize the relationship between the sympathetic and parasympathetic part of the autonomic nervous system.
2. Within the segments treated, it helps 'normalize the circulation between organs and organ systems and other tissues belonging to that segment'.
3. Locally it improves the blood supply of the surface tissues in the area under treatment, and in particular the connective tissue element.

The treatment stroke provides a stimulus that bears **little result** if it is too weak, **harmonizes** if it is adequate, and **overemphasizes** the sympathetic side of the autonomic nervous system if it is too strong. It is this overemphasis which produces the rather unpleasant and occasionally dramatic side-effects alluded to earlier.

Examination

The haphazard application of CTM in an undisciplined and unsystematic way and without prior examination can only enhance criticism of this convincingly effective procedure. In addition to any standard examination required, the patient must also be inspected for the presence of connective tissue zones before CTM is instituted.

Generally, the patient is examined and treated in the sitting position with back straight, hips and knees at right angles, feet comfortably supported and the hands resting on the thighs. The trunk and buttocks should be adequately exposed (Figure 18.8). The slight postural contraction necessary to maintain this position allows freer movement of the skin on the subcutaneous tissues. If the patient's condition makes it necessary, both investigation and treatment positions can be adjusted accordingly.

Visible Investigation

Visible connective tissue zones are not always apparent to the untrained eye, and only become obvious when changes have taken place in the deeper layers between subcutis and fascia. Visible zones typically appear as band-like drawn-in areas,

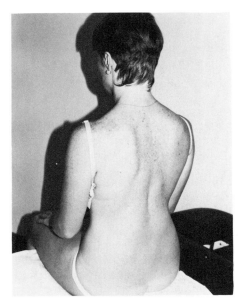

Fig. 18.8 Patient position.

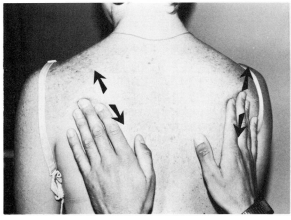

Fig. 18.9 Palpation of the superficial layers. The arrows indicate the direction of the small pushes (see text).

or flattened planes of tissue over the back and buttocks (see Figure 18.1). Thus in venous/lymphatic disturbances of the legs, a drawn-in band can be observed passing from the middle third of the sacrum, parallel to the iliac crest laterally and forwards over the gluteus medius. The patient may report frequent swelling of the legs and feet when hot, cramps in the calf, varicose veins or even a past history of phlebitis. If the tendency is

present in both legs, the zones are present on both sides, otherwise they are present only on the affected side. The severity of the drawn-in area indicates the more severely affected side (Ebner, 1975).

Manual Investigation

Three techniques of palpation are used to confirm the presence of zones. Zones not sufficiently developed to become visible are often detected while palpating. The more superficial skin layers are palpated using both hands applied simultaneously on either side of the back. The physiotherapist's slightly flexed fingers of both hands gently engage the body surface using just sufficient pressure to obtain adherence between the finger tips and the patient's skin (Figure 18.9). Small to and fro pushes are then used to displace the subcutaneous tissues against the fascia. These are performed sequentially over the connective tissue zones so as to obtain information about them. Palpation generally begins in the buttock and sacral regions moving upwards over the low back towards the zones between and over the scapulae.

The examiner should also bear in mind that areas of hypersensitivity (Head's zones) and increased muscle tone (Mackenzie's zones), if found to be present are informative, and can add further weight to any conclusions already drawn. It is thus vital for the operator to be conversant with the segmental supply of the various organ systems.

The deeper layers are palpated by pulling away a skin fold from the fascia (Figure 18.10). The technique is carried out beginning at the lower costal margin and progressing upwards to the shoulder region, always comparing right and left sides and relating significant tightness to the known connective tissue zones. Suspicions aroused on examination are frequently confirmed when strong resistance to the CTM stroke is met during treatment.

Details of the visible and palpable connective tissue zones should be adequately recorded for 'diagnostic' and later comparative purposes.

Finally, the so-called **diagnostic stroke** (Bischof and Elmiger, 1963) reveals the vascular skin reaction, the tissue tension, tissue density and tissue sensitivity over the immediate paravertebral area on the right and left from L5 to C7 (Figure 18.11). This stroke is, in effect, a **long stroke** passing the length of the back, and therefore through many of

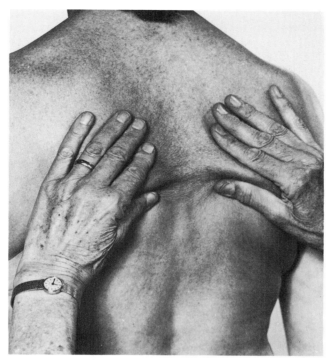

Fig. 18.10   Picking up the deeper layers.

the connective tissue zones. While the physiotherapist performs the diagnostic stroke, the patient is asked to report the sensation he feels. Proportional changes in sensation, tissue resistance and vascular response can be equated to provide ever-increasing support for a confident assessment of zonal tension. Appropriate, but carefully worded questioning, should be undertaken to ascertain the patient's condition with regard to the suspected organ malfunction. For example, in a patient with obvious buttock contour changes suggestive of 'arterial leg disturbance' (see Figure 18.1), the physiotherapist might casually ask if he has any difficulties walking. A typical picture of gradually worsening intermittent claudication may emerge. Details of walking distance before onset of pain, what he does to relieve it, how long it takes to subside, and how far or long he can continue walking is vital information on which the future effect of treatment may be gauged. In such a patient, assessment of the peripheral pulse strength provides a further means of monitoring progress.

The temptation to enthusiastically overemphasize examination findings should be avoided, as it may unduly worry a patient who has not been referred for the problem revealed.

Zones frequently present without any 'pathological background' (Bischof and Elmiger, 1963). The patient may have suffered the indicated disturbances earlier in life, or he may have a tendency to suffer them under conditions of stress. These zones are referred to as **mute** or **silent zones**, and attention to them in treatment is seen as of vital importance to the overall success of the massage (Terich-Leube, 1957).

Treatment

It is known empirically (Luedecke, 1969) that the connective tissue zones have connections with each other, thereby setting up feedback circuits. The therapeutic influences of the stroke may reach the organ, nerves and vessels innervated from the same segmental level, but also be received by other connective tissue zones, and affect other zones via these. For example, paraesthesia of the hands often disappears while treating caudal areas, and frozen

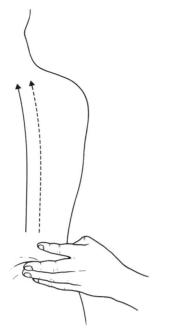

Fig. 18.11   Diagram to illustrate the diagnostic stroke. (After Bischof and Elmiger, 1963.)

shoulders frequently show dramatic increases in range of movement following similar caudal treatment. It may help the understanding of this effect if the reader recalls the 'tight sheet' explanation used on p. 215.

The observation that these intersegmental connections existed and that only after tension in the caudal section had been removed was it possible to work successfully elsewhere, was found at an early stage of CTM development.

As a general rule, nearly all treatments should start in the sacral area of the back and work slowly and systematically towards the area of the complaint. Ultimately, all regions which show positive zonal signs must be included if the final aim of CTM treatment specified by Ebner (1975) is to be upheld. That is:

> To normalize within the limit of still functioning vascular pathways the tension over the whole body surface.

The treatment areas on the trunk are divided into **sections**. These, and strokes performed over the limbs, head and anterior trunk, have been described in detail elsewhere (Ebner, 1975). The importance of the caudal or **basic section** (Figure

18.12) cannot be overstressed, as it is clear from experienced workers in Europe and in the English-speaking countries of the world that:

1. A degree of success can often be obtained from treatment of this area alone.
2. Normal tension and normal responses (subjective and objective) in the basic section must be achieved if any degree of success in other regions of the body is to occur.
3. If any undesirable reactions appear during treatment, it is likely that insufficient attention has been given to the basic section, and that the physiotherapist should immediately return to it to overcome the reaction.

It is important that the CTM strokes are not performed in a haphazard way over the body surface. Strokes tend to follow dermatomes, direction of muscle fibres and muscle fascia, tendons and at right angles to intermuscular septa and fascial borders. Special 'stretching manipulations' (Ebner, 1975) are used in the axilla, elbow, palm and foot, which provide a final stretch to the connective tissue when tension has already been relieved by the stroking technique.

During treatment, comforting flat-handed **release strokes** are performed routinely at the termination of the basic and thoracic sections.

As treatment progresses away from the basic section, it is not uncommon to encounter areas where local and general responses occur that are inappropriate and cannot be altered, even with strict attention to the basic section and operator technique. General patient discomfort, local tickling combined with a lack of the normal scratching sensation, or visible circulatory response while treating the thoracic region is a typical example. The use of rapid, and consequently very sharp, stimulatory strokes to appropriate 'trigger points' (Ebner, 1975) usually provides the correct response when treatment is resumed. Trigger point strokes are thought to provide a strong 'circulatory stimulus' (Ebner, 1975), and are found:

1. In a triangle formed by the external abdominal oblique, latissimus dorsi and the superior border of the iliac crest.
2. On the posterior aspect of the greater trochanter.
3. At the angle between the lateral end of the clavicle and the spine of the scapula.
4. In the adductor hiatus of the thigh.
5. In the popliteal space behind the knee.

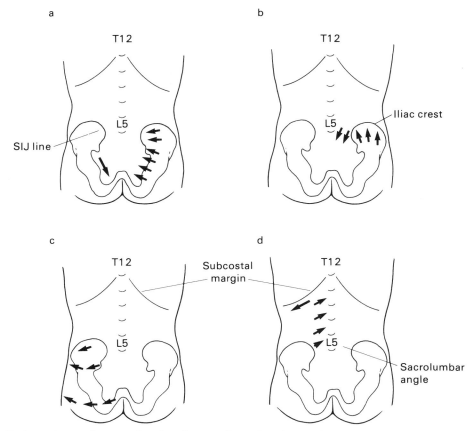

Fig. 18.12   Basic section; *a*, first set of strokes; *b*, second set of strokes; *c*, third set of strokes; *d*, fourth set of strokes. (After Ebner, 1975.)

The reader should note that these are not related to the well-known myofascial trigger points described by Travell and Simons (1983).

Application and Treatment of Pain

The role of CTM in the treatment of pain may be difficult to visualize in the light of the foregoing discussion. It will be recalled that CTM started as a therapeutic procedure, attempting to influence deep-seated pathology. The early German physiotherapists enjoyed a unique relationship with their medical colleagues, who referred patients with pathologically affected organs in order to observe the results. They noted beneficial effects in the following: heart diseases; respiratory conditions; disorders of the digestive system (stomach, intestinal tract, liver and gallbladder); diseases of the urinary system; gynaecological and obstetric conditions; many neurological conditions and in particular, circulatory disorders of the extremities. It is unlikely that many physiotherapists encounter such relationships with medical practitioners today. However, it was only through treatment of patients with disorders classically amenable to physiotherapy (who coincidentally had some of the above conditions) that the beneficial results of CTM on organ pathology have been verified, and the pleasing effect on the referred condition was discovered. Thus, spinal and peripheral joint problems (whether benign or of traumatic origin), sciatica, neuralgia, nerve root pain, osteoarthritis and rheumatoid arthritis are a few examples that have been found to respond well. The rationale underlying the successful application of CTM in musculoskeletal disorders is based on the assumption that increases in local circulation to pathologically

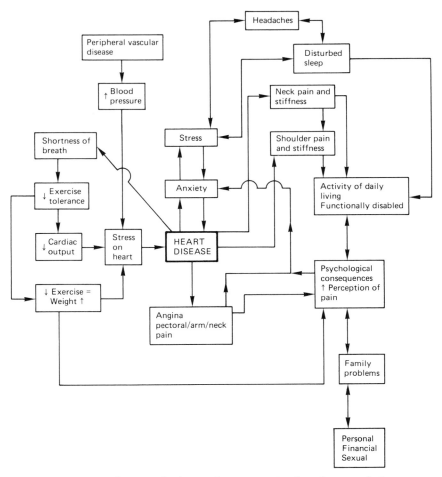

Fig. 18.13   A theoretical scheme of events issuing from heart pathology.

tense connective tissues helps to rebalance their depressed fluid content, and thereby increase extensibility. Additionally, in conditions where circulatory stasis has resulted in abnormally high concentrations of unwanted metabolic byproducts, the benefits of increasing local blood flow are self-evident. This may be a mechanism by which CTM has a direct effect in the alleviation of pain. There is some evidence that CTM is as effective as epidural injection, and more effective than pethidine in the treatment of persistent post-sympathectomy pain (Frazer, 1978).

A large proportion of patients seeking help from physiotherapists for painful disorders of the musculoskeletal system also endure minor and sometimes major disturbances of other body systems. The relationship of 'organ' pathology and musculoskeletal pain has perhaps been underestimated. CTM, in conjunction with standard examination procedures, provides a unique opportunity for the evaluation of such relationships, as well as providing a successful physical alternative to traditional management.

The commonly held aetiological association between heart disease and frozen shoulder (DePalma, 1973) serves as a useful example of the type of 'thinking processes' involved when tackling a patient's problem with CTM. Figure 18.13 illustrates a theoretical, but none the less plausible scheme of events issuing from a pathological heart disorder. Examination of this patient would reveal typical patterns of pain and restriction associated with the

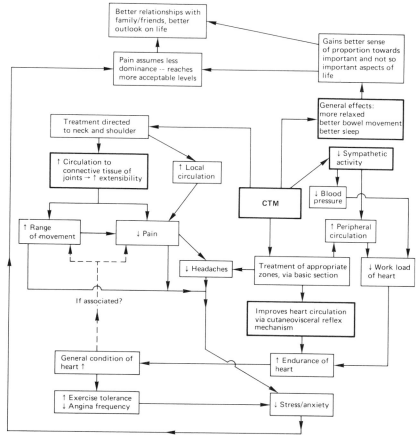

Fig. 18.14 Postulated mechanism of how CTM benefits a patient with neck, shoulder and heart problems.

neck and shoulder problems for which he had been referred. The inclusion of an examination for connective tissue zones may reveal relevant heart, peripheral arterial, headache zones and perhaps silent zones. Figure 18.14 illustrates the way in which CTM is thought to influence this patient's problem.

There are many clinical presentations which can be fitted into this broad scheme and to which CTM can be usefully applied. Thus, in middle-aged and elderly patients with low back pain, the physiotherapist may encounter such problems as intermittent claudication or migraine headaches. Women during the menopause frequently suffer musculoskeletal problems and are often found, via CTM, to suffer a wide variety of bizarre physical, mental and personal complaints that they had been understandably anxious about revealing. It is the authors' experience that these patients receive

considerable help through the physical pathway of CTM combined with sympathetic and confident consideration of their stressful state.

In attempting to answer the following questions, it might help the reader, who may be thinking of a particular presentation, in deciding whether CTM would be an appropriate avenue of treatment.

1. Would an improvement in circulation to the symptomatic region be beneficial? All disorders involving the circulation benefit from CTM, provided the pathology has not reached an irreversible situation. The authors have achieved success in the alleviation of Raynaud's disease, intermittent claudication, varicose ulcers and gangrene. The latter two conditions should be treated without entering the affected areas, as the skin is excessively fragile.

2. Does the physiotherapist think that the general

condition of the patient, both physical and mental, may be contributing to the presentation. If so, CTM examination is likely to be revealing and treatment beneficial.

3. Will the patient find this form of treatment acceptable? It is not easy to explain to a patient that treatment of his neck should begin over his buttocks! The patient must be taught that treatment areas, and areas which cause discomfort and show pathological symptoms, are not always the same. It may help if the patient understands that for treatment to be effective, the buttock and low back regions must be treated first. Patients easily accept the confidence and skill of an experienced physiotherapist.

Contraindications

Although possibly self-evident, it should still be stated that CTM is contraindicated in conditions where any increase in circulation is likely to be detrimental. Of particular note are: malignancy; acute inflammatory conditions; closed abscesses; during menstruation and the final trimester of pregnancy. In patients with notably low blood pressure, a degree of caution should be exercised as the massage can produce quite dramatic peripheral dilatation. The operator should progress treatment slowly and be vigilant for early signs of shock.

It is hoped that this short chapter has provided some interest and new thoughts for those who have already discovered CTM, as well as for those to whom it is unfamiliar. CTM has a fascinating history, and differs quite markedly from trends in manual therapy today.

Over the years quite significant numbers of physiotherapists have been taught the technique, yet most have done little more than experiment enthusiastically with it for a few weeks during postcourse euphoria! Others have simply been unable to approach their patients with CTM. This is not meant to be a criticism of these physiotherapists, as their difficulties and evaluation of CTM are understandable. However, it does serve to highlight several points that are vital for the future survival of CTM (see below). It also underlines the loopholes that these clinicians have found, and which need to be overcome before more widespread use of the technique is likely to occur. Thus:

1. It is paramount that a physiotherapist understands the nature and background of a technique before being able to apply it confidently and effectively to patients. CTM has a dated and questionable scientific foundation which badly needs re-evaluating and researching.

2. It is only an effective modality if undertaken in the logical and carefully controlled way described. The emphasis must be on scrupulous examination and reassessment, precision of technique, and informed observation of the patient and his tissues. Just as manipulative therapy has gained attention via its widespread use and excellent results, so must CTM. Once it becomes more widely recognized as a valuable clinical tool, CTM may attract the scientific attention it so desperately needs.

3. Attention can be focused on CTM via:
   (a) the favourable results of treatment;
   (b) the more widespread teaching of the technique, which in the authors' opinion, should extend to undergraduates;
   (c) the recognition of its value by referring medical colleagues.

References

Bischof, I. and Elmiger, G. (1963) Connective tissue massage. In *Massage, Manipulation and Traction* (ed. S. Licht), Baltimore: Waverly Press, pp. 57–83

DePalma, A.F. (1973) *Surgery of the Shoulder*, 2nd edn, J.B. Lippincott, Philadelphia

Dicke, E. (1954) *Meine Bindegewebsmassage*, Marquardt, Stuttgart (cited by Bischof and Elmiger, 1963)

Ebner, M. (1968) Connective tissue massage: therapeutic application. *NZ J. Physiother*, 3(14), 18–12

Ebner, M. (1972), *Connective Tissue Massage, Uses and Contraindications in Obstetrics and Gynaecology*. Newsletter No. 32, The Obstetric Association of Chartered Physiotherapists, London

Ebner, M. (1975) *Connective Tissue Massage. Theory and Therapeutic Application*, R.E. Krieger, New York

Ebner, M. (1978) Connective tissue massage. *Physiotherapy* 64(7), 208–10

Frazer, F.W. (1978) Persistent post-sympathetic pain treated by connective tissue massage. *Physiotherapy*, 64(7), 211–12

Hall J.M. (1979) An analysis of connective tissue massage. In *Aspects of Manipulative Therapy* (ed. R.M. Idczak)., Proceedings of a multidisciplinary international conference on manipulative therapy, Melbourne, Australia

Head, H. (1893) On disturbances of sensation with especial reference to the pain of visceral disease. *Brain*, **16**, 1–133

Kohlrausch, W. and Leube, H. (1953) *Hochergymnastik*, Fischer, Jena (cited by Bischof and Elmiger, 1963

Leube, H. and Dicke, E. (1944) *Massage Reflektorischer Zonen im Bindegewebe bei Rheumatischen und Inneren Erkrankungen*, Fischer, Jena (cited by Bischof and Elmiger, 1963)

Luedecke, U. (1969) History, basis and technique of connective tissue massage. *Aust. J. Physiother.*, **15**(4), 141–8

Mackenzie, J. (1909) *Symptoms and their Interpretation*, Shaw and Sons, London

Sato, A., Sato, Y., Shimado, F. and Torigata, Y. (1975) Changes in gastric motility produced by neuceptive stimulation of the skin in rats. *Brain Res.*, **87**, 151–9

Stoddard, A. (1962) *Manual of Osteopathic Technique*, 2nd edn, Hutchinson, London

Stoddard, A. (1969) *Manual of Osteopathic Practice*, Hutchinson, London

Terich-Leube, H. (1957) *Grundriss der Beindegewebsmassage*, Fischer, Stuttgart (cited by Bischof and Elmiger, 1963)

Travell, J. and Rinzler, G.H. (1946) Relief of cardiac pain by local block of somatic trigger areas. *Proc. Soc. Exp. Biol. Med.*, **63**, 480–7

Travell, J.G. and Simons, D.G. (1983) *Myofascial Pain and Dysfunction: The Trigger Point Manual*, Williams and Wilkins, Baltimore, Md.

Volker, R. and Rostovsky, E. (1949) Ueber den therapeutischen wert der BGM bei gefaess-stroerunger der gliedmassen. *Z. Rheumaforsch*, **8**, 192 (cited by Ebner, 1975)

19 Hydrotherapy

ALISON T. SKINNER and ANN M. THOMSON

Introduction

The term hydrotherapy is derived from the Greek *hydor* meaning water and *therapeia* meaning to heal. Hydrotherapy was first used by the Greeks in the time of Hippocrates (460–375 BC), who treated disease with hot and cold water, diet, rest and as few drugs as possible. Following the Greek influence, the Romans began building baths (1st century AD) for both recreational and curative purposes. During the Dark Ages there was little use of therapeutic baths, but in the reign of Elizabeth I they came back into fashion. Then, in 1697, Sir John Flayer published a paper entitled *An enquiry into the right use and abuse of hot, cold and temperate baths in England*. His views, however, were not well supported in England, but in Germany tepid baths were used extensively for the relief of muscle spasm and in the treatment of hyperexcitable patients. During the late nineteenth and early twentieth centuries, mineral baths and spas increased in popularity throughout Europe and the United States.

Gradually, hydrotherapy has become a widely accepted therapeutic modality used by physiotherapists in the treatment of a variety of patients with many different diseases or disorders.

The physical properties of water and pain relief

Water has certain physical properties which have a direct bearing on pain relief. These are: *buoyancy*, *hydrostatic pressure*, *turbulence* and *temperature*.

Buoyancy

This is a force acting in the opposite direction to the force of gravity and is experienced as an upthrust. The force of buoyancy can thus provide weight relief, the extent of which is dependent on the proportion of the body below water level.

Approximate weight relief achieved at different levels is (Harrison and Bulstrode, 1987)

Immersion to ASIS level	– 54% males, 47% females.
Immersion to xiphisternum	– 35% males, 28% females.
Immersion to C7	– 8% males and females.

Pain due to weight-bearing can thus be relieved in a hydrotherapy pool. The patient, therefore, may be treated in various modifications of standing and sitting. The normality of movement restored is a factor in the maintenance of pain relief after the patient has left the pool. Buoyancy, with or without floats, can provide complete support for the body in supine floating. This position enables the patient to relax, thus easing muscle tension or spasm with the consequent relief of pain. There is no localized pressure on the patient's bony prominences when floating, and this is very comfortable for patients who have lost body tissue after a debilitating disease.

When the body is supported by buoyancy, the arms, legs and trunk may be moved just under the surface of the water and parallel with it. This freedom of movement can help to regain a full range of movement in joints with the result that synovial fluid may sweep across the cartilage bringing nutrition and lubrication back to the joint surfaces. The movement also facilitates fluid movement through the tissue and fascial planes helping to drain the metabolic products which have accumulated and which act as a noxious stimulus.

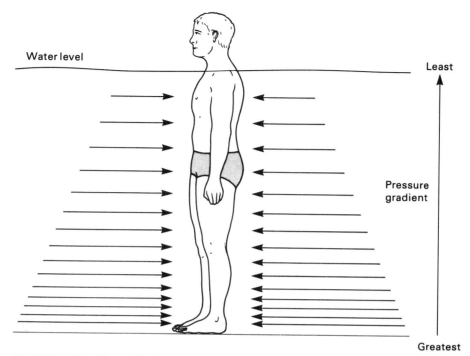

Fig. 19.1   The effects of hydrostatic pressure when the patient is standing in the water.

Hydrostatic Pressure

This property of water provides an even pressure on all surfaces of an immersed limb or body at any one given depth. However, the pressure is greater deeper in the water and less nearer the surface (Figure 19.1).

For each foot of water in which the body is immersed the pressure increases by 22.4 mmHg. Cardiac volume has been shown to be increased by approximately 180 ml during immersion up to the suprasternal notch in the upright position (Hall *et al.*, 1990).

The pressure gradient therefore aids the flow of venous blood and lymph in an antigravitational direction when the patient is standing in the pool, and this may help reduce oedema in the foot and lower leg. Thus where oedematous fluid creates tensions and distortion within the tissues with consequent pain, the effects of the hydrostatic pressure may be utilized for pain relief.

Turbulence

This is an irregular movement of water molecules. Within a hydrotherapy pool, turbulence may be created by an underwater douche, which is a jet of water from a hose pipe. The douche is used to apply a pressure on the tissues and may be moved around a painful area. It is, therefore, like a deep soft tissue manipulative technique without contact between the physiotherapist's hand and patient's skin. Patients report dramatic pain relief from this modality, and it is interesting to postulate that this may be due to pressure and the stretching of tight tissues and movement of fluid through the various fascial planes as well as the stimulation of mechanoreceptors. Turbulence may also be created by the physiotherapist moving through the water. When the patient is lying in the floating position (float lying), and turbulence is created just beyond the patient's head, the effect is that the patient moves through the water (Figure 19.2). This has a relaxing effect and may be used to ease muscle tension or spasm especially in the neck and shoulder girdle area.

If a patient has difficulty in walking through the resistance of the water and this causes discomfort, the physiotherapist may walk in front of the patient so that a wake is created for the patient to walk in (Figure 19.3). This makes walking easier and therefore reduces the discomfort.

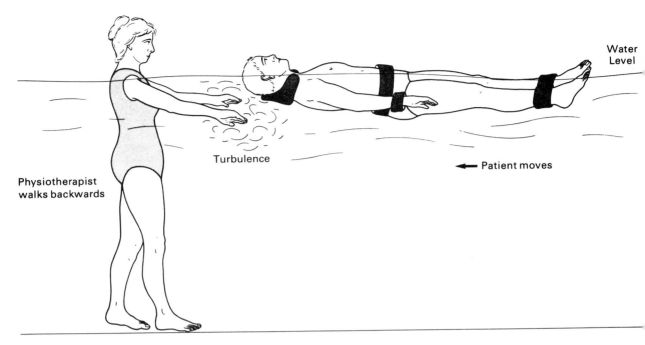

Fig. 19.2   The application of turbulence with the patient lying in the floating position.

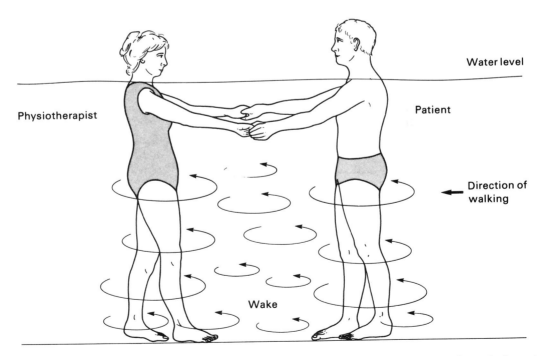

Fig. 19.3   The application of turbulence with the physiotherapist and the patient walking through the water.

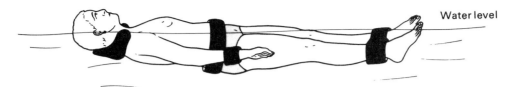

Water level

Fig. 19.4   Float lying.

Temperature

The water in a hydrotherapy pool is generally maintained at a temperature of between 35°C and 36°C. Therefore during the time a patient is being treated, the whole body is warmed. This induces relaxation of muscle spasm, promotes increased flow of circulation and facilitates movement of joints. The effects of heat in pain relief have been discussed in Chapter 16. The temperature of the water should be reduced when patients perform activities such as an exercise circuit, e.g. 32°–33°C. Where there are groups of people performing activities the temperature may be reduced to 30°C.

Techniques associated with pain relief in the hydrotherapy pool

Relaxation Techniques

Conscious relaxation

The patient is in float lying and is encouraged to feel that the floats and water are supporting the body totally. The suggestion of floating and 'letting go' encourages the patient to relax.

Contrast relaxation

The patient is again in float lying (Figure 19.4). Instructions are given so that the patient tightens the muscles which increase in tone, then relaxes with a consequent lengthening effect on the muscles. For example, where the back extensors are to be relaxed, the patient is instructed to lift the pelvis up out of the pelvic float, hold and then relax. Where the knee flexors are to be treated the patient is instructed to push the foot down against the float into the water, hold and then let go. The knee is then straightened by buoyancy and the flexors relax.

Passive movements and relaxation

With the patient supported in floats, the physiotherapist stands behind the patient's head and places a hand on either side of the chest wall, to straighten and support the upper trunk. The patient's upper trunk is then moved rhythmically from side to side so that the pelvis and legs move reciprocally in an easy and relaxed manner. The pelvis can also be held by the physiotherapist and the trunk, head and arms moved in a similar way. The physiotherapist may hold the patient's feet together and produce a side-to-side or figure-of-eight movement, which produces a rhythmical reciprocal movement of the whole body.

Oscillatory Passive Movements

The use of these procedures is developing in pool therapy. Localized and regional manipulation (Chapter 17) may be adapted for use in the pool. The oscillations are slower due to the resistance of the water and there is less localization due to the difficulties of fixation. Examples of procedures used are:

1. Posteroanterior pressures to the spine with the patient in float lying,
2. Longitudinal oscillations to the shoulder and the hip.
3. Cervical spine rotation where the patient is in float lying with the neck fixed on the physiotherapist's shoulder and the thorax is rotated.
4. Lumbar spine rotation where the patient may be either on a half plinth or holding the bar across the corner of the pool. The legs are supported by the physiotherapist and the pelvis rotated.
5. Caudad gliding of the humeral head can be applied with the patient in float lying and the arm in abduction.

The therapeutic effects are similar to those

indicated in Chapter 17. The warmth of the water assists in relaxation of muscle spasm and the freedom of movement can enable the patient to join in actively, e.g. in lumbar spine rotation or glenohumeral abduction.

Hold–relax technique (see also Chapter 12)

This technique is used to increase range of movement at a joint or to lengthen muscles where increased muscle tension associated with pain is the limiting factor. The muscle group is made to contract strongly against resistance (hold phase) applied by the physiotherapist and this is followed by a relaxation phase during which there is a lenghtening effect in the muscle. Generally the patient's position is chosen so that buoyancy assists movement into the new range. This helps to break up the pain – spasm – pain cycle.

A float may be used to provide the resistance to the 'hold' phase. The resistance of the float is varied according to the strength of the muscles treated. During the 'relaxation phase' the float provides a stretch on the muscle.

Repeated contractions (see also Chapter 12)

This technique involves applying maximal resistance to the agonist muscles involved in a movement making the muscles work isotonically, then isometrically, then isotonically with consequent lengthening due to reciprocal inhibition of the antagonists. In the pool, the resistance can be applied by turbulence, with or without buoyancy. Isotonic work is generated when the patient performs a movement through the water and isometric work is generated when a position is held by the patient who is moved by the physiotherapist through the water. As with hold–relax, there is breaking up of the pain – spasm – pain cycle with the added benefit of strengthening the agonist muscles.

Exercises

Exercises are directed towards improving coordination, increasing joint range, strengthening muscles and improving function. Buoyancy may be counterbalanced, assisting or resisting with the added effect of floats, bats, or flippers. While these exercises may not be of direct obvious benefit in relieving pain, the restoration of normal function is usually associated with pain relief.

Breathing exercises

The patient lies in the water on a half-stretcher with the legs moved to one side, which stretches the chest wall muscles and trunk side flexors of the opposite side. The physiotherapist gives the instruction to the patient to breathe in deeply on the stretched side and then to breathe out. Just prior to the inspiratory phase, the physiotherapist applies slight stretch to the patient's legs and pelvis which stretches the intercostal muscles and at the same time applies manual pressure on the thorax to encourage inspiration. This technique is of value in the treatment of patients who have had a thoracotomy or have ankylosing spondylitis. Patients appear to find deep breathing and trunk mobility exercises easier after this technique of breathing exercises and these are thus of value in pain control.

Posture training

Many patients who have pain arising from tissues of the neuromusculoskeletal systems have an underlying postural defect which predisposes these tissues to injury or prolonged stress. Retraining of postural awareness and a sound basis for movement must be an integral component of any treatment programme. For example, if a patient has an excessive lordosis in the lumbar spine backward pelvic tilting is taught until the patient can register the feeling of a balanced pelvis. As a guide the pelvis is well balanced when the ASIS and the PSIS are on the same horizontal plane with the patient in standing. In this position the patient performs activities such as holding a float in each hand and pushing each hand alternately into the water with trunk side flexion; holding floats as above trunk turning – progressing to holding a bat in both hands to increase the resistance. If the patient has difficulty in tilting the pelvis backwards then it may be necessary to lengthen the hip flexors, or the back extensors, to start the exercise with the knees slightly flexed or to apply soft tissue massage to mobilize tight soft tissue over the lumbar spine. To be effective in pain relief, these principles must be applied before and during activities performed by the patient in the pool.

Water fitness – long term relief

Exercises in water can help in both maintaining and improving physical fitness. The exercises are normally performed rhythmically to music. The programme is designed to stretch and strengthen muscles, move joints through full range together with improving heart and lung function. The warmth of the water and the weight relief provided allows muscles and joints to be exercised without pain or damage. Generally people are taken in groups of eight to ten. People wishing to participate in these exercise programmes on a continuing and regular basis may find suitable classes in a local leisure centre.

Smit and Harrison (1991) in a pilot study found that patients with chronic lower back pain had pain relief at the end of a course of hydrotherapy but after three months pain levels had returned to pre-treatment levels. The patients did, however, feel much better in general terms. It would appear that some form of continuing programme is required and this may be obtained by the patients joining a water fitness class.

Swimming

Many patients are advised to take up swimming for the relief of spinal pain. It is essential that this advice is based on a sound assessment of the patient's clinical problems. Breaststroke, butterfly and front crawl all tend to increase the lumbar lordosis and extensor muscle activity. Therefore, patients whose problems arise from flattening of the lumbar spine generally do benefit from these strokes, but patients with an increased lordosis often have an increase in pain. Patients who derive benefit from rotation techniques, may benefit from performing the front or back crawl. Where a patient has a scoliosis a special exercise programme tailored for the individual is required and symmetrical swimming strokes may be contraindicated. People who swim for pleasure and who have degenerative changes in the neck develop pain in the neck and shoulder girdle area if they hold the head out of the water as they swim, especially on breaststroke. This happens particularly in women who like to keep their hair dry. The leg action in breaststroke involves a forced valgus position of the knee which can lead to stretching and strain of the medial collateral ligament with resultant pain. Patients with knee pain therefore should be advised to avoid the breaststroke action. Costill *et al* (1992) state that up to 60% of elite competitive swimmers complain of shoulder pain. Patients with shoulder pain, therefore, should have a programme of exercises in water and swim only when there is no risk to the shoulder particularly in the presence of a rotator cuff lesion. Swimming is an excellent form of exercise for gaining fitness but clearly must be used therapeutically with careful attention to the biomechanics of the patient's problem.

Conditions which are appropriate for pain control or relief by pool therapy

Rheumatic disorders

Rheumatoid arthritis

Patients with this disease benefit from the effects of weight relief particularly on the joints which are recovering following an active stage in the disease. In the warmth and support of the water, patients are able to exercise in a pain reduced state increasing muscle strength, maintaining or increasing joint movement and improving stamina and general fitness.

Osteoarthritis

Patients with osteoarthritis of the spine, hips, knees or shoulders benefit from hydrotherapy. Where there is bilateral osteoarthritis of the hips or knees, the weight relief allows for muscle strengthening and re-education of gait in the presence of pain relief with resultant functional improvement. With the patient on a half-stretcher, longitudinal oscillatory passive movements applied in the long axis of the femur help to control pain in patients with advanced osteoarthritis of the hip. The hold–relax technique is of particular benefit for relaxing spasm in the hip adductors and flexors and in the knee flexors where appropriate. The spasm of the lumbar spine extensors associated with osteoarthritis of the spine also responds to relaxation techniques. Mobility and pain relief in the lumbar spine may be obtained by treating the patient in float lying. The physiotherapist places her hands under the patient's lumbar spine and performs an oscillatory movement in a posteroanterior direction, thereby encouraging relaxation of the lumbar spine extensors.

Ankylosing spondylitis

The nature of this condition results in pain being present in many joints at one time. The buoyancy and warmth of the water therefore help to reduce this widespread pain. Relaxation techniques and breathing exercises, together with spinal mobility and extension exercises, are all-important for the control of pain in patients with this condition. Barefoot advocates the use of group therapy for patients with AS so that the pain relief obtained can be continued. Groups are organized under the auspices of the National Ankylosing Spondylitis Society. Stretching of tight structures, particularly flexor muscles, and maintenance of range is ensured by stretching techniques incorporating the principles of hold–relax technique (PNF) with floats to apply the resistance and the stretch (Bulstrode and Barefoot, 1987; see also Barefoot, 1988). There appears to be some indication that hydrotherapy has a prophylactic effect in ankylosing spondylitis. In this instance, patients attend for hydrotherapy at 6-monthly intervals to ensure that the joints are kept mobile, muscle strength is maintained and good posture is practised. Thus the pain associated with joint stiffness and soft tissue contractures can be prevented or lessened.

Spondylosis

Patients with cervical spondylosis report benefit from relaxation techniques where the pelvis is moved by the physiotherapist and the trunk, head and arms swing reciprocally. This helps to ease the tension in the neck and shoulder muscles which is associated with this condition. The neck extensors may be strengthened by the patient pushing against the neck float with the chin tucked in. This also stretches tightness of the upper cervical spine extensors, which is so often associated with spondylosis. The pain of lumbar spondylosis responds to relaxation and to repeated trunk rotation exercises, especially when the upper trunk is fixed and the pelvis rotates.

Patients with these conditions tend to have exacerbations and remissions of pain. Hydrotherapy is indicated after the initial acuteness has settled, because it affords relief of severe pain. This then allows for the restoration of mobility and progress towards the restoration of function.

Orthopaedics and Trauma

Fractures of the lower limb

Fractured neck of femur

Elderly patients who have sustained fractured neck of femur are usually treated by internal fixation and early mobilization. Walking on land is painful because these patients find it difficult to keep weight off the limb even with a frame or crutches. The weight relief afforded by buoyancy (Harrison *et al.*, 1992) restores the patient's confidence in an otherwise painful walking pattern. Rising from a chair is also difficult, and this movement can be practised in the pool with the assistance of buoyancy. Thus hydrotherapy helps to accelerate the rehabilitation of these elderly patients.

Fractures of the femoral and tibial shafts

Patients with these fractures often have pain and stiffness in the knee. Hold–relax technique, repeated contractions and progressive exercises for strengthening the muscles that control the knee given in the warmth of the water enable these patients to recover mobility and function.

Fractures of the upper limb

Fractured neck of the humerus with or without a dislocated shoulder

Patients with these injuries are often elderly and are afraid to move the arm because of the pain. The patient sits on a stool or stands in the pool with the shoulders under the water and is encouraged to relax so that buoyancy may raise the arm and flex the shoulder joint. The warmth of the water reduces the pain, and the patient regains confidence in moving the arm. This approach facilitates the re-education of reversed humeroscapular rhythm. If there is spasm of the adductors, hold relax technique may be used to regain abduction. Once the patient is confident in moving the arm up to 90° from the chest wall, the starting position is changed to float lying, in which position the arm can be assisted into full elevation.

Back pain following trauma or operation

Following operations such as laminectomy or fenestration patients may begin pool therapy approximately 10–12 days after the operation. Following trauma to the back, the patient is often given a period of bed rest immediately after which pool therapy may begin. In these patients, the back extensors are often in spasm and it is important to break the pain–spasm–pain cycle. Relaxation techniques, general at first and then localized to the area of greatest spasm, relieve the pain and enable the patient to feel freedom of movement within the spine. Where the patient is afraid of pain on spinal movement, encouragement is given in moving the arms and legs. These activities make the muscles controlling the trunk act as fixators which helps to accelerate the circulatory flow through spinal structures removing inflammatory exudate and relieving pain.

Knee surgery

Patients who have reparative surgery for a knee injury often have a history of long-standing knee pain. These patients benefit from pool therapy by the weight relief, by techniques such as oscillatory distraction, which reduces intra-articular friction and by having the strength of the quadriceps increased with progressive exercises. These patients have a daily programme of part hydrotherapy and part dry-land rehabilitation. Where pool therapy is given first, patients report relief of pain which improves their performance and function in dry-land rehabilitation.

Running in Deep Water

This has been advocated by Sarah Rowell (n.d.) for maintaining or restoring fitness during recovery from injury. The patient is maintained in an upright position using a flotation aid in the form of a belt or a life jacket in water at a depth such that the patient's feet are off the floor. A running action is performed with arms and legs. It is especially useful for patients who have sustained a fracture or severe injury of the lower limb because there is no impact stress on the limbs as would be associated with weight-bearing. The same principle would apply to restoration of mobility in a spine that has been injured.

Amputation

Patients with lower limb amputations sometimes develop painful contractures over the flexor aspects of the hip and/or knee. Passive stretching is applied to the tight structures with the patient lying on a half-stretcher in the water. The discomfort of the stretching is reduced by the warmth of the water and therefore the effect is more quickly obtained than on land. Buoyancy may be used to assist the stretching, e.g. if the patient is lying prone on a half-stretcher buoyancy will assist hip extension and help stretch the tight flexors and associated soft tissue contractures.

The patients enjoy swimming, and the freedom of movement afforded by the water contributes to the overall sense of well-being.

Neurological Conditions

Multiple sclerosis

Patients with this condition often suffer back pain, which is relieved in water due to a combination of warmth and support. It is worth trying passive movements and relaxation to reduce spasticity, which will further relieve pain and this may then be followed by passive stretching of structures contracted due to prolonged sitting in the later stages of the condition.

While hydrotherapy may not have any effect on the course of the disorder, patients report several days of comfort and easier movement following pool treatment. The management of these patients should employ six to eight treatment sessions at approximately 6-monthly intervals. A careful watch should be kept for the occasional patient with multiple sclerosis who does not like the humidity and warmth of the pool and becomes very tired as a result. Such a patient may not be suitable for this type of treatment.

Hemiplegia

The painful shoulder associated with hemiplegia can be treated with some success. The patient sits on a stool with buoyancy assisting the affected arm up to 90° flexion. If the physiotherapist then supports the patient's arm with one hand, and helps to protract the patient's shoulder girdle with the other hand, tightness of the retractors is eased and the patient finds shoulder movement easier. If flexion and extension of the shoulder are then encouraged in the horizontal plane just under the water surface, there is reduction of pain which has a carry-over into functional activities on land.

Polyneuropathies

In the early stages of recovery from these conditions, the comfortable handling of the patient is difficult because of hypersensitivity of the patient's skin. Treatment in the pool with relaxation in float lying reduces the hypersensitivity so that re-education techniques for the recovering muscle groups are more comfortable for the patient. Initially, the patient needs to be lowered into the water and taken out again in a sheet to avoid handling of the skin.

Aqua-natal classes.

It is generally reccommended that women who wish to attend these should wait until the 20th week of pregnancy and six weeks after the birth of the baby. The main muscle groups of the body are exercised in a safe supportive medium. The buoyancy of the water provides weight relief which is particularly helpful during the later stages of pregnancy to relieve backache. Both buoyancy and the warmth of the water help the women to learn to relax which can have a carry-over effect during labour. It may also help the women to sleep better and possibly improve bowel function. The improvement in general well-being enables the women to cope better with pain.

Postnatally the abdominal and pelvic floor muscles can be strengthened. In the upright position buoyancy assists pelvic floor contractions and reduces postnatal pain associated with pelvic floor stretch or damage.

Aqua-natal exercises improve general fitness by working the respiratory, cardiovascular and musculoskeletal systems. As muscle power and general fitness improve, the onset of pain is diminished.

Respiratory Disorders

Thoracotomy

Following thoracotomy, patients may have a combination of pool treatment and dry-land exercises. The humidity in the pool room is high, therefore when the patient breathes in there is water vapour in the inspired air. This helps to loosen secretions and makes coughing less painful. The warmth of the water surrounding the chest wall also reduces pain and thoracic mobility improves. This effect carries over from one day to the next so that the patient finds arm movements and breathing exercises on land more comfortable. Patients may be treated in the pool two days after the operation with the wound covered by a plastic dressing. According to Boyd (1976), patients benefit from daily treatment in the pool and may participate in a group programme. A patient who had this regime following a second thoracotomy had a more speedy recovery than after the first thoracotomy, the postoperative management of which did not include pool therapy.

Haemophilia

Pain in this condition arises from a bleed into joints or muscles, which if untreated, results in contractures and loss of functional movement patterns. Passive stretching exercises given to the tight muscles are much more comfortable with the patient in a pool rather than on dry land. Joints are treated with mobilizing exercises and selective muscle strengthening designed to restore muscle balance. Osteotomy of the femoral or tibial bones is often necessary where repeated bleeding has caused loss of joint cartilage with consequent deformity. Patients have pool treatment when the stitches have been taken out after 10 days, and although full joint range may not return, there is restoration of pain-free function.

Summary

That pain relief is a therapeutic entity of hydrotherapy is undisputed in terms of patients' reports. It is interesting to consider why there may be this pain relief. The water is at 35°C, therefore the whole body is immersed in a medium, the temperature of which is above that of the skin (33.5°C); this, therefore, affords relaxation which in turn reduces muscle tension and the pain–spasm–pain cycle is broken. The warmth of the medium also produces a redistribution of circulation so that there is an increase of blood flow through the superficial tissues. The activity of sweat glands is increased following pool therapy because the body loses heat gained during treatment by evaporation of sweat. There is also an increased rate of circulation through the vessels of the working muscles during exercises performed in the pool. These effects may produce chemical changes within neurons and result in pain relief which lasts longer than the pool therapy.

There is no doubt that patients find movements easier in the warm pool than on dry land and are therefore able to perform activities through a greater range of movement. Muscles are therefore shortening and lengthening and joint surfaces are moved through a greater range than on land. This must move synovial fluid across articular cartilage, and tissue fluid through tissue spaces which improves nutrition and may restore chemical balance within the tissues with consequent pain relief.

Patients who are unable to move well on land derive great pleasure from the freedom of movement in the pool. This applies particularly to patients with rheumatoid arthritis, ankylosing spondylitis, multiple sclerosis and acute pain associated with degenerative disorders of the joints both peripheral and spinal. These patients leave the pool room with a sense of well-being and achievement. It is probable therefore, that some of the pain relief reported by patients is due to a raising of the pain tolerance level which enables the patient to manage the pain although it may well be still present.

Overall, therefore, pool therapy has a place in the number of skills available to the physiotherapist in the relief or control of pain in patients.

References

Barefoot, J. (1988) *Stretch Relax and a Little Bit More. Exercises for Ankylosing Spondylitis*, Georgian Music Desktop Publishing, Bath

Boyd, J.M. (1976) A new programme for thoracotomy patients. *Physiotherapy* [*Canad.*], **28** (5), 274–6

Bulstrode, S., Barefoot, J. *et al.* (1987) The role of passive stretching in the treatment of ankylosing spondylitis. *Br. J. Rheumatol*, 2640–2

Costill, D.L., Maglischo, E.W. and Richardson, A.B. (1992) *Swimming*, Blackwell Scientific P; Oxford, ch. 19, p. 187

Hall, J. Bisson, D. and O'Hare, P. (1990) The physiology of immersion. *Physiotherapy*, **76** (9), 517–20

Harrison, R.A. and Bulstrode, S.J. (1987) Percentage weight-bearing during partial immersion in the hydrotherapy pool. *Physiotherapy Practice*, **3**, 60–3

Harrison, R.A., Hillman, M. and Bulstrode, S. (1992) Loading of the lower limb when walking partially immersed. *Physiotherapy*, **78** (3), 164–6

Rowell, S. (n.d.) Running in deep water. *Athletics Weekly and Coaching Focus*.

Smit, T. and Harrison, R.A. (1991) Hydrotherapy and chronic lower back pain. A pilot study. *Aust. Physiother.*, **37** (4), 229–34

Further reading

Davis, B.C. and Harrison, R.A. (1988) *Hydrotherapy in Practice*, Churchill Livingstone, Edinburgh

Farrell, R.J. (1976) A hydrotherapy program for high cervical cord lesions. *Physiotherapy (Canad.)* **28(1)**, 8–12

Golland, A. (1981) Basic hydrotherapy. *Physiotherapy*, **67**(9), 258–62

Reid Campion, M.J. (1985) *Hydrotherapy in Paediatrics*, Heinemann Medical, London

Reid Campion, M.J. (1990) *Adult Hydrotherapy*, Butterworth Heinemann, London

Skinner, A.T. and Thomson, A.M. (1983) *Duffield's Exercise in Water*, 3rd edn., Baillière Tindall, London

20 *The management of postoperative pain*

ALEXANDRA HOUGH

What is so surprising is that this deplorable state of affairs has persisted and continues to persist in many hospitals, despite considerable advances in the pharmacology of analgesic drugs.

Smith, 1991

Introduction

Postoperative pain is notorious for being widespread and unnecessarily severe. Possible reasons for this 'deplorable state of affairs' are the following:

1. An attitude that pain is unimportant, inevitable and to be borne with fortitude, especially in cultures which see stoicism as a virtue and distress as a weakness.
2. Lack of knowledge. Lavies (1992) found that doctors did not realize that there is less than one chance in 3000 of patients becoming addicted to postoperative analgesics, and indeed 82% of doctors admitted to being ill-educated in pain control.
3. Inexperience, tradition and overwork (Justins and Richardson, 1991).
4. Wide and unpredictable variations in patients' perception of pain and response to drugs.
5. Patients failing to ask for or expect adequate pain relief.
6. Rudimentary pain assessment, leading to health staff not knowing how much pain their patients are experiencing.

Some staff have only a limited understanding of the subjective nature of pain. McCaffery and Ferrell (1992) found that half of the nurses in their study doubted patients' reports, and it is common to hear criticism of patients for having a 'low pain threshold' or being 'naughty' for complaining of pain. Pain is more than a sensation, it is the perception and reaction to that sensation. It is a personal experience, not something that can be judged by someone else. The only sure definition of pain is that it is what the patient says hurts. We do not serve our patients well if we allow ourselves to lose our sensitivity and become part of a system that shames or tranquillizes patients who express pain.

> 'Whose pain should the physician control: The patient's? That of the relatives? Or his own, generated by his inability to help the patient? (Szasz, 1968)

Pain and breathing

The commonest postoperative pulmonary complication is atelectasis, and the commonest cause of atelectasis is pain (Simpson *et al.*, 1992). The relation between pain and atelectasis is illustrated in Figure 20.1, and this can be understood readily by anyone trying to take a deep breath when in the dentist's chair.

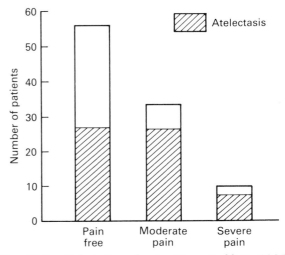

Fig. 20.1 Atelectasis and pain. (From Embling, 1985, by permission.)

Pain from thoracic or abdominal surgery leads to guarding spasm of trunk muscles, inhibition of breathing, and inevitably some degree of atelectasis. This is exacerbated by immobility, which is greater if there is pain.

Pain also causes hypertension, tachycardia, excess oxygen consumption, sleep deprivation and delayed hospital discharge (Carron, 1989). It creates a vicious cycle of muscle spasm and reflex sympathetic activity.

Closed alveoli are harder to inflate than partially open alveoli. Therefore, for both pain management and respiratory care, prevention is better than cure. This begins before surgery.

Preoperative management

Preoperative advice enhances cooperation and reduces the anxiety that exacerbates pain perception. It is time well spent, and has been shown to lessen postoperative complications (Cupples, 1991), reduce analgesic requirements by half, and lead to discharge nearly 3 days earlier than in patients not given this form of preparation (Egbert et al., 1964). It is especially important for children, elderly people and patients expecting to wake up in the intensive care unit.

The preoperative visit should be carried out as early as possible because anxiety at impending surgery inhibits receptivity (Cupples, 1991). Reduction of anxiety is not a luxury because the stress response is thought to contribute to muscle breakdown, delayed healing, immunosuppression and other postoperative complications (Salmon, 1992).

The preoperative visit includes:

1. Explanations about the importance of maintaining activity preoperatively and resuming it as soon as possible postoperatively.
2. Advice to feel free to ask for pain killers postoperatively if drugs are not to be given automatically.
3. Information specific to the operation. Some patients like to know everything about the wound, drips, drains and what it will feel like, while a few make it clear that they want to know the minimum. People undergoing complex procedures may benefit from visits by patients who have had similar surgery.
4. Discussion of the patient's previous experiences of pain, their expectations and preferences for pain management, plus liaison with other team members.
5. For high-risk or anxious patients, practice in how to roll, deep breathe, use the incentive spirometer, sit up and cough with minimum pain.

Patients who are particularly worried can be taught relaxation to reduce the perception of pain (Miller and Perry, 1990). Tapes and books are available as adjuncts. A modified form of relaxation can be done in a few minutes with the help of the following suggestions:

- Take up your most comfortable position.
- Imagine that you are in a place that you find peaceful, such as a beach or sunny meadow.
- Breathe in slowly and deeply.
- As you breathe out, feel the tension draining out of your body and into the floor.
- Use a relaxed abdominal breathing pattern (Hough, 1991).
- To help focus on your breathing and prevent your attention wandering, count slowly and silently to three as you breathe in, and slowly and silently to four as you breathe out.

This can be done at any time of day in order to fit into the busy hospital schedule. Rhythmic breathing should be maintained throughout the procedure, and imagery can be incorporated if appropriate.

Although relaxation decreases anxiety, mindless reassurance does not engender trust and can impair the 'work of worry'. This 'work' is a natural and necessary part of anticipating a stressful event, and helps in the process of adjustment to the operation and its outcome. Postoperative distress is related to lack of preoperative anticipation of pain and discomfort (Salmon, 1992).

The tradition of prolonged food and fluid fasting is now considered unjustified. This practice causes distress, dehydration and can contribute to morbidity and mortality. Fluid fasting can be physiologically harmful and a dry mouth makes it difficult to expectorate postoperatively. A light meal and clear fluids by mouth should be allowed up to 3 hours before surgery (Hung, 1992; Strunin, 1993).

Pre-emptive analgesia reduces postoperative pain by preventing noxious impulses from gaining entry into the central nervous system. Injury provokes prolonged change in CNS function, which influences the response to subsequent afferent inputs. This 'memory' of pain can be prevented by, for example, adding anti-inflammatory drugs to the premedication or using nerve blocks. Drug

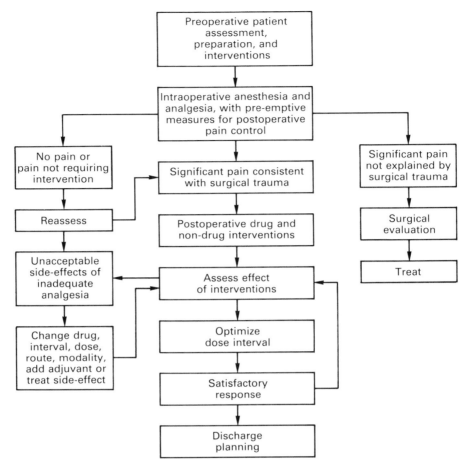

Fig. 20.2   Pain management flowchart. (From Jacox *et al*. 1992, by permission.)

dosage to prevent pain is many times less than that required to abolish pain after it has occurred (Katz *et al*., 1992). Post-amputation pain syndromes can be either reduced by neurolytic sympathectomy, which relieves preoperative ischaemic pain, or eliminated by epidural analgesia up to 3 days preoperatively (Cousins, 1989).

Postoperative assessment

Accurate assessment of patients in relation to their pain and respiration allows logical decisions to be made about appropriate management, and prevents unnecessary interventions such as asking a patient with no secretions to cough.

Postoperative pain should be assessed and recorded on the patient's chart in the same way as any vital sign, preferably 2-hourly on the first postoperative day, with a named nurse being responsible to ensure accountability. A pain flow chart helps to monitor management (Figure 20.2). The method of assessment depends on patient preference, many patients finding a visual analogue scale (VAS) easiest. More detailed assessment can include anxieties and fears related to pain, and the strategies that patients normally use to relieve their own pain.

Pain assessment is also a right for people who are cognitively impaired or do not speak English, not just those who can complain in a way that is easy to understand. If verbal report is not possible, pain is suspected in the presence of restlessness, agitation, pallor, sweating, shallow breathing or breath-holding. Family members can be involved in assessment if appropriate.

Reduction in the perception of pain

Perception of pain varies with factors that physiotherapists cannot modify, such as the type of incision, operative technique and method of suturing, discomforts such as drainage tubes and nasogastric tubes, and the patient's upbringing and past experience. In addition, social class and education affects the expression of pain perception (East, 1992). Pain perception also varies with factors that physiotherapists can modify, such as the following side effects of surgery.

Nausea is experienced by 30% of patients and is particularly common after lengthy surgery, if there is pain or dizziness, and in patients who are anxious or obese. It can be reduced by drug review (Watcha and White, 1992), hydration, pain relief, or acupressure using a comfortable finger-kneading technique on the mid-anterior wrist three-fingers-breadth above the distal skin crease (Barsoum *et al.*, 1990).

Discomfort is minimized by sensitive positioning and handling. A rope attached to the foot of the bed encourages independent bed mobility and improves comfort.

Anxiety is reduced by giving preoperative information, encouraging autonomy and preventing sleep fragmentation.

Depression may occur if surgery causes mutilation or altered body image, for example colostomy or mastectomy. An understanding ear or referral to other members of the health team or a self-help group may prevent a sense of loss degenerating into depression.

Fatigue can be minimized by negotiating with patients rather than imposing a postoperative programme on them, and by encouraging frequent short walks rather than infrequent long ones.

Urine retention and *flatulence* increase pain and impair excursion of the diaphragm. Urine retention can be helped by acupressure at the hollow proximal to the mid-transverse arch of each foot. Flatulence can be relieved by pelvic tilting and knee rolling in crook-lying.

Postural hypotension may be an early sign of mild unrecognized hypovolaemia. Such patients should avoid any sudden motion or position change.

Hiccups may be inhibited by acupressure at the tip of each eleventh rib.

Handling patients in pain

Pain works subversively, undermining one's self-confidence and self-control. The sense of anticipation is honed, to hysteria almost, and one quickly learns to be thoroughly suspicious of the well-meant: 'this won't hurt'.

Brooks, 1990

Physiotherapists should be seen as experts in the relief of pain rather than its perpetrators. The essence of physiotherapy is skilful handling, and we are well equipped for this with a combination of physical dexterity, knowledge of physiology and a holistic approach to the needs of each individual.

Certain guidelines are fundamental to handling patients in pain:

1. Most importantly, patients must be assured that they are in control. Control reduces anxiety and physiological arousal, and increases tolerance for pain (Gil *et al.*, 1990).
2. Analgesia should be given automatically before physiotherapy, instead of first 'checking' to see if treatment causes pain, a strategy known as shutting the stable door after the horse has bolted. Hurting patients reduces cooperation.
3. Unnecessary handling should be avoided, the degree of activity being decided after assessment.
4. The patient should be informed of why, how and when each movement will take place. Words to avoid are 'just relax', which signals to any seasoned patient that they are about to be hurt, or 'sorry' after an unexpected movement instead of clear explanations before the movement.

The principles of the following techniques are to offer patients advice and support, and allow them to move themselves as much as possible, rather than be moved by someone else.

Long-sitting to lying (Figure 20.3).

Patients are asked to push back against the physiotherapist's hand and forearm so that they are actively using their back extensors and therefore reciprocally relaxing their abdominal muscles. Reassurance is needed so that patients push back hard enough to eliminate eccentric abdominal muscle work. Physiotherapists need the support of their fist and knee on the bed to protect their own back.

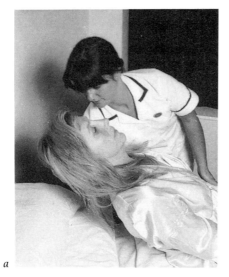

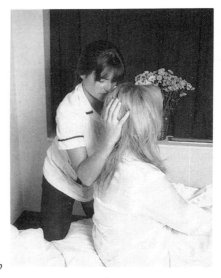

a   *b*

Fig. 20.3*a, b*   Long-sitting to lying. Some physiotherapists like to use two arms for extra support.

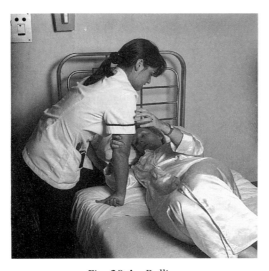

Fig. 20.4   Rolling.

Rolling (Figure 20.4)

Patients are asked to first bend their knees, then remain in supine but shift away from the physiotherapist to leave room to manoeuvre. They then hold on to the physiotherapist's arm or a bed rail, push with their knees and roll towards the physiotherapist in one piece. They are encouraged to emphasize pushing with the legs rather than pull-ing with the arms in order to inhibit abdominal muscle work.

Sitting up over the edge of the bed (Figure 20.5)

From the side-lying position, patients are asked to move to the edge of the bed, hold the physiotherapist closely and allow themselves to be supported until sitting up so that abdominal muscle work is minimized. The physiotherapist presses her fist into the bed to protect her back. Suggested instructions to the patient are, 'let me take your weight and we'll come up together on a count of 3'. Patients who have had chest surgery should hold their arms across their chest rather than over the physiotherapist's shoulder.

Supported cough (Figure 20.6)

Patients may prefer to remain in side-lying, but if they are willing, sitting over the edge of the bed is mechanically most efficient for coughing, and the physiotherapist is well positioned to give supportive, firm and accurately timed manual assistance. When patients are alone, they may find a pillow, towel or cough belt helpful. Reassurance can be given that the stitches will not burst, which only happens if the wound is infected, and then rarely.

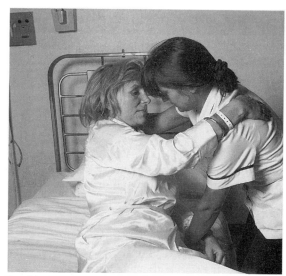

Fig. 20.5   Sitting up over the edge of the bed.

Medication

Doctors prescribe and nurses administer analgesic drugs, but physiotherapists need to understand them and be an active member of the team so that their postoperative care is effective.

Analgesic drugs, like other forms of pain relief, should be given before rather than after pain occurs.

Morphine remains the favourite opioid analgesic.

Side-effects include nausea, constipation, hypotension and elimination of spontaneous sighs. In large doses it depresses respiration. A breathing rate below 11 bpm defines hypoventilation but is an unreliable and late sign of respiratory depression. Drowsiness is not synonymous with respiratory depression. Oximetry is more reliable.

An exaggerated fear of respiratory depression or opioid dependence often leads to inadequate dosage. Depression of respiration is reversible by the opiate antagonist naloxone without loss of analgesia. Opioid dependence is rare unless administration is continuous in a patient who has no pain (Aitkenhead, 1989). A new opioid called tramadol is thought to avoid the side-effect of respiratory depression (Vickers, 1992). Analgesic drugs are discussed in detail in Chapter 11.

The effectiveness of postoperative analgesia varies not only with the patient's perception of pain, but also with that of health staff. Patients may receive only a quarter the dose prescribed (Rosenberg, 1992), male doctors tend to assume that patients feel less pain than female doctors, and senior nursing staff often allow patients less medication than juniors (Pitt and Healey, 1989).

The uptake, distribution and elimination of a drug varies between individuals. Blood concentration after intramuscular injection varies by at least a factor of 5, and even if this variable is overcome, the concentration at which each individual becomes painfree varies by a factor of 3 or 4 (Justins and Richardson, 1991).

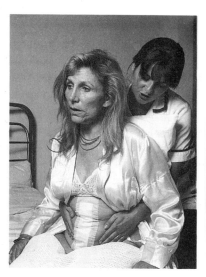
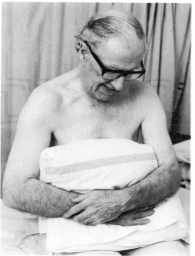
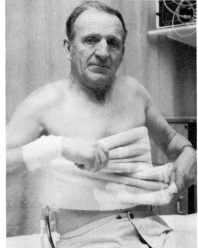

Fig. 20.6 *a, b, c*   Supported cough.

Patients in severe pain, or those who have had chronic pain before surgery, will need a combined approach of opioid, NSAID and local anaesthetic (Cousins, 1989).

Drugs are delivered by a variety of routes, each with their own advantages and disadvantages.

Intramuscular route

Use of the time-honoured 'p.r.n.' intramuscular injection is widespread despite it being the least effective mode of pain relief. This 'as required' analgesia has no rational basis, is usually interpreted as 'give as little as possible', produces wide fluctuations in blood levels, leaves pain unrelieved in half the patients (Jacox et al. 1992) and augments a vicious cycle of anxiety and pain, especially in patients who do not want to appear demanding. Although berated in the literature, it is popular because it is considered, mistakenly, to be the safest regime.

Regular intramuscular prescription is more effective than the p.r.n. routine because it takes less drug to prevent pain from occurring, but dosage may still be 'spectacularly ineffective', due to wide variations in individual response (Hull, 1988).

Intravenous route

The intravenous route gives superior pain relief, offering reliable uptake by the systemic circulation and rapid onset so that the dose can be titrated for each patient. A continuous infusion allows smoother pain relief than intermittent bolus doses, but a combination provides control of both background pain and acute episodes.

Patient-controlled analgesia (PCA) delivers a preset dose of drug by a syringe pump when the patient presses a button. This accommodates to individual needs, encourages mobility, reduces sleep disturbance, is preferred by patients for the autonomy it allows, and requires half as much drug to achieve the same pain control (Hill et al., 1990). A preprogrammed lock-out interval is a safety measure and ensures that each dose achieves peak effect before the next dose is released. Some machines provide a background infusion which can be altered in response to the number of demands made by the patient. Respiratory depression is rare, but monitoring by oximetry is advisable if the patient has limited understanding and

staffing levels are low (Rosenberg, 1992). PCA does not reduce the incidence of nausea, and antiemetics may be needed. Relatives should be warned not to press the button.

Fluctuations in plasma drug levels can now be smoothed out by computer-assisted infusion technology (Biddle, 1992).

Regional analgesia

Transmission within the peripheral nervous system can be blocked by regional analgesic techniques. These act locally and do not befuddle the entire central nervous system, cause less nausea, and many have no central depressant effect on respiration or consciousness. Individual nerves such as digital, wrist, ankle, ilioinguinal, penile and femoral can be blocked with local anaesthetic. Other techniques are described below.

Intercostal

Intercostal nerve blocks are useful after unilateral abdominal incisions, thoracotomy or rib fractures. They are administered by repeated injections into multiple nerves, or more comfortably by continuous infusion. Extrapleural infusion is a further advance in comfort (Majid, 1992). Respiration is not depressed, but pneumothorax is a risk, and the X-ray should be scrutinized if any positive pressure techniques such as intermittent positive pressure breathing or manual hyperinflation are anticipated.

Epidural

The epidural route alters spinal processing by delivering drugs to the epidural space, the catheter being left in situ. Opiates, local anaesthetic or both are used. They work directly on the opiate receptors along the spinal cord, and can control pain originating anywhere below the cranial nerves. Lumbar and thoracic routes are commonly used, but caudal injections are useful after pelvic or perineal surgery. In increasing order of efficacy, administration is available by intermittent blockade, continuous infusion or PCA (Owen et al., 1993).

Advantages are legion: prolonged pain relief, improved lung function, decreased oxygen consumption, reduced incidence of deep vein thrombosis and infection, and hospital stay shortened by an average of a week (Smedstad, 1992). There is also an increase in graft blood flow after vascular surgery (Cousins, 1989).

Disadvantages are partial sensory or motor loss from the local anaesthetic, leading sometimes to weak legs, and blockade of sympathetic outflow, especially noticeable in hypovolaemic patients. Patients should therefore lie flat for 30 minutes after a top-up to avoid hypotension. High blocks are mainly associated with hypotension, while low blocks may cause urinary retention. Delayed respiratory depression can occur, and some form of observation or monitoring is advisable for up to 24 hours after the final dose. Respiratory depression and urinary retention are reversible with naloxone. Hypotension may require fluids, postural change and vasopressor therapy. Other side-effects of the epidural route are nausea and paralytic ileus.

Intrathecal

Another spinal technique is to deliver opioids to the subarachnoid space by intrathecal analgesia (Grace and Orr, 1993), producing profound analgesia without motor, sensory or sympathetic block. Side-effects include 'spinal headache' due to dural puncture; if this occurs during mobilization, the patient should be returned to bed.

Paravertebral

A combination of the effects of epidural and intercostal routes is provided by paravertebral block, by which analgesics are injected into the paravertebral space, an extension of the epidural space (Lönnqvist, 1992). It is suitable for one-sided incisions such as cholecystectomy or thoracotomy. Pneumothorax is a risk.

Intrapleural

Upper abdominal surgery, thoracic surgery or multiple rib fractures are indications for continuous intrapleural infusion of local anaesthetic. This technique has few side-effects and gives better pain control with less respiratory depression than intravenous analgesia (Mann et al., 1992).

Plexus block

Continuous infusion through a catheter inserted near the brachial or lumbar plexus provides analgesia after limb surgery.

Topical analgesia

Up to 24 hours' postoperative analgesia is provided by local anaesthetic sprays, ointments, wound infiltration, or, for knee surgery, intra-articular infusion (Joshi et al., 1993).

Other routes

Subcutaneous

The advantages of subcutaneous injection are simplicity and, when given by infusion, effectiveness. The disadvantage of unpredictable uptake is reduced if administered by PCA (White, 1990).

Oral

The oral route can be used several days after surgery if acute pain has subsided. Advantages are simplicity and pain-free administration. Disadvantages are limited and unpredictable effect due to variability of metabolism by the liver. Limitations are postoperative gastric stasis, vomiting and inability to swallow.

Transdermal and transmucosal

The skin and mucus membranes provide imaginative routes of administration. Skin patches provide trauma-free, safe, but slow-acting analgesia or anti-emesis (Biddle, 1992). Local skin anaesthesia is produced by applying EMLA (eutetic mixture of local anaesthetics) cream to the skin, and no child or neonate should now be submitted to venepuncture, lumbar puncture or any injection without prior application of this 'magic cream'. Adults also benefit (Ralston, 1993).

Mucus membranes are less of a barrier than the skin and allow speedy drug absorption, as cocaine abusers have discovered. More happily, PCA can now be administered sublingually (Jorgensen et al., 1988) and children delightedly anticipate their postoperative fentanyl lollipops.

Nitrous oxide

Rapidly effective and short-lived analgesia can be administered by 5–10 minutes' inhalation of a 50% mix of nitrous oxide and oxygen (Entonox, or in the United States, Nitronox), delivered from a cylinder via face mask and demand valve. Side-effects on the cardiovascular and respiratory systems are minimal (Jones and Hutchinson, 1991), but the patient may feel light-headed, nauseous or giggly, hence its alternative name of laughing gas. A gratifying side-effect is the maintenance of normal lung volume, which in narcotic-treated patients is reduced by an average 22% (Kripke *et al.*, 1983). High doses and continuous use are associated with bone marrow suppression or blood toxicity, but this is not a problem with the doses used before and during physiotherapy.

Nitrous oxide is contraindicated in the presence of acute head injury or low cardiac output (because of peripheral vasodilatation) and subcutaneous emphysema or pneumothorax (because nitrous oxide is more soluble than nitrogen and readily diffuses into sealed pockets of air). The X-ray of a patient with fractured ribs should be checked before using Entonox in case of pneumothorax.

Despite its 175-year history, and its benefits for both adults and children over 4 years of age, Entonox is still not used for the many minor but painful hospital procedures for which it is ideal. It must be medically prescribed, which usually needs a suggestion from the physiotherapist.

Cryoanalgesia

Reversible cold-induced nerve lesions are a form of neural blockade. Cryoanalgesia is an open procedure in which an instrument called a cryoprobe is applied directly to a nerve, freezing it to $-70°C$ (Carron, 1989). This destroys nerve axons without damaging the sheath, creating total pain relief by rendering the relevant area anaesthetic. The nerve regenerates and sensation returns after a period lasting between 2 weeks and several months. Thoracotomy allows direct access to the intercostal nerves and is therefore particularly suited to this form of pain control.

Cold packs are a less exotic means of applying cryoanalgesia but are useful over intact skin to inhibit the peripheral response to rib fracture pain.

Transcutaneous electrical nerve stimulation (TENS)

TENS is underused in postoperative care. It is least effective when used as a last resort, and high-risk patients should be identified early.

Effects

TENS does not depress the respiratory system, is non-invasive, non-toxic, cheap, and produces mobile and happy patients. It is usually used as an adjunct rather than a replacement for medication, but Bayindir (1991) has reported that 95% of postoperative patients using TENS required no narcotics. It has also been claimed that TENS enhances bone healing (Cimino and Hugar, 1980). Agreeable side-effects include reduction in nausea and paralytic ileus (Hymes *et al.*, 1974).

Technique

Details are described in Chapter 14. Specific postoperative modifications are described below.

Four electrodes are normally placed close to each corner of the incision as soon as possible after surgery, avoiding areas of anaesthetic skin. If sterile electrodes are available, two long electrodes are applied in the operating room, one each alongside the wound and under the dressing, with the controls set at a level determined before surgery (Figure 20.7).

As patients become more awake, they can set the controls, and decide how many days to use the machine and whether to use it at night. Liaison with nursing staff and daily skin checks and washes are needed,

Following heart surgery, TENS electrodes should be placed as far away from ECG electrodes as possible to reduce interference with the monitor. TENS is contraindicated in people using a demand or synchronous pacemaker.

TENS has also shown some success in treating long-term wound pain. This rare complication varies from mild localized tenderness to continuous aching and burning along the scar, and is thought to be due to neuroma formation following nerve damage. It is also reduced by effective management of pain in the acute phase (Cousins, 1989).

Acupuncture

Acupuncture (Chapter 13) can provide postoperative pain relief equivalent to medication, with the added advantage of maintaining vital capacity because it does not depress respiration (Facco *et al.*, 1981). Disadvantages are staff time for application, and a 3–4 hour wait for peak intensity.

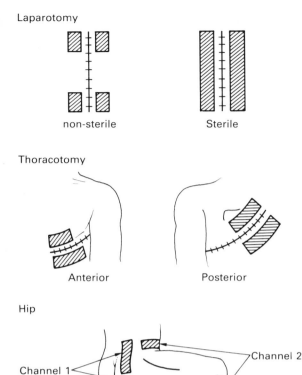

Laparotomy

non-sterile   Sterile

Thoracotomy

Anterior   Posterior

Hip

Channel 2

Channel 1

Fig. 20.7 Electrode placement for postoperative TENS.

Breathing exercises

Effective pain control allows early mobilization, which renders breathing exercises redundant in uncomplicated cases (Dull and Dull, 1983; Jenkins *et al.* 1990). If for surgical or medical reasons the patient is bed-bound, or if breathing exercises are necessary for other reasons, they should be done in a position that achieves a balance between comfort and optimal ventilation/perfusion matching (Hough, 1991).

Cilia are temporarily paralysed by general anaesthesia, but secretions are usually cleared by muco-ciliary transport in the immediate postoperative period. Superficial secretions in the throat may be the only problem and are easily removed by throat clearing. Early mobility helps to prevent secretions accumulating and becoming infected. Coughing and other forced expirations should be done only if indicated, not routinely, because expiration beyond resting lung volume is painful and causes airway closure which is not easily reversed in postoperative patients.

Postural drainage, percussion and vibrations cause pain, diaphragmatic splinting and loss of lung volume. They are rarely necessary after surgery.

Pain after abdominal surgery

Analgesia tends to be taken less seriously after abdominal surgery than chest surgery, but laparotomy often causes more pain than sternotomy. Vertical incisions create twice the distracting force on the wound and are a greater hindrance to mobilization than transverse incisions (Garcia-Valdecasas *et al.*, 1988).

Pain after chest surgery

After thoracotomy, side-lying on the non-operated side is not only the most comfortable position, but optimizes ventilation/perfusion matching. After thoracotomy or sternotomy, shoulder and postural exercises should be started as soon as pain allows. Pain that is caused by stretching thoracic joints during surgery can be eased by mobilizations of the joints at the spine (Dickey, 1989).

Pleural surgery is particularly painful because the pleura is well-endowed with nerve endings. Pleurodesis entails the introduction of irritant chemicals into the pleura, which sets up a sterile inflammation so that every breath causes the raw surfaces to rub together. Introduction of local anaesthetic to the pleura during surgery eases this pain.

If deep breathing or incentive spirometry are necessary after sternotomy, some patients find that manual support of the wound on inspiration improves comfort and allows greater chest excursion. Shoulder elevation should be performed bilaterally to avoid a shearing stress on the sternum. If the sternum is heard or felt to click on movement, a cough belt is needed for support.

When moving patients with chest drains, the tubing should be held against and in alignment with the patient's chest to minimize discomfort.

When leaving patients after treatment, the drains must be fixed in such a way that they do not drag on the wound.

Pain after head and neck surgery

If the sternomastoid has been cut during head and neck surgery, the patient's head needs manual support during postoperative handling. If the spinal accessory nerve has been damaged, pain and limited shoulder abduction are a risk, so that patients should adhere scrupulously to an exercise regime, postural correction and advice such as avoiding traction on the brachial plexus. Patients are often nil-by-mouth for some time, and mouthwashes should be freely available.

If head and neck surgery causes a combination of disfigurement and loss of speech, it can be a devastating experience for the patient. Comprehensive multidisciplinary support helps to limit the frustration and ease the grief that can augment pain and hinder rehabilitation.

Pain in the intensive care unit

Treatment for pain, anxiety and insomnia is interwoven in the intensive care unit. Pain is more easily managed in mechanically ventilated than spontaneously breathing patients because respiratory depression is less relevant. Prior to physiotherapy treatment, a bolus of intravenous analgesia is often indicated, but Entonox is particularly useful, administered by a doctor or respiratory technician directly through the ventilator before and during treatment.

Sedation and analgesia are required for most ventilated patients, but are not a substitute for the primary task of explanations and relief of physical discomfort. If anxiety stems from realistic perceptions, drugs that cloud consciousness can cause delusions and hallucinations.

Muscle relaxants such as atracurium may be given to ventilated patients in order to induce paralysis and prevent resistance to ventilation. They act as a form of chemical restraint, obliterating the only means by which patients can indicate discomfort. They should be accompanied by sedation or analgesia, and explanations that the drug will make them feel weak. Paralysed patients are conscious and can feel, hear and think normally.

Pain in children and neonates

The traditional attitude which leads to poor pain management in adults is exaggerated in children and even more so in infants. Eland (1985) surveyed 2000 children after major surgery or with burns, and found that two-thirds received no analgesia at all. Procedures such as intubation and chest drain insertion are often performed without medication, and some infants have undergone heart surgery with no analgesia or even anaesthesia (Anand et al., 1985).

The reasons that children are treated in a way that would bring prosecution if applied to animals are thought to be the following:

- Children's pain is often not believed or taken seriously, and health staff tend to rely on intuition, assumptions and personal beliefs when assessing children's pain (Beyer and Byers, 1985),
- Children's analgesia needs careful prescription.
- Children may not express pain in terms that are easily understood by adults, and their coping strategies may include sleeping, playing and activities which do not communicate the experience of pain to adults.
- Children may minimize complaints because of fears of the dreaded injection.
- Children are easily held down by force.
- Some health staff do not realize that children are able to feel pain from birth.

Pain intensity is thought to be greater in babies than in older age groups. Immature neurons are particularly sensitive to damage (Tyler et al., 1991), and premature neonates have a lower threshold to pain than full-term infants (McIntosh et al., 1993). In addition, childhood pain may form the basis for lifetime pain processing, and the psychological impact may be long term and profound (Beyer and Byers, 1985)

The experience of childhood pain is embedded in the broader experience of being frightened. Fear of pain is compounded by fear of separation and fear of the unknown. Fears are not usually communicated, and many children find it difficult to ask for help (Alex and Ritchie, 1992), which means that active intervention is advisable to correct misconceptions, and analgesic administration should not be determined only by request.

The perception of pain is greater in children who have been sensitized by frequent painful procedures. Children's distressed behaviour increases over time if there is no intervention (Broome, 1990).

Assessment

The best indicator of a child's pain is the child. If he or she is able to count to four, it is better to ask the child rather than parent about the pain, especially as this gives an indication of the associated fear (Manna *et al.*, 1992). For younger children, the parent's assessment is more accurate than that of health staff. Assessment varies with the age of the child, but an absence of crying does not indicate an absence of pain. Methods include the following, which are described in more detail by Beyer and Byers (1985):

- For those over 3 years, a modified VAS such as the Oucher, which allows children to choose one out of six expressive photographs representing various degrees of distress.
- For 4- to 7-year-olds, a Hurt Thermometer, which is a picture of a thermometer with a red elastic representation of mercury, which the child stretches to choose from 0 to 4 degrees of pain.
- For children over 7 years, a VAS graded from 'no hurt at all' to 'worst hurt'.
- For 4- to 8-year-olds, a Poker Chip Tool, in which children, using four white poker chips, indicate how many pieces of hurt they are feeling.
- Preoperative ranking of colours according to the perception of pain intensity, followed by postoperative selection of the colour of their pain.

Pain charts (Sparsholt, 1989a) may be used for prelingual and non-verbal children, who can also be observed for signs of withdrawal, face and body reactions, behaviour change such as irritability, pallor, momentary breath-holding, prolonged sleeping and in older babies who have been subjected to traumatic procedures over some time, an expression of frozen watchfulness similar to the abused child (Sparsholt, 1989a). If assessment is based on observation of behaviour, this must be accurate, consistent and distinguish between pain and other forms of distress.

Physiological measures such as changes in respiratory rate, heart rate, blood pressure and oximetry can be used as adjuncts but are not specific as indicators of pain.

Management

Preoperative explanations can be augmented with pictures, books, rehearsals and encouragement to discuss the experience with children who have had the same operation. It should not be assumed that the parents have explained the operation to the child. Physical sensations should be described, and the reason for the sensations explained. Truth is essential to maintain the child's trust and minimize fear. Young children cannot always distinguish cause and effect, and in the absence of explanations may build up frightening and bewildering fantasies because the boundary between reality and fantasy is blurred.

Postoperatively, any method used for adult pain relief can be adapted for children (Rice, 1989), usually by a painless route. If respiratory depression occurs, it can be reversed by naloxone. Children benefit particularly from TENS (Fowler-Kerry, 1990) and, for children over 8 years, patient-controlled analgesia (Irwin *et al.*, 1992). The rectal route is not advisable because absorption is slow and variable, it can be seen as abusive by children and there has been one known fatality (Gourlay and Boas, 1992). For discomfort, paracetamol, codeine or a combination of both are useful, but aspirin is contraindicated because of its association with Reye's syndrome.

Children should be asked what they feel will best help them. Methods to reduce pain perception include:

- Most importantly, according to 99% of children, the presence of a parent (Broome, 1990).
- Information on what will occur and what it will feel like (Broome, 1990).
- Distraction with toys, physical stroking, stories, games or television.
- Rhythmic breathing patterns such as 'ha-who' breathing, in which the child inhales, then says 'ha' on expiration, followed by an inhalation and 'who' on expiration.
- Imagery, for example combining 'ha-who' breathing with visions of a train.
- Encouragement to practise relaxation by going 'limp as a rag doll'.
- Being listened to, believed and empowered, so

that children have some control over what is done to them.

- Unstressed parents who have been informed and fully involved throughout.

Children like to be touched as little as possible after surgery. If coughing is necessary, they prefer to splint the incision themselves by leaning forward with their arms crossed or hugging a teddy bear. Siblings, grandparents and if possible pets should be welcomed. Children must not be discouraged from crying nor told to be brave.

Choonara (1989) argues that there is some evidence for children under 6 months being extrasensitive to opiates, especially if premature or ill, but he explains that other authorities show how these drugs are not only safe but can actually reduce complications. Monitoring is advisable, either by oximetry or other means (Barrier and Wren, 1989; Anand et al., 1985).

Local anaesthetic techniques such as wound infiltration, peripheral nerve blocks, plexus blocks and epidurals are well suited to neonates. Pacifiers, rocking, holding and swaddling are comforting, but are not a substitute for meticulously prescribed analgesia.

Relieving the pain of preterm infants speeds their recovery. The perception of pain is reduced by an appropriate environment. Dimmed lights at night allow more sleeping and weight gain, and reduced noise reduces episodes of desaturation, rapid breathing, crying and intracranial hypertension. Beneficial influences are the mother's voice and a soft blanket to lie against which prevents the insecurity of feeling exposed (Sparsholt, 1989b).

Booklets and advice on children's pain can be obtained in Britain from Action for Sick Children, Argyle House, 29–31 Euston Road, London NW1 2SD.

Pain in elderly people

Elderly people are at risk of undertreatment with analgesics (Jacox, 1992). Accurate prescription is often hampered by impaired absorption, distribution, metabolism and elimination of drugs. Older people tend to be stoic about reporting pain, and may harbour the misconception, sometimes shared with health staff, that 'I thought it was just because I was getting old'. Pain is not a natural part of the ageing process.

Confusion or postoperative delirium in the elderly can be a sign of pain, or can indicate other problems such as hypoxia, dehydration, infection, over-medication, disturbed sleep or disorientation caused by admission to hospital.

Perception of pain is increased by:

- Depression, often unrecognized, which is a common outcome of the helplessness associated with admission to hospital.
- Constipation, due to drug therapy, change of diet or the immobility of illness and hospitalization.
- Loss of autonomy, which can be minimized by respecting patients' senior status, experience and wishes regarding management.
- Patients being expected to spend longer than is comfortable slumped unhappily in hospital chairs.
- Distress and discomfort caused by incontinence, which can be minimized by maintenance of mobility and ready access to the bathroom.
- Disorientation.

Practical ways to maintain orientation in elderly people are to avoid using first names uninvited (Williamson, 1984), advise patients to get dressed whenever possible, use leg bags rather than undignified catheter bags, and encourage patients to bring to hospital as much clutter of personal possessions as practical.

Without accurate pain control, postoperative physiotherapy may be at best a waste of time and at worst damaging to the patient. The keys to success are active involvement of the patient, and close teamwork with other health staff. The talents of anaesthetist, nurse, physiotherapist, clinical psychologist and pharmacist are best utilized by setting up an Acute Pain Service (Lavies, 1992).

Effective pain control brings real benefit in both morbidity statistics and individual well-being, as best described by John Dryden:

> 'For all the happiness mankind can gain
> Is not in pleasure but in rest from pain'.

Acknowledgements

Many thanks to Bernadette Henderson and Clare Pain for their invaluable advice.

References

Aitkenhead, A.R. (1989) Analgesia and sedation in intensive care. *Br. J. Anaesth.*, **63**, 196–206

Alex, M.R. and Ritchie, J.A. (1992) School-aged children's interpretation of their experience with acute surgical pain. *J. Pediatr. Nurs.*, **7**, 171–80

Anand, K.J.S, Brown, M.J., Causon, R.C. *et al.* (1985) Can the human neonate mount an endocrine and metabolic response to surgery? *J. Pediatr. Surg.*, **20**, 41–8

Barrier, G. and Wren, W.S, (1989) Acute pain of neonates and children in surgery and intensive care. *Int.Care Med.*, **15**, S37–9

Barsoum, G., Perry, E.P. and Fraser, I.A. (1990) Postoperative nausea is relieved by acupressure. *J. R. Soc. Med.*, **83**, 86–9

Bayindir, O. (1991) Use of TENS in the control of postoperative chest pain after cardiac surgery. *J. Cardiothorac. Vasc. Anaesth.*, **5**, 589–91

Beyer, J.E. and Byers, M.L. (1985) Knowledge of paediatric pain: state of the art. *Childrens Health Care*, **13**, 150–9

Biddle, C. (1992) Transdermal and transmucosal administration of pain-relieving and anxiolytic drugs. *Heart Lung*, **21**, 115–24

Brooks, D.H.M. (1990) The route to home ventilation: a patient's perspective. *Care Crit. Ill*, **6**, 96–7

Broome, M.E. (1990) Preparation of children for painful procedures. *Pediatr. Nurs.*, **16**, 537–41

Carron, H. (1989) Extension of pain relief beyond the operating room. *Clin. J. Pain*, **5** (Suppl.1), S1–S4

Choonara, I.A. (1989) Pain relief. *Arch. Dis. Child.*, **64**, 1101–2

Cimino, A.B. and Hugar, D.W. (1980) Transcutaneous neural stimulation. *J. Foot Surg.*, **19**, 12

Cousins, M.J. (1989) Acute pain and the injury response. *Reg. Anesth.*, **14**, 162–79

Cupples, S.A. (1991) Effects of timing and reinforcement of pre-operative education on knowledge and recovery of patients having coronary artery bypass graft surgery. *Heart Lung*, **20**, 654–60

Dickey, J.L. (1989) Postoperative osteopathic manipulation of median sternotomy patients. *J. Am. Osteopath. Assoc.*, **89**, 1309–22

Dull, J.L, and Dull, W.L. (1983) Are maximal inspiratory breathing exercises or incentive spirometry better than early mobilization after cardiopulmonary bypass? *Phys. Ther.*, **63**, 655–9

East, E. (1992) How much does it hurt? *Nurs. Times*, **88**, 48–9

Egbert, L.D, Battit, G.E, Welch, C.E. *et al.* (1964) Reduction of postoperative pain by encouragement and instruction of patients. *N. Engl. J. Med.*, **270**, 825–7

Eland, J.M. (1985) The role of the nurse in children's pain. In *Perspectives in Pain* (ed. L.A.Copp), Churchill Livingstone, New York

Embling, S.A. (1985) Incidence, aetiology and implications of pulmonary atelectasis following cardiopulmonary bypass surgery. MSc dissertation, University of Southampton

Facco, E., Manani, G., Angel, A. *et al.*, (1981) Comparison study between acupuncture and pentozocine analgesic and respiratory postoperative effects. *Am. J. Chin. Med.*, **9**, 225–35

Fowler-Kerry, S.E. (1990) An evaluation of TENS with children. *Pain*, Suppl.5, S9

Garcia-Valdecasas, J.C., Almenara, R., Cabrer, C. *et al.* (1988) Subcostal incision versus midline laparotomy in gallstone surgery. *Br. J. Surg.*, **75**, 473–5

Gil, K.M., Ginsberg, B., Muir, M. *et al.* (1990) Patient-controlled analgesia in postoperative pain. *Clin. J. Pain*, **6**, 137–42

Gourlay, G.K. and Boas, R.A. (1992) Fatal outcome with use of rectal morphine for postoperative pain control in an infant. *Br. Med. J.*, **304**, 766–7

Grace, D. and Orr, D.A. (1993) Continuous spinal anaesthesia in acute respiratory failure. *Anaesthesia*, **48**, 226–8

Hill, H.F., Chapman, C.R., Kornell, J.A. *et al.* (1990) Self-administration of morphine in bone marrow transplant patients reduces drug requirement. *Pain*, **40**, 121–9

Hough, A. (1991) *Physiotherapy in Respiratory Care – a Problem-Solving Approach*, Chapman and Hall, London

Hull (1988) Control of pain in the perioperative period. *Br. Med. Bull.*, **4**, 341–56

Hung, P. (1992) Pre-operative fasting. *Nurs. Times*, **88**, 57–60

Hymes, A.C., Yonehiro, E.G., Raab, D.E. *et al.* (1974) Electrical surface stimulation for treatment and prevention of ileus and atelectasis. *Surg. Forum*, **25**, 222–4

Irwin, M., Gillespie, J.A. and Morton, N.S. (1992) Evaluation of a disposable patient-controlled analgesia device in children. *Br. J. Anaesth.*, **68**, 411–13

Jacox, A., Carr. D. and Chapman, C.R. (1992) Clinician's quick reference guide to postoperative pain management in adults. *J. Pain Sympt. Management*, **7**, 214–28

Jenkins, S.C., Soutar, S.A., Loukota, J.M. *et al.* (1990) A comparison of breathing exercises, incentive spirometry and mobilization after coronary artery surgery. *Physiother. Theory and Practice*, **6**, 117–26

Jones, A.Y.M. and Hutchinson, R.C. (1991) A comparison of the analgesic effect of TENS and Entonox. *Physiotherapy*, **77**, 526–9

Jorgensen, B.C., Schmidt, J.F., Hertel, S. *et al.* (1988) Patient-controlled analgesic therapy by sublingual buprenorphine. *Clin. J. Pain*, **4**, 75–9

Joshi, G.P., McCarroll, S.M., Brady, O.H. *et al.* (1993) Intra-articular morphine after anterior cruciate ligament repair. *Br. J. Anaesth.*, **70**, 87–8

Justins, D.M. and Richardson, P.H. (1991) Clinical management of acute pain. *Br. Med. Bull.*, **47**, 561–83

Katz, J. *et al*, (1992) Preemptive analgesia. *Anesthesiology*, **77**, 439–46.

Kripke, B.J., Justice, R.E. and Hechtman, H.B. (1983) Postoperative nitrous oxide analgesia and the FRC. *Crit. Care Med.*, **11**, 105–9

Lavies, N. (1992) Identification of patient, medical and nursing staff attitudes to postoperative opioid analgesia. *Pain*, **48**, 313–19

Lönnqvist, P-A., (1992) Continuous paravertebral block in children. *Anaesthesia*, **47**, 607–9

Majid, A.A. (1992) Pain control after thoracotomy. *Chest*, **101**, 981–4

Mann, L.J, Young, G.R. and Williams, J.K. (1992) Intrapleural bupivacaine in the control of post-thoracotomy pain. *Ann. Thorac. Surg.*, **53**, 449–52

Manne, S.L., Jacobsen, P.B. and Redd, W.H. (1992) Assessment of acute pediatric pain. *Pain*, **48**, 45–52

McCaffery, M. and Ferrell, B.R. (1992) Does the gender gap affect your pain control decisions? *Nursing*, **92**, 49–51

McIntosh, N., Van Veen, L. and Brameyer, H. (1993) The pain of heelprick and its measurement in preterm infants. *Pain*, **52**, 71–4

Miller, K.M. and Perry, P.A. (1990) Relaxation techniques and postoperative pain in patients undergoing cardiac surgery. *Heart Lung*, **19**, 136–46

Owen, H., Kluger, M.T., Ilsley, A.H. *et al.* (1993) The effect of fentanyl administered epidurally by patient-controlled analgesia, continuous infusion or a combined technique. *Anaesthesia*, **48**, 20–5

Pitts, M, and Healey, S. (1989) Factors influencing the inferences of pain made by three health professions. *Physiother. Pract.*, **5**, 65–8

Ralston, S.J. (1993) Use of EMLA cream for skin anaesthesia prior to epidural insertion in labour. *Anaesthesia*, **48**, 65–7

Rice, L.J. (1989) Management of acute pain in pediatric patients. *Clin. J. Pain*, **5**, Suppl. 1, S42–50

Rosenberg, M. (1992) Patient-controlled analgesia. *J. Oral Maxillofac. Surg.*, **50**, 386–9

Simpson, T., Wahl, G., DeTraglia, M. *et al.* (1992) The effects of epidural versus parenteral opioid analgesia on postoperative pain and pulmonary function. *Heart Lung*, **21**, 125–40

Salmon, P. (1992) Surgery as a psychological stressor. *Stress Medicine*, **8**, 193–8

Smedstad, K.G. (1992) Postoperative pain relief and hospital stay after total esophagectomy. *Clin. J. Pain*, **8**, 149–53

Smith, G. (1991) Pain after surgery. *Br. J. Anaesth.*, **67**, 233–4

Sparsholt, M. (1989a) Pain and the special care baby unit. *Nurs. Times*, **85**, 61–4

Sparsholt, M. (1989b) Minimising discomfort in sick newborns. *Nurs. Times*, **85**, 39–42

Strunin, L. (1993) How long should patients fast before surgery? *Br. J. Anaesth.*, **70**, 1–3

Szasz, T.S. (1968) The psychology of persistent pain. In *Pain* (ed. A. Soulairac) Academic Press, London

Tyler, D., Fitzgerald, M., McGrath, P. *et al.* (1991) Second international symposium on pediatric pain. *Pain*, **47**, 3–4

Vickers, M.D. (1992) Tramadol: pain relief by an opioid without depression of respiration. *Anaesthesia*, **47**, 291–6

Watcha, M.F. and White, P.F. (1992) Postoperative nausea and vomiting. *Anesthesiology*, **77**, 162–84

White, P.F. (1990) Subcutaneous PCA. *Clin. J. Pain*, **6**, 297–300

Williamson, C. (1984) What's in a name? *Nurs. Times*, **80**, 30–1

21 *A rehabilitation approach for chronic disabling low back pain*

FIONA JONES AND GILLIAN THOMAS

Introduction

A programme for the management of chronic back pain has been in existence at the Wolfson Medical Rehabilitation Centre (WMRC) since 1987. Other similar programmes exist and are being developed in the UK and abroad (Edwards 1992). This particular programme recognises the principle of **chronic pain** and its association with **illness behaviour** together with the theory of **locus of control**. Also incorporated are the benefits of **behaviour modification through physical exercise, education** and **retraining** with the advantages provided by a group setting.

It is a three week intensive programme for people with long-standing back pain, aimed at enabling the person to self manage their pain, gain confidence once more in their abilities and be weaned from the reliance on the medical model which has so far failed to provide relief.

The individual's physical limitations are identified and how they impact their work and leisure environment. Through a structured exercise programme, to improve fitness and mobility, together with support and advice on back care management, it aims to allow the patient to apply the approach in their normal life.

There are a wide range of psychological issues which accompany the problem of chronic pain. These issues are recognized by all the clinicians involved and behavioural management forms an extensive part of the programme.

The team, which operates as an integral functioning unit, is **multi-disciplinary**, comprising medical staff, physiotherapists, occupational therapists, clinical psychologists, with additional support from nursing staff and a dietician.

This chapter aims to explore in part the nature of the problems these patients present with as a result of their chronic back pain and examine the principles by which the team operates **highlighting the physiotherapeutic input to this particular approach**.

The chronic pain process

To understand the philosophy that enables a multi-disciplinary programme such as ours to facilitate a change to a more normal and productive way of living, it is necessary to have an awareness of the **psychological behavioural patterns** that become linked with the presenting physical symptoms.

The ways in which an event of low back pain affects an individual's life are diverse. Progression from the initial occurrence through to chronic back pain and in some cases the development of chronic illness behaviour has been widely researched.

4 out of 5 of the population suffer from an episode of back pain at some time, 80 to 90% of these recover comfort and function within 3 months (Hazard, 1989.) However 5 to 10% of all individuals suffering a low back pain episode ultimately become chronic patients and this small minority is responsible for upwards of 80% of medical costs for all back treatment (Polatin, 1988).

The WMRC back programme accepts those with a history of back pain defined as chronic. Traditionally 'chronic' was defined as a pain that was present 6 months post onset. Phillips (1991) found that chronic sufferers exhibit a large degree of behavioural adjustment to their continuing pain. Although the larger adjustment occurs in the first 3 months, a continuing adjustment occurs right up to the 6 months' assessment. The largest shift in the pain problem occurs between the acute and sub-chronic points confirming the decision of the International Association of Pain (1986) to change the term chronicity to **3 months post onset**.

This definition of chronic pain defines the cross-section of patients referred to the WMRC programme with the majority of patients having a history of greater than 3 months and a percentage having suffered with back pain for some years.

The patients seen demonstrate the full range of behavioural responses to their pain. Approximately 50% exhibit distress and illness behaviour although all of our patients have had their normal pattern of life disrupted as a result of the pain.

Waddell (1984) states the need to clearly distinguish the symptoms and signs of illness behaviour and it is defined as 'observable and potentially measurable actions and conduct which express and communicate the individual's own perception of disturbed health'. The need therefore for therapists to accept and understand the behavioural components of chronic back pain is paramount as this forms the basis for our approach for all our patients.

How the individual responses vary could be due to a variety of factors. Past beliefs and experiences, bitterness at the failure of the medical model of assessment and treatment and a cycle of pain, reduced function and loss of self esteem all may lead the original injury to become a source of control. The predisposition of an individual to the development of illness behaviour is one aspect. There are some indications that pain, response to pain, compliance to treatment and self-care are dependent on the patient's **attitudes, beliefs and cognitions** (Harkapaa, 1990).

As the chronic back pain becomes increasingly dissociated from the original physical basis then the behaviour manifested is exaggerated. Overt pain behaviour such as guarding, grimacing and bracing have been shown to be related to concurrent level of function and treatment outcome (Conally, 1990).

Signs such as severely impoverished movement, loss of normal speed rhythm and functional disability are coupled with **overt pain signals**, the most common being the hand clasped permanently on the low back. In the acute phase of the patient's injury, various avoidance behaviours such as limping are effective in reducing pain or suffering from nociception. With chronic patients it may be the **anticipation of suffering** and not the suffering per se, that provides the persistence of avoidance behaviours (Fordyce, 1981).

Assessment or interview is based around the functional problems which are apparent as a result of the pain. Clinical examination frequently gives rise to an overstatement of symptoms with copious adjectives used to describe the nature of the pain and suffering. The knowledge of the basis for these responses and that through physical activity the unravelling can begin, is a great challenge for the therapist.

How does Chronic Pain Impact Functional Capacity?

Pain is no longer regarded as merely a physical sensation of noxious stimulus and disease. Distress, illness behaviour and ultimately the sick role which clouds the original pain source testify to its more complex nature. However, the way an individual responds to pain is no doubt dependent on many factors, not least their pre-existing attitudes and beliefs. Fordyce distinguished 2 types of sufferers – **'pacers'**, i.e. those who carry on regardless of their knowledge that what they are doing will make the pain much worse, and secondly the **'recliners'** who avoid everything for fear it may make the pain worse. All those on the WMRC programme have a **reduced functional capacity** but to varying levels, giving a spectrum of response falling between the 'pacer' and the 'recliner', with consequences in some cases of an **inability to work, have a social life, have leisure interests, and maintain normal family relationships**. Chronic pain can have the effect of curtailing life to its barest essentials, with ordinary obligations evaded or cut to a minimum and even the simplest of diversions eliminated. Life is centred around the pain and frequently it is a focus of distress for other family members.

One of the most significant factors that people complain of is the inability to work and the conseqences which arise. Prolonged time away from work in itself makes recovery and return to work less likely to occur. The strain of financial problems, the stress which this causes within the family and a **change of role and status** as a result can be extremely detrimental to normal family life.

The emotional significance of chronic pain as represented by the work, leisure and social repercussions are closely linked to the physical impairments the person describes. There is no doubt that inactivity in a general sense has a physical effect in terms of fitness, with almost unequivocal findings that chronic low back pain patients have rather **low levels of activity** compared to their pre-pain levels or to normal controls (Linton, 1984). Flexibility and strength will, as a consequence, also be compromised. So despite what the diagnosis or reason for the chronic pain and degrees of illness behaviour, one can always look as a therapist at the physical implications and use them to impact the other intricate behavioural and socio-economic factors. Indeed many of our clients have had prolonged bedrest with disastrous effects and this negative response of bed rest has been widely documented, ranging from a catabolic state and general malaise (Bortz, 1984) to decreased physical fitness (Mayner, 1985). Reports of the damaging outcome and consequent **loss of confidence** in moving and performing even simple daily tasks, are stated with desperation at the initial interview and are a common theme of conversation amongst clients during the first few days of the programme.

Frequently there is a **great deal of effort** expended to perform the most simple of tasks; this may be for a variety of reasons such as the **immense fear of reinjuring** or just the loss of the feeling of smooth and coordinated movement, with each task being associated with negative experiences.

The reduction in functional capacity is therefore vast and diverse requiring an immediate and comprehensive effort by therapists and clients to begin to instigate a programme which will lead to change.

The Locus of control.

Health **locus of control** is a **theoretical construct** which has been used in health research. It refers to a **person's belief in control over illness**. Many, but not all, studies show that a good outcome is more positive in people who strongly believe in their internal control over illness, and, as already mentioned, negative emotional reactions may well predict a poorer response to treatment in patients with low back pain, whether they are receiving surgical intervention, conservative treatment or multimodal treatment.

The association with distress, that in the past has been brought about by exercising needs to be acknowledged. Patients who do not believe in personal control over their back pain and are still waiting for the all important 'cure' may disregard

given instructions and subsequently gain less from treatment. Usually by the end of week one of the **WMRC** programme these issues would have been identified and the onus of management begin to shift from the therapist to the patient. The clinical assumption that an increase in activity causes an increase in pain should be debated and there is evidence that the development and maintenance of chronic pain suggests that the subsequent reduction in activity may not be due to **nociception** but to a variety of **learned factors**. Hence a stress type reaction involving fear, anxiety and muscular tension may well be a learned stereotypical response, where the patient believes that participating in a given activity will result in pain.

The stronger belief in personal control over back pain was significantly associated with **more frequent exercising** (Harkapaa et al., 1990) Thus reinforcing the value of physical exercise in addressing the need for patients with long-standing back pain to having internal control over their 'illness'.

The growing accepted trend in the management of chronic low back pain is that in order to obtain the best response, the patient should be actively encouraged to take **greater personal responsibility** for their back care. However, many patients with this nature of problem, have gone through a series of attempts to control their pain, with little result. Bearing in mind the often low level of personal control and the negative experiences that may be associated with attempts in the past, the challenge lies with the therapist who is asked to be innovative in a completely 'hands off' context and, importantly, be subtle with providing the new learning process attempted by the WMRC programme given that further failure even at an early stage in the programme can mean the chance is lost.

Why Might the Medical Model have Failed?

One of the criteria for assessment for the WMRC Chronic Back Pain Programme is that **all outstanding medical investigations and any other therapeutic intervention is to be carried out by the referring agencies, prior to referral**. There are two reasons for this, **firstly** that we can then be sure as therapists we are not dealing with a problem that could be solved relatively easily by surgery or traditional outpatient physiotherapeutic measures, and **secondly** that the patient holds no doubt that everything else has been tried and has so far failed.

Why the medical treatment has failed the patient

may be due to a number of factors. The medical model has often a simplified view of cause and effect in physical illness, and has subsequently come under attack from social and behavioural scientists over the past decade or two. Failed treatment and repeatedly **negative investigations** (e.g. X-rays, which can give no clue to prognosis) often gear the patient to the passive invalid role, with little or no expectation that he/she can influence the course of his/her disability. This simple organic/functional dichotomy has led to accusations of malingering, not only by the medical profession but also by the patient's family (Main, 1987). Waddell (1984) states that the fundamental error is sometimes in the assumption that all signs and symptoms of the disease can be explained in terms of the **physical disease**. Although the holistic ethos is often quoted, invariably the tendency is to follow the path of treating only the disease or the impairment.

Patients very often still believe that the answer to their problems lies with the doctor and a diagnosis of their continuing predicament. Selecting those patients who have **not** gained satisfaction through this **conventional method** gives the possibility that a broad and intensive programme provided over a period of three weeks, as opposed to a fifteen minute consultation, can go some way to changing the **negative behavioural responses** (associated in many cases but to different degrees) and thus **optimise the potential for improvement.**

Entry into the Rehabilitation Environment

WMRC is a rehabilitation unit which runs its back programme and neurological programmes concurrently, therefore when the back pain patient first enters into the rehab environment they will see and meet a variety of other patients with a diversity of problems.

Some rehabilitation units claim positive effects of the back programme patients being in the same therapeutic environment as severely neurologically impaired patients with the premise that it is advantageous to someone worse off than oneself. We have found that by keeping the 2 sets of patients separate it enables the feel and atmosphere of the back programme to be more easily controlled with the aim of creating an 'upbeat' gym, fitness and health care set-up

We also feel that many of those patients who show chronic illness behaviour are not ready on

admission to be affected by those that they see around them but have to come through a series of changes themselves.

The word 'rehabilitation' can conjure up a variety of images, many of which have been alien to the patient since their initial injury and displacing the fear and anticipation that the pain may be made worse is a primary objective.

A great deal of importance is placed on the relationship that is formed between the therapist and the patient. Initially there may be hostility and lack of faith that yet another attempt to improve their current situation is underway.

An environment that is non-confrontational, where the therapist accepts without question the patient's report of their symptoms is the basis on which we would wish the recovery process to begin. The necessity to move from the **'parent-child trap'** to an **'adult to adult'** association begins from day one.

Why is there a need for an integrated team?

An integrated team is vital to promote change within such a defined time frame (only 3 weeks). To be able to address all the various components of the client's problem demands different skills from not only the team, but also the patient, who is considered to be an integral member of the team.

As in any successful team, different roles are adopted by different players; an educational role, a counselling role, a motivator and challenging role, a role to create a sufficiently secure environment to reduce fear and promote self-confidence and a facilitator of relaxation, self-pacing and self-management.

The team operation has to be quite structured to be efficient, promoting early communication and commitment to the client to gain an effective outcome.

The process of change

This is thought of as a **journey**, through which the patient has to undergo a series of alterations in their behaviour and consequently their physical functioning.

Patients are told by the therapists and indeed by patients further into the programme that **the pain will initially get worse.**

Once this has been established then it becomes

all right for the patients to wince and moan and complain because we all expect it.

After the initial increase in pain comes the sense, for the first time in many cases, of being able to carry out some form of exercise. The fear that is associated with movement can begin to be eroded by seeing others within the programme that are carrying on despite their pain, with the only adverse effects being stiffness associated with having carried out some exercise, an **accepted type of pain**.

Physiologically exercise can facilitate a release of endorphins which with its analgesic effect enables some improved functional capacity.

The feeling of success, however small, and the support and encouragement from others, gives the motivation to continue to strive for greater goals.

The process of **positive reinforcement** given when functional goals are met and the gradual process of gaining more confidence can take a varying amount of time depending on the entrenchment of patterns of illness behaviour.

Usually by the middle of the second week the patient takes on a slightly different role within the group, **gaining esteem** by being able to offer support to those just beginning the programme.

The status that goes with someone that has 'survived' the strenuous physical exercise and is now taking the challenge of gaining control of their lives is satisfying and inspiring to other patients.

There is no end point to the journey. However, by the third week the patients usually feel comfortable with the constraints of the programme and may be beginning to feel anxious about carrying on the improvements after discharge. This is a **critical time** and frequently patients can show signs of resuming some of their previous behaviours. The relationship that has formed between the therapist and patient should be one whereby support is given but not so much that the patient feels they cannot cope alone. The process must give the patient a feeling they are able to cope with setbacks, which are inevitable, without sinking back into the sort of despair that was previously so apparent.

At time of discharge we would hope not to be involved much at all in the advising and supportive role but to have slowly withdrawn with the patient making decisions and goalsetting independently.

The **self-reward and individual motivation** is the ultimate aim of the programme.

The means for change

The process of affecting behavioural responses through the use of physical exercise is not new and its beneficial affects are well documented.

Patients entering the WMRC back programme have an initial interview and clinical assessment with the physiotherapist.

All aspects of the history of their back pain are examined and discussed. We try to give the patient the feeling that we are there to listen to all that has happened, to empathise, not to contradict what they may be recounting and to gain an overall picture of the effects that the pain has had on their lives.

The clinical examination is centred on gaining a set of baseline levels of fitness, strength and mobility, with a standard functional scoring that is used to form a set of outcome measures.

The emphasis is on gaining **measurements** which the patient can identify with and which can be used throughout the programme to **demonstrate change**. Therefore, the patient is fully involved with the recording and scoring and encouraged to take an active part in the collection and retention of data.

The first impressions gained by the patients are vital. Information about the philosophy of the programme is given to all patients and the emphasis is on **good communication** between the team and the patient, an open and friendly atmosphere that the patient can slip into easily.

The relationship between the therapist and the patient is one of adult to adult, the therapists are not there to bully or persuade the patient into trying to perform but for the patient to decide for themselves that they are going to take up the challenge.

The programme consists of a 5 hour day, three 40 minute physiotherapy sessions, two 40 minute occupational therapy sessions and individual counselling from a clinical psychologist as appropriate.

Patients are admitted in a 'rolling' programme which means that every week there are 4 new patients admitted, with a total of 12 patients on the programme at any one time.

Physiotherapy input is based around hydrotherapy, group activities and a session where the patients work on their own individual programme. It has been found to be more successful **not to tailor programmes too much to individual problems** but instead use a **broad and extensive mobilizing and strengthening regime** which includes a variety of standard fitness equipment. The purpose of this is to create a **normal gym type environment** rather than the therapeutic and clinical atmospheres which have been associated with failure in the past.

By using not only our physiotherapeutic skills but our skills of behaviour modification, the patient is presented with a climate where he/she is on the same level as the therapist, and can hopefully begin to realise that constant reports of pain do not serve any purpose and that far greater attention and satisfaction can be gained from having **achieved small successes**.

Success and knowledge of results being so important in the process of change from illness to wellness, all methods possible are employed to **demonstrate change** to the patient. There is use of circuits in the gym and in hydrotherapy (even noticing the amount of water that has splashed out of the pool as a measure of increased exuberance the patients are showing!).

The **group dynamics** help to give encouragement to the patient by noticing and praising when they are doing well and this peer support is strongly encouraged.

The third week progresses some of the group activities to those which the patient may feel inspired to continue with **after discharge**, e.g. badminton, volleyball, swimming, walking longer distances, and planning is undertaken as to how the improved level of fitness can be continued after discharge, given that exercising alone at home is not easily sustained.

No formal follow-up system is in place as it is felt this only continues the reliance on the 'system' but much is made of the fact towards discharge of how the patient no longer needs therapeutic help and advice. The actual discharge, if the programme has been successful, is carried out with a **confirmation** of all the improvements made with a **discussion and demonstration of all the improved scores** which can often be dramatic and sometimes act as inspiration to those entering the programme.

Measurement of change

Whilst no formal evaluation of the programme has yet been undertaken fully at WMRC, the measures used invariably demonstrate change on an individual basis. The most valid physical measure used is the **10 metre walk**. Also incorporated are the 40 metre run, gross flexion and extension measure-

ment, ability to squat, ability to bridge, as well as the gym and hydrotherapy circuit scores. These are aimed at addressing flexibility, muscle strength and exercise tolerance.

Occupational therapy uses a **scoring system** for posture movement, problem solving, and sitting and standing tolerances (both subjective and observed). Clinical psychology measures **anxiety, depression, self-confidence, locus of control and use of coping strategies**. Also the **patient's individual goals** are identified on admission and documented if attained at discharge. A group study of the WMRC back Pain Programme is currently being set up.

Conclusion

If we support the emphasis of change in the management of low back pain as being aimed at the **restoration of function** as well as the **relief of pain**, what can we do as a profession? how can we constructively reinforce the change?

Whilst ensuring that we as physiotherapists are clear in our own minds about the importance of reinforcing the restoration of function as well as the relief of pain, we should also be clear in what **environment this is most realistically achieved**.

Currently our approach within the profession is performed in different settings; individual patients receiving 'hands on' treatment behind curtains, group education in busy outpatient departments or intensive group activity and education in a rehabilitation unit, which is geared to the reduction of disability whatever the cause.

Should we be raising the 'public and medical profession' awareness of the advantage of the different settings and the diversity of our skills and approaches, or should we be changing our own practice as physiotherapists? Certainly this is happening in many areas.

Ultimately, a more effective **evaluation of our current approaches is vital for us to make any informed decision**.

References

Barnes, Smith, Gatchell and Mayer (1989) Psychosocio-economic predictors of treatment success/failure in chronic low-back pain patients. *Spine*, **14**

Connally and Sanders (1991) Predicting low back patients' response to lumbar sympathetic nerve blocks and interdisciplinary rehabilitation: the role of pretreatment overt pain behaviour and cognitive coping strategies. *Pain*, **44** 139–46

Edwards, Zusman, Hardcastle, Twomey, O'Sullivan and McLean (1992) A physical approach to the rehabilitation of patients disabled by chronic low back pain. *Med. J. Austral.* **156**

Fordyce, Shelton and Dundore (1982) The modification of avoidance learning pain behaviours. *J. Behav. Med.* **5**

Frank (1993). Regular Review – Low back pain *BMJ*, **306**

Härkäpää, Järvikoski, Mellin, Hurri and Luoma. (1991) Health locus of control beliefs and psychological distress as predictors for treatment outcome in low-back pain patients: results of a 3-month follow-up of a controlled intervention study. *Pain*, **46**, 3–41

Hazard, Bendix and Fenwick (1991) Disability exaggeration as a predictor of functional restoration outcomes for patients with chronic low-back pain. *Spine*, **16**

Hazard, Fenwick, Kalisch, Redmond, Reeves, Reid and Frymoyer (1989) Functional restoration with behavioural support – a one-year prospective study of patients with chronic low-back pain. *Spine*, **14**

Linton (1985) The relationship between activity and chronic back pain. *Pain* **21**, 289–94

Mechanic and Volkart (1960) Illness behaviour and medical diagnoses. *J. Hlth Hum. Behav.* **1**, 86–94

Mooney (1987) Where Is the Pain Coming From? – Presidential Address International Society for the Study of the Lumbar Spine, Dallas 1986, *Spine*, **12** 754–9

Nicholas, Wilson and Goven (1991) Operant-behavioural and cognitive-behavioural treatment for chronic low-back pain. *Behav. Res. Ther.* **29**, 225–38

Oland and Tveiten (1991) A trial of modern rehabilitation for chronic low-back pain and disability – vocational outcome and effect of pain modulation. *Spine*, **16**

Philips and Grant (1991) The evolution of chronic back pain problems: a longitudinal study. *Behav. Res. Ther.* **29**, 435–41

Polatin, Gatchel, Barnes, Mayer, Arens and Mayer (1989) A psychosociomedical prediction model of response to treatment by chronically-disabled workers with low-back pain. *Spine*, **14**

Waddell (1987) A new clinical model for the treatment of low-back pain. *Spine*, **12**

Waddell, McCulloch, Kummel and Venner (1980) Non-organic physical signs in low-back pain. *Spine*, **5**

Waddell, Bircher, Finlayson and Main (1976). Symptoms and signs: physical disease or illness behaviour? *BMJ*, **289** 739–41

Williams (1989) Illness behaviour to wellness behaviour – The 'school for bravery' approach. *Physiotherapy*, **75**

22 *The management of cancer pain in terminal care*

BETTY O'GORMAN

Introduction

A dictionary definition of pain is 'a bodily or mental suffering, distress, ache, penalty or punishment, sensation of acute discomfort or emotional suffering or grief'. In caring for the terminally-ill patient, it must be remembered that any combination of these factors may be present. 'Pain is what the patient says hurts' (IASP Subcommittee on Taxonomy, 1980).

Pain is either acute or chronic, and this chapter is concerned with chronic pain. In a hospice situation, some 70% of patients admitted are complaining of chronic pain. This is not necessarily their only symptom. Chronic pain is unrelenting and distressing for the patient, but it can sometimes be worse for the onlookers, the carers, family and friends; there is so little that they can do to help except be supportive. They feel useless. In these circumstances, where care extends for a family over 24 hours, the resulting stress can be devastating. Similarly, the nurse who cares on a continuous 8-hour shift can suffer in the same way as the family. The physiotherapist, who comes and goes, is likely to bring a measure of relief and in turn can be supportive to the rest of the team.

A patient's attitude to pain is influenced by past memories of how that pain was dealt with, and bad experiences lead to apprehension and anxiety. It has been acknowledged for some time that anxiety and stress lead to an increase in pain felt. The problems caused by pain are the same whether the patient is cared for at home or in hospital.

The multidisciplinary team

The combined skill of the multidisciplinary team is much needed, with the appropriate disciplines being involved with the patient. In order to employ the correct member of the team in caring for the patient, a careful assessment of the patient must be made by the doctor, nurse and physiotherapist.

Physical pain is normally predominant and can be helped by medication and physiotherapy. Mental, emotional and spiritual factors can be present in varying degrees and will also need to be considered. Mental and emotional pain can be helped by counselling by the social worker or bereavement counsellor and spiritual pain by the appropriate minister's counsel.

Causes of cancer pain (Baines, 1985)

Bone Pain

This is one of the more common causes of pain in advanced malignant disease. It is often severe and can be difficult to control. Patients' description of their pain is very variable. It may be termed 'a dull ache', 'red-hot' or even 'stabbing', and is frequently exacerbated by movement or by pressure.

It is thought that prostaglandins are liberated by tumour deposits in bone (Editorial, 1976) causing resorption of surrounding bone and sensitization of nerve endings to painful stimuli. Bony metastases may therefore cause pain when they are relatively small, and as they enlarge they may cause stretching of the well-innervated periosteum, and eventually result in distortion of the bone under stress and pathological fracture.

Liver Pain

The pain is usually described as a constant dull ache in the right upper abdomen exacerbated by leaning forward, but some patients report a sudden stabbing pain over the liver coming in bouts and lasting for a few minutes once or twice a day. Tumours of the bronchus, pancreas, stomach, large bowel and breast are common causes of liver metastases.

Pelvic Pain

Pain originating in the soft tissues of the pelvis is usually felt in the rectum, even if this has been previously removed at operation. It is less commonly referred to the low back, hypogastrium, perineum and genitalia. It is often exacerbated by sitting down and sometimes by constipation. It may be described as rectal fullness 'like a tennis ball' or as a severe shooting pain 'like a red hot poker'. The great majority of patients with pelvic pain have primary tumours in the rectum, colon or (if female) in the reproductive tract. Such tumours may remain localized in the pelvis for long periods. In a survey of 40 patients with terminal disease, one-third had experienced pelvic pain for over a year (Baines and Kirkham, 1984).

Chest Pain

Pain from the thoracic viscera and true chest wall pain are both felt in the chest wall, but visceral pain is referred to the area supplied by the upper four thoracic nerve roots. Thus a complaint of pain in the lower chest usually indicates local disease, but upper chest pain may be caused by disease deeper in the chest. In a series of 78 patients with chest pain, it was usually described as 'an ache in the ribs' or a 'tightness'.

Intestinal Colic

This may occur in abdominal or pelvic malignancy where there is complete or partial (subacute) bowel obstruction. The most common primary tumour to cause obstruction is carcinoma of the ovary. Colic is felt centrally in the umbilical or hypogastric regions. The pain usually comes in paroxysms and can sometimes be relieved by local heat or pressure.

Nerve Compression Pain

Pain may be caused by compression or, less commonly, by infiltration of nerve roots, plexuses and peripheral nerves by tumour tissue. Such pain is experienced in the corresponding dermatome, i.e. the area of the body where pain is felt if the nerve is stimulated. Nerve compression pain is often described as 'aching' or 'burning', less often as 'shooting'. The pain is often associated with weakness, sometimes with paraesthesiae and numbness. As both cranial and peripheral nerves can be involved by tumour at any site along their lengths, there is a great variety of pain syndromes. Probably the most important are the painful arm due to metastases in the cervical spine or involvement of the brachial plexus, and the painful leg due to metastases in the lumbosacral spine or pelvis.

Headaches

These are due to raised intracranial pressure.

Non-malignant Causes of Pain

A considerable proportion of cancer patients report pains that are not directly related to the disease process. These may be caused in three ways:

1. **Related to treatment.** A thoracotomy scar may continue to be painful for months or years following surgery. Other surgical procedures also occasionally cause persistent pain. Bladder spasm is sometimes caused by a catheter. Constipation and dyspepsia can be due to medication.
2. **Associated with debilitating disease.** Patients with advanced cancer are often bed- or chair-bound and experience aches and pains as a result of being relatively immobile. Bedsores may develop and constipation be made worse by anorexia and lack of exercise.
3. **Due to other diseases.** Many elderly patients suffer with osteoarthritis, rheumatoid arthritis, haemorrhoids and other painful conditions.

Symptom Control

In order to be able to achieve the best care for the patient, the physiotherapist must have an understanding of the appropriate drug regime and the principles of symptom control.

According to Baines (1987), there are five basic principles of symptom control and these are as follows.

1. Analyse the Cause

An attempt should always be made to establish the cause of each symptom, but this should involve a clinical history and physical examination with the minimum of investigations. The cause should be sought under the following headings:

(a) Anatomy – Where is the lesion causing this symptom?
(b) Pathology – What pathological process is at work?
(c) Biochemistry – Is the symptom caused by some biochemical disturbance?
(d) Psychology – Could the symptom be aggravated or even caused by some psychological problem?

2. Modify the Disease Process

Modify the disease process that is causing the pain by radiotherapy, chemotherapy or hormonal manipulation. Palliative radiotherapy has an important part to play in the relief of pain from bone metastases. The relief usually begins within a few days of starting treatment and maximum effect is reached 2–4 weeks after completion.

3. Interrupt the Pain Pathways

Certain cancer pains are localized and are mediated by nerves which can be blocked without causing unacceptable side-effects. The most useful nerve blocks have proved to be the following:

(a) Coeliac plexus block for upper abdominal pain.
(b) Paravertebral block for chest wall pain.
(c) Lumbosacral intrathecal block for perineal pain.
(d) Lumbar sympathetic block for tenesmus.
(e) Brachial plexus nerve block for severe arm and shoulder pain.
(f) Hip block, injecting the nerve to quadratus femoris and the obturator nerve for painful metastases involving the hip joint.

4. Understand the Drugs

This involves an understanding of the site of action of the drugs used. Analgesics can be divided into those with a mainly central action, such as paracetamol, and the narcotic analgesics. Pain from bony metastases is thought to be caused by the production of prostaglandins which sensitise free nerve endings. The non-steroidal anti-inflammatory drugs inhibit prostaglandin synthesis and their use may avoid the need for morphine, or allow the effective dose to be lower.

Symptom control also involves an understanding of the length of action of the drugs used. For example, oral morphine in solution has a plasma half-life of 2.5 h, so it needs to be given 4-hourly to maintain a constant plasma drug concentration in the therapeutic range. Other analgesics, with differing durations of action, require differing dose intervals. The dose given in every case should be the lowest compatible with pain control. It can be increased every 24 h and more frequently if pain is severe.

An understanding of drug side-effects is also needed so that concurrent laxatives and antiemetics can be given if necessary.

Oral medication is preferable to injection and tolerance is a minor problem which is usually self-limiting after a few weeks. Addiction to drugs does not occur in the cancer patient.

Analgesic drugs

Paracetamol

This is preferable to aspirin for the control of mild pain, unless the specific anti-inflammatory effect of aspirin is required, e.g. in pain from bone metastases. Paracetamol does not cause gastric disturbance, and up to 1 g 4-hourly may be given.

Morphine

If cancer pain is not controlled with non-narcotic and weak narcotic analgesics, and if appropriate adjuvants have already been introduced, a change should be made to a strong narcotic. Morphine remains the most useful strong narcotic. It is well absorbed by mouth, and has a plasma half-life of about 2.5 h. It should be given 4-hourly as this maintains an adequate blood level for analgesia and minimises toxic side-effects. Both morphine sulphate and morphine hydrochloride are widely available and are interchangeable.

Morphine is usually prescribed in chloroform water as this acts as an antimicrobial preservative. A typical prescription might read:

'morphine hydrochloride 20 mg; chloroform water to 10 ml; to take 10 ml 4-hourly'.

If pain has just escaped control by paracetamol and codeine/dextropropoxyphene, morphine 10 mg 4-hourly will probably be adequate. The dose can be increased every 24–48 h, or more frequently if pain is severe. Suggested doses are 10, 20, 30, 45 and 60 mg (90, 120 and 150 mg are only rarely needed). If changing from paracetamol alone, a 5 mg dose may suffice. MST-Continus is a controlled release preparation of morphine sulphate which can be given 12-hourly; 10, 30, 60 and 100 mg tablets are available. Patients appreciate the simple twice-daily regime, but titration of dose is less easy. Severe pain is probably better controlled with 4-hourly morphine solution, at least initially.

Diamorphine

Diamorphine remains the drug of choice for injection because of its great solubility. Injections are required if the patient is vomiting, unable to swallow or semicomatose, but very rarely simply to control pain. A battery-operated syringe driver is manufactured by Graseby Medical and gives a continuous subcutaneous infusion. It is a convenient way of giving diamorphine, it can be reloaded every 24 h by the nurse and 4-hourly injections are avoided.

Oxycodone

Analgesic suppositories are of value, especially in the home, in the situation where injections would otherwise be needed. Oxycodone suppositories 30 mg are available: 15–60 mg 8-hourly is the usual dose. (Oxycodone 30 mg 8-hourly rectally is equivalent to morphine 15 mg 4-hourly orally.)

Phenazocine

A small number of patients have persistent nausea with morphine or dislike a liquid preparation. Phenazocine 5 mg is equivalent to morphine 25 mg and it can be given 6–8-hourly.

Dextromoramide

This has a short duration of action, about 2 h, and is sometimes useful to 'boost' analgesics, e.g. before a painful procedure such as wound dressing.

Adjuvant medication

This includes the non-steroidal anti-inflammatory drugs. Tumours in bone (and possibly elsewhere) liberate prostaglandins which sensitize nerve endings to painful stimuli. Anti-inflammatory drugs inhibit prostaglandin synthesis and are therefore effective at the site of the pain, whereas narcotic analgesics act centrally. They are the treatment of choice in bone pain and are occasionally used with benefit in other types of pain. There is no general consensus as to the most effective drug, probably a first-line treatment should be aspirin or a propionic acid derivative such as flurbiprofen or ketoprofen. Indomethacin, with its wider range of side-effects, is indicated for more intractable pain. These drugs are occasionally of use in pelvic pain and in the pain from cutaneous metases.

Glucocorticosteroids

These are widely used in the control of many types of pain in the cancer patient. The common factor in 'steroid responsive' pain is that it is caused by pressure from tumour plus peritumour inflammatory oedema. Corticosteroids reduce the inflammatory response and thus diminish pain. The following are examples of steroid use:

(a) Headaches due to raised intracranial pressure. Dexamethasone 16 mg/day is given.
(b) Nerve compression pain. Most patients will require narcotic analgesics but adjuvant steroids using dexamethasone 4–6 mg/day may help in intractable pain.
(c) Visceral pain, especially hepatomegaly and pelvic pain.
(d) Lymphoedema, caused by pelvic tumour.
(e) Bone pain. Corticosteroids are less effective than non-steroidal anti-inflammatory drugs but are occasionally of value if the latter are not tolerated or are not giving relief.

In all these situations, there is no guaranteed response and a week's trial of a corticosteroid is recommended. The drug can be discontinued if

ineffective or reduced to an acceptable maintenance dose if pain control is achieved.

Muscle relaxants

(a) Diazepam or baclofen are used for muscle
spasm secondary to anxiety, bone metastases
or in spastic paraplegia.
(b) Smooth muscle relaxants such as hyoscine and
the antidiarrhoeal loperamide are used to control intestinal colic in patients with inoperable
bowel obstruction. Emepronium is of value
in bladder or urethral spasm secondary to
tumour, infection or catheter.

Antibiotics

(a) Pleural pain is often caused by secondary infection rather than malignant involvement of the
pleura.
(b) Deep infections, especially in the pelvis, increase pain as well as causing an offensive
discharge. Metronidazole is used, often in combination with a broad spectrum antibiotic.
(c) Superficial infections, such as fungating breast
tumours, rarely benefit from antibiotics unless
there is considerable surrounding cellulitis.
Local applications, such as povidone-iodine
with liquid paraffin, are more effective.

There is much discussion about the use of psychotropic drugs in the management of cancer pain. It
is generally recognized, however, that anxiety and
depression increase the experience of pain. It is
preferable to treat these with non-drug methods:
emotional support from staff, diversional therapy,
physiotherapy and relaxation. If such methods are
inadequate then psychotropic drugs should be prescribed, usually diazepam for anxiety and amitriptyline for depression.

5. Emotional, Social and Spiritual Factors

Symptom control in terminal illness is not just a
technique of using drugs correctly. It involves attention to the whole personality of the patient, his
hopes, his fears, his family, his philosophy of life.
Unless these are taken into account, the likelihood
of good symptom control is small.

Physical management

It is only because of good pain control that physiotherapy can be practised in terminal care. Primary
pain relief is due to medication and not to physiotherapy. Total cooperation between the medical,
nursing and physiotherapy staff is needed to
achieve this. This cooperation and effort must not
be undermined by inefficient physiotherapy that
could cause pain. There are no pain barriers to be
pushed through in this field.

Efficient physiotherapy must be sensitive to the
patient's needs and must rationalize each individual's potential. Patients goals are often simple
(and not necessarily those of the physiotherapist):
the desire to sit out of bed, to mobilize independently to the bathroom, or to walk in a garden with
the family. These goals must of necessity be short-
term and flexible, oscillating as the patient does
between improvement and deterioration.

The physiotherapist must understand the disease
process, not just the diagnosis, and must have a
comprehensive knowledge of the drugs used and
their dosage so that an appropriate contribution
can be made to the overall management of the
patient.

General Principles of Physiotherapy

In all treatments the following essential guidelines
should apply:

1. Commence treatment as soon as possible and
on a daily basis.
2. Consider the patient totally.
3. Consider the safety of the patient.
4. Do not make false promises.
5. Take care at all times. Inappropriate, vigorous
physiotherapy could cause distress, an increase
in pain or even a pathological fracture.
6. Listen to the patient's own observations of his
symptoms: they could indicate a pathological
fracture or an incipient paraplegia as pain-
relieving drugs may mask a new pain.
7. Do not make a patient's deterioration obvious
to them by their physiotherapy. Do not take the
patient off treatment while they are aware.
Scale the treatment down to their capabilities.
8. Be prepared to counsel the patient.
9. Consider the relatives, involve them in the
patient's treatment and goals and share their
achievements.

Rehabilitation programmes cannot be drawn up but treatment must be given on a day-to-day basis and short-term goals set and achieved.

Exercise

Preventive treatment

Regular exercise, either active, active-assisted, self-assisted active or passive, is needed to prevent joint and muscle stiffness possibly leading to contractures. All paralysed or partially paralysed limbs must be exercised and instruction given to the patient, nursing staff and relatives on how to perform them. Deformities must be prevented as they lead to unnecessary discomfort and distress, making even simple nursing procedures difficult.

Many patients suffer from multi-pathology. This can be a mixture of malignant or non-malignant conditions that may well have pre-dated the malignancy or consist of multiple pathology entirely from malignancy. Patients with a variety of different conditions can be assisted with exercise. Patients with the following conditions will all need appropriate exercise in order to maximize mobility and maintain independence:

brain tumours – primary or secondary – leading to hemiplegia, hemiparesis or ataxia depending on the site of the tumour;
spinal tumours – primary or secondary – that lead to possible paraplegia or paraparesis;
lung tumours and tumours of the bronchi;
sarcomas and bony metastases that may have sustained a pathological fracture needing operative repair.

Similarly appropriate exercise is needed for any non-malignant condition that the patient has, e.g. osteoarthritic joints or spine, rheumatoid arthritis, neurological conditions – multiple sclerosis or previous polio, amputations, etc. If the patient has sustained a pathological fracture with or without operative repair, appropriate exercise will be needed.

Mobilization of stiff joints

Regular exercises are needed to attempt to mobilize stiff joints. Occasionally, radiant heat pads, ice, or (if there are no metastases present) ultrasound may be used on the affected joint plus appropriate manual therapy techniques, e.g. the gentler 'mobilization' procedures.

General mobilization of patient

Many patients lose their ability to be mobile as a result of various factors. Uncontrolled symptoms, pain, loss of appetite, nausea, vomiting, diarrhoea or constipation can all lead to immobility and therefore weakness. The physiotherapist is not necessarily treating the condition from which the patient is suffering, merely the consequence. If the patient is allowed to remain inactive he is quite likely to suffer general aches and pain and the risk of pressure sores will be increased.

Almost inevitably the patient will have weakened legs and so an active scheme of leg exercises is taught. These are kept simple and the patient is encouraged to repeat them – two to three times in the day. These often need to be written down because of a poor short-term memory and also to involve the relatives. When the quadriceps contract against gravity, standing with assistance (if necessary) will be attempted, followed by walking. When the patient is mobile, attention can be paid to any other weak areas and they can then be exercised accordingly. Rollator walking frames are particularly useful for the generally weak patient (Figure 22.1) or those with pathology in the arms, thorax or upper spine, as they allow the normal walking pattern to continue without the need to lift a walking frame. Those patients who remain only just mobile need encouragement from a physiotherapist, sometimes a scheme of active leg exercises and possibly assessment for a walking aid. If generalized weakness or dyspnoea remains a problem, the provision of an electric wheelchair will afford a degree of independence and mobility.

Positioning

The physiotherapist needs to advise the nursing team on the positioning of patients in bed, reclining armchairs and wheelchairs. Small pillows and cushions, often custom-made, are far more effective than large conventional pillows for supporting limbs and head (Figure 22.2). Bed cradles are necessary to relieve the pressure on the legs and also allow the patient some freedom of movement.

Limbs that are paralysed, grossly oedematous, fractured, affected by osteoarthritis or rheumatoid arthritis, etc. will need maximum support in a good anatomical position. Particular attention needs to be paid to keeping the ankle joint at a right angle and abducting the arm away from the trunk at approximately a 15°–20° angle.

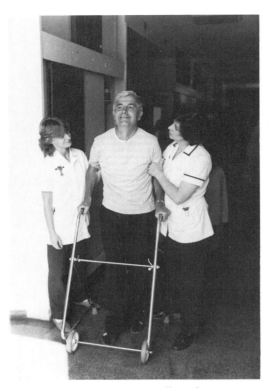

Fig. 22.1   Rollator walking frame.

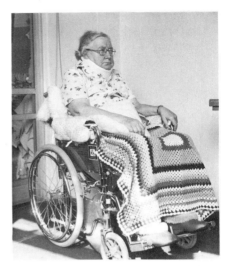

Fig. 22.2   Small, custom-made pillows used to support the patient's arm.

When there are primary or secondary lesions in the spine, collars and/or spinal supports may be needed. The position of the trunk and head in relation to gravity needs to be considered. A mattress variator or adjustable electric bed (see section on ADLs) will help positioning.

In order to minimize the effect of gravity on the body the patient should be inclined back from the vertical (Figure 22.3). By doing this, either in bed or in a reclining armchair or wheelchair, the line of gravity will then pass in front of the head and neck through the thorax. A further advantage to the patient of being placed in the semi-reclining position is the relief of pressure of the thorax on the abdomen. This allows the diaphragm to work more efficiently and so aid breathing. This is relevant when the spine is collapsing due to pathological changes.

Aids to daily living (ADLs)

If ADLs are to be of benefit, they need to be provided speedily and can be updated regularly.

Lightweight orthoses and lively or rigid splints may be needed but their value needs to be carefully assessed in order that they do not inconvenience the patient more than they help.

A gutter sling (Figure 22.4) is useful for supporting a fractured or oedematous arm. Soft collars, or occasionally lightweight rigid ones, sometimes help pain in the cervical region, although positioning plus the use of small neck pillows are often of more help. The provision of a mattress variator or bed with an electric facility to adjust the back and foot position will give the patient independence over position and also aid comfort.

General relaxation

The teaching of general relaxation is particularly valuable in the patient suffering from emotional pain or anxiety. If relaxation is taught in conjunction with a tape recording, the patient can practise while alone and, when proficient, use the tape during times of acute anxiety or attacks of pain. Occasionally, several patients will benefit from relaxation therapy in a group.

Massage and bandaging

This can play a small part in helping to reduce oedema in limbs. It can also help in the treatment

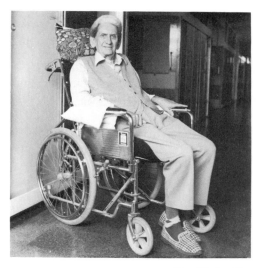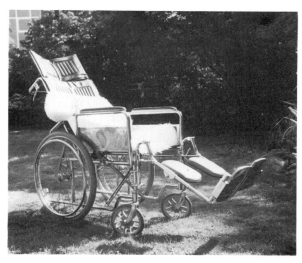

Fig. 22.3   The semi-reclining wheelchair.

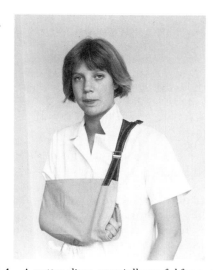

Fig. 22.4   A gutter sling, especially useful for supporting a fractured or oedematous arm.

of acute stiff necks and low back pain in conjunction with gentle mobilization of the affected area. Sometimes massage is used when a patient has local pain but also has the need for a one-to-one contact treatment (see Chapter 17). The control of postural oedema can be aided by massage, positioning and elastic support.

The patient with a lymphoedematous limb secondary to cancer is often told 'nothing can be done'. The limb – arm or leg – can be effectively treated with a daily regime of massage, multi-layered compression bandaging and exercise, usually for a 2- to 3-week period. Following a reduction or containment in the size of the limb, an elastic compression garment will need to be provided and worn constantly in order to contain the size of the limb. For the terminal care patient, it may be that treatment will oscillate between bandaging, a compression garment and at times the combination of both in order to contain, if not to reduce, the swelling as the patient deteriorates.

The regime of treatment is complex, and the reader is referred to Regnard *et al.* (1988), Gray (1987) and Badger and Twycross (1988) for complete details.

Breathing exercises

Pain in the chest is not necessarily relieved by physiotherapy, but discomfort can be helped by the use of breathing exercises, light clapping and shaking or expiration and the teaching of efficient coughing. Similarly, correct positioning and support of the patient in conjunction with teaching local relaxation of the head, neck, shoulder girdle and thorax will all help patients with chest pain and discomfort.

Primary or secondary lesions may be present in the lungs or bronchus with possibly a superimposed infection. Some patients are going to die from a chest condition. It is quite inappropriate to attempt to clear secretions from the chest of a dying patient with postural drainage.

When a patient is referred for treatment with either chest pathology and/or an infection, the physiotherapist needs to know whether the treatment is to be active or palliative, otherwise they may well question their own efficiency. If the treatment is to be active, the patient will be on an antibiotic, possibly a mucolytic, maybe nebulization, and with light clapping and shaking and the teaching of efficient coughing, an attempt will be made to clear the chest of secretions. If the treatment is to be palliative there will certainly be no antibiotic, and if the patient is sleeping it is not so important to disturb them for treatment. Sometimes what begins as an active treatment changes to a palliative one if the patient does not improve.

Physiotherapy will continue as long as the patient is being helped. If secretions in the upper areas of the lung fields become a problem, causing distress and noisy respiration, then the appropriate medication will be given. An opiate such as diamorphine 2.5 mg – 5 mg and hyoscine 0.4 mg – 6 mg will reduce the secretions and act as a sedative and amnesic.

Dyspnoeic patients are often anxious; to be short of breath for any length of time is frightening. General relaxation, if taught and practised with the aid of a tape, will often help. The patient needs to be taught efficient use of their chest by practising breathing exercises and how to improve their exercise tolerance. They should be instructed to undertake one activity at a time, not to walk and talk, to stop and rest before they become very breathless, to speak in shorter sentences with rests in between. The provision of an electric wheelchair may assist the dyspnoeic patient to have a degree of freedom.

If secretions are present, helping to clear them will aid air entry, and again this may be achieved with light clapping and shaking and teaching efficient coughing.

Pain control and its assessment

It is the physiotherapist who must assess whether a patient is pain-controlled or not. Many patients are judged, quite accurately, to have no pain at rest. However, on mobilization this might not be so. Patients suffering from bony metastases may well be pain-relieved at rest but on attempted

ambulation, especially where the bony metastases are in the lower limb or spine, will often experience pain. It is here that the physiotherapist must use skills of assessment and report back to the team. The use of transcutaneous electrical nerve stimulation (TENS) can be of great benefit in relieving the control of chronic pain (see Chapter 14).

Counselling

It is often during the course of treatment that the patient will seek more knowledge or advice about his condition from the physiotherapist. As part of a team, the physiotherapist must feel able to seek help from whichever discipline is best suited to deal with the patient's needs. If it is the physiotherapist who provides the relevant information, it is essential that not only do the family and patient receive it, but that the rest of the team know also.

Conclusion

Very few terminally ill patients decline physiotherapy. Being able to offer a non-invasive positive treatment to weak and ill patients is welcomed by them and their families. More often than not, they are able to achieve much more than their expectations would allow them to believe possible.

Acknowledgements

The author wishes to thank Dr Mary Baines for her help in allowing her work on drug control of common symptoms to be used in this chapter, and Miss Pauline Watford for typing the text.

References

Badger, C. and Twycross R. (1988) *Management of Lymphoedema: Guidelines*, Sir Michael Sobell House, Churchill Hospital, Oxford

Baines, M.J. (1985) Cancer pain. *Postgrad. Med. J.*, **60** (710), 852–7

Baines, M.J. (1987) *Terminal Illness. Textbook of Medical Treatment* (eds R.H. Girdwood and J.C. Petrie), Churchill Livingstone, London

Baines, M.J. and Kirkham, S. (1984) Clinical aspects of diseases in which pain predominates – carcinoma. In

Textbook of Pain (ed. P.D. Wall), Churchill Livingstone, London

Editorial (1976) Ostolytic metastases. *Lancet*, **2**, 1063

Gray, R. (1987) The management of limb oedema in patients with advanced cancer, *Physiotherapy*, **73** (10), 504–506

IASP Subcommittee on Taxonomy (1980) Pain terms: a list with definitions and notes on usage. *Pain*, **8**, 249–52

Regnard, C., Badger, C. and Mortimer, P. (1988) *Lymphoedema: Advice on Treatment*, Beaconsfield Publishers, Beaconsfield, Bucks

23 *Pain relief in obstetrics and gynaecology*

MARGARET POLDEN

Pain or discomfort due to 'female' reasons will probably be experienced by almost all women in one form or another during their lifetime. This can include period pains or dysmenorrhoea, pelvic pain, caused by pelvic inflammatory disease or endometriosis; the discomforts of pregnancy, labour and its aftermath; the unpleasant sensations of prolapse (descent of the pelvic organs), and the pain of osteoporosis, which is directly linked to the hormonal changes of the menopause. MacArthur *et al.* (1991) draw attention to the long-term health problems beginning for the first time soon after childbirth. These include backache, headaches, musculoskeletal symptoms, stress incontinence, urinary frequency, haemorrhoids and depression. They found that many women did not consult a doctor with their postpartum symptoms; only 31% of those with backache went to a doctor; 48% of those with depression/anxiety; 48% of those with frequent headaches; and 14% of those who had stress incontinence. The reason for non-consultation was not known, but, the authors proposed it may have been due to perceptions of available treatment or to the severity of the symptoms. Could it also be that the women perceived these discomforts, which adversely affect their quality of life, as part of a 'woman's lot'; a natural sequel to child-bearing, and as such something to be accepted?

Disability, pain and discomfort in women will directly affect the families they care for as well as inconveniencing and distressing the sufferers themselves. If physiotherapists can understand the reasons for pain of obstetric and gynaecological origin, they will be better able to use safe physical agencies to improve the quality of life, in both the short and long term, of their clients.

Pregnancy

Pregnancy is a natural physiological event, most commonly experienced by normal young women who are fit and healthy. In spite of this, and because of the huge range of physical changes experienced in the nine months of pregnancy, many women suffer discomfort and pain, sometimes acute. Although the huge hormonal changes will affect the cardiovascular, respiratory, alimentary and renal systems (to create the best possible environment for the growing fetus), the major changes likely to involve the obstetric physiotherapist, and which frequently lead to pain, will be those affecting the musculoskeletal system and the genital tract. The so-called 'minor ailments' of pregnancy which are a direct result of these changes, are often dismissed by carers as being of no importance, and, from the pathological point of view, this is probably correct. However, simple advice and treatment is often all that is needed to make the expectant mother's life more comfortable and to relieve her anxieties.

The commonest pain problems likely to be encountered in the antenatal period are:

- Backache and pelvic girdle pain
- Osteitis pubis: pubic diastosis
- Costal margin pain
- Carpal tunnel syndrome
- Pelvic floor discomfort
- Cramp
- Uterine ligament pain
- Disintegrating fibroids

Backache and pelvic girdle pain

As the fetus grows, so the mother's body changes in shape. This is largely due to the dramatic increase in the size of the uterus and its contents. Normally the uterus is a small pear-shaped pelvic organ, weighing approximately 50–60 g. At term it will have grown into a large muscular sack,

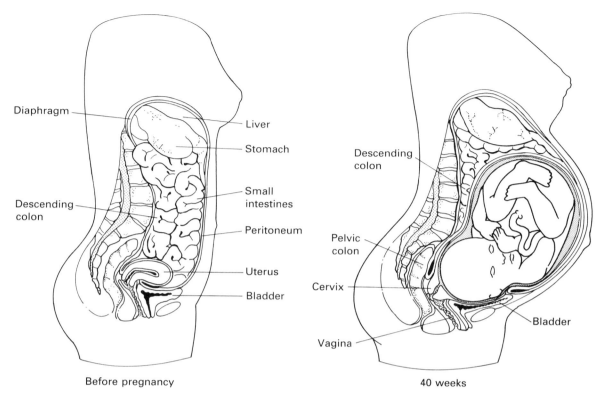

Diaphragm

Liver

Stomach

Small intestines

Descending colon

Peritoneum

Uterus

Bladder

Before pregnancy

Descending colon

Pelvic colon

Cervix

Vagina

Bladder

40 weeks

Fig. 23.1

reaching the xiphisternum at 36 weeks and weighing about 1000 g. The fetus will probably weigh 3–3.5 kg and the placenta will weigh approximately one-sixth of this amount. In addition, the uterus will also contain a quantity of amniotic fluid. As the uterus grows it forces the abdominal muscles to stretch and frequently the recti abdominis muscles will separate (diastasis recti abdominis).

As long ago as 1934 relaxation of the symphysis pubis, beginning in the first half of pregnancy and increasing during the last months, was noted (Abramson *et al.*, 1934). Hormonally mediated 'remodelling' of ligaments and connective tissue leads to a generalized increase in joint laxity and range of movement (Polden and Mantle, 1990). This is significantly increased in women having their second baby compared to those who are pregnant for the first time, although further increase in elasticity does not develop in subsequent pregnancies. The purpose of this change in extensi-

bility is to permit the mother's musculoskeletal system to adapt to her change in shape and to allow movement in her pelvic joints as the fetus passes through her pelvis in labour. These ligamentous changes reach their maximum at 38 weeks, and full recovery is only achieved 4–5 months after the birth of the baby (Calguneri *et al.*, 1982).

The posture of most pregnant women alters during pregnancy to compensate for their changing shape and, thus, their changing centre of gravity (Figure 23.1). How this happens will depend on individual factors such as joint range, muscle strength and fatigue. This will usually involve an increase in the lumbar and thoracic curves. It used to be thought that there was an alteration in the pelvic tilt, but Bullock *et al.* (1987) have suggested that this is not the case.

Another factor in the alteration of joint function in the final three months of pregnancy is an increase in fluid retention. Many women develop

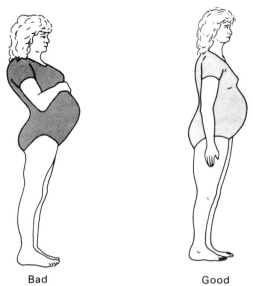

Fig. 23.2 Using pelvic tilting to hold the fetus in the pelvis as long as possible and to maintain good posture.

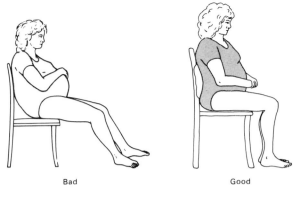

Fig. 23.3 Using a pillow or lumbar roll to support the back when sitting is more comfortable.

oedema in their extremities which reduces joint range. Finally, it should be borne in mind that, because of the increased abdominal load, women may have difficulty in performing simple activities, such as bending and lifting, safely, particularly if leg and other muscles are not capable of coping with the increase in body weight.

Back and pelvic girdle pain is probably one of the most commonly experienced 'minor ailments' of pregnancy and should be of interest and concern to all physiotherapists. Unfortunately, the lack of importance which midwives and doctors frequently attach to what could be major discomfort is often reflected in the policy of physiotherapy departments. 'You've got backache because you're pregnant; you'll have to wait until your baby is born for it to be treated' is a comment frequently reported by women. In the hierarchy of importance for urgent physiotherapy treatment, back pain in pregnancy is often relegated to 'the bottom of the pile', so that women, who may be coping with a job outside the home as well as having to care for a family including other children, struggle on without expert diagnosis and help.

It has been shown that about 50% of pregnant women report pain which is severe enough to affect their lifestyle (Mantle *et al.*, 1977, 1981; Nwuga, 1982; Fast *et al.*, 1987; Berg *et al*, 1988). It can occur at any stage in the pregnancy, but often the first episode is between the fourth and seventh months; and although it can involve any part of the spine, it tends to be experienced at a slightly lower level in the pregnant as opposed to the non-pregnant woman.

Prevention of back pain

Mantle *et al.* (1981) showed that early pregnancy back care advice was instrumental in preventing some back pain and reduced the intensity of that which was experienced. Many hospitals are now offering an evening class at 12–16 weeks and physiotherapists should be involved in these. Good back care habits will not only benefit women during the months of their pregnancies but will stand them (and their families) in good stead for the rest of their lives. Some adaptation of back care principles will be necessary for pregnant women (Polden and Mantle, 1990) but should include information on lying, sitting, standing, walking, bending and lifting. It is advisable for a short illustrated leaflet to be provided, including a contact telephone number for the physiotherapist should it prove necessary. This leaflet should provide 'reminders' for postural correction (Figures 23.2, 23.3), daily activities (Figures 23.4, 23.5) and good back usage.

Management of back and pelvic girdle pain

It is most important for a full examination and assessment to be carried out in all women presenting with back pain in pregnancy, which is interfering with their lifestyle (Polden and Mantle, 1990), and time for this must be built into the daily

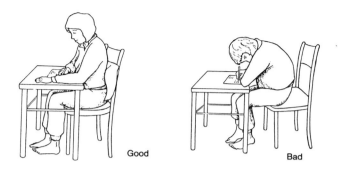

Fig. 23.4   Back care when sitting and working.

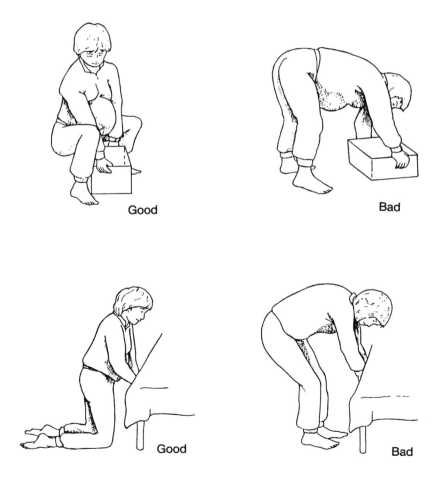

Fig. 23.5   Back care during daily activities.

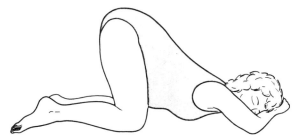

Fig. 23.6   Resting in this position can relieve backache.

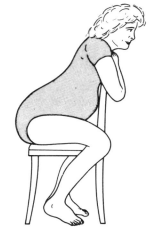

Fig. 23.7   Sitting astride a chair is less likely to lead to a stiff, aching back.

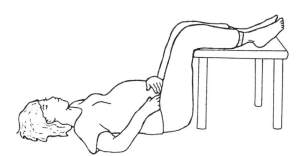

Fig. 23.8   Relief of a tired, aching back.

workload of obstetric physiotherapists. Specifc pain syndromes will emerge. These include:

- Low back pain.
- Sacroiliac dysfunction.
- Sciatica.
- Coccydynia.
- Thoracic spine pain.
- 'Postural' backache.
- Osteitis pubis; diastasis (separation) of the symphysis pubis.

Physiotherapy techniques which can usefully be used include gentle mobilizations, heat, massage, ice packs, ultrasound and TENS. Full and clear advice as to what the woman can and cannot do and how she should move in and out of bed should be part of each consultation.

Many women will find suggestions for alternative positions of rest helpful (Figures 23.6–23.8). 'Self-help' pelvic tilting exercises can be useful for relieving low backache (Figure 23.9), lumber extension (Figure 23.10), can also be included. Where the sacroiliac joint is involved women often find relief by adopting the following positions at home (Figures 23.11–23.13). A sacroiliac support designed to be used in pregnancy frequently enables women to carry on with their daily routine in comfort. Several manufacturers now provide these and, because of the difference in price, it is worth making inquiries before ordering them!

Although suppliers of TENS equipment usually make the proviso that it should not be used in pregnancy before 38 weeks, its use as a symptomatic means of pain control has been described (Mannheimer, 1985; Fisher and Hanna, 1987; Mantle, 1988). Its use may be more acceptable to women than pharmacological analgesia.

Osteitis pubis; diastasis symphysis pubis

The very painful and distressing separation of the symphysis pubis can occur as early as 22 weeks gestation and is often associated with sacroiliac dysfunction. When severe the mother may be unable to walk and turning over in bed can be excruciatingly painful. Hagen (1974) found that there was a tendency for symptoms to be repeated in subsequent pregnancies and for the condition to occur earlier and with increasing intensity. The old remedy of binding the hips with a roller towel or the use of a trochanteric belt may give relief. Bed rest, with appropriate advice as to moving in bed, may be necessary initially (the mother should keep her knees bent and pressed together). A walking frame or sticks may be useful; ice packs could give relief when applied over the tender symphysis pubis.

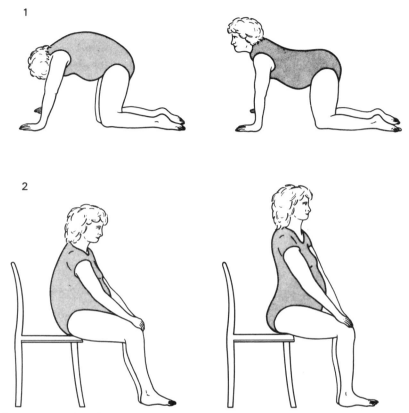

Fig. 23.9   Pelvic tilting in prone kneeling and sitting with careful and controlled 'humping and hollowing'.

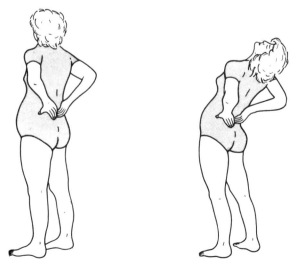

Fig. 23.10   Repeated lumbar extension in standing can give pain relief.

Costal margin pain

As the uterus rises in the abdomen, the rib cage 'flares' out sideways, and the circumference of the chest wall may increase by as much as 10–15 cm. This is often associated with pain or a bruised feeling along the costal margin. Side flexion *away* from the pain, with the arm of the affected side raised over the head, or stretching with both arms raised above the head with the hands clasped, may give relief.

Carpal tunnel syndrome

Fluid retention in the final trimester of pregnancy can lead to compression of the median nerve as it passes under the flexor retinaculum at the wrist. Paraesthesia and pain (at night) and clumsiness and the inability to hold things can result. It has

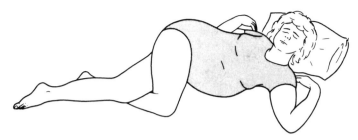

Fig. 23.11   Lying flat, rotate the pelvis away from the pain. Rock gently in this position.

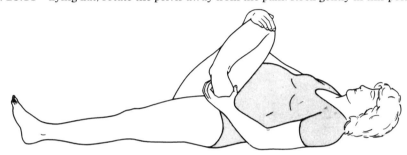

Fig. 23.12   Draw the knee up towards the shoulder and the heel towards the opposite groin, then hold the position for a few moments.

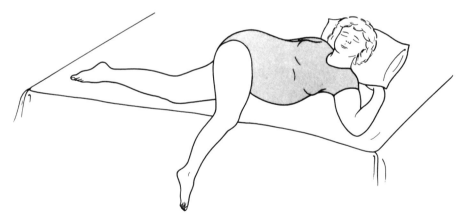

Fig. 23.13   Allow the leg to hang comfortably over the edge of the bed.

been reported that between 2.5% and 50% of women (Melvin *et al.*, 1969; Gould and Wissinger, 1978; Voitk *et al.*, 1983; Ekman-Ordeberg *et al.*, 1987) will experience symptoms. Wearing a wrist splint at night has been shown to relieve symptoms in 46 out of 56 women (Ekman-Ordeberg *et al.*, 1987). Wrist and hand exercises in elevation; ice packs and ultrasound are techniques which can be used where the symptoms persist; most resolve following delivery and the subsequent diuresis. A similar condition, the so-called T-4 syndrome

(McGuckin, 1986) may arise from the thoracic spine. Where this is present, passive mobilization techniques for the thoracic spine, directed to the appropriate thoracic level, may give relief.

Pelvic floor discomfort

At the end of the pregnancy women frequently complain of 'pressure' or a 'dropping out' sensation due to the weight of the uterus and its contents on the pelvic floor. This discomfort will be compounded where there are vulval varicose veins and haemorrhoids. Pelvic floor contractions and resting with the hips raised on pillows can be helpful. Adopting the position shown in Figure 23.6 temporarily reduces intrapelvic pressure and sometimes gives relief.

Cramp

Calf cramp frequently disturbs sleep during pregnancy. The exact pathophysiological mechanism is as yet unknown; lack of calcium, salt or vitamin D have all been suggested as causes as well as ischaemia and nerve root pressure. It is often triggered by the woman stretching in bed with her feet plantar flexed. Prevention is often possible if she remembers to dorsiflex her feet while stretching. A spasm can be relieved by active or passive dorsiflexion of the foot with extension of the knees. Vigorous foot exercises for 20–30 seconds following a spasm, plus calf massage, can ease the severe 'bruised' sensation which often remains.

Uterine ligament pain

The woman who is pregnant for the first time is often alarmed by sharp 'shooting' pains or a dull ache low in the abdomen. Reassurance that she is *not* in labour may be all that is needed. An explanation that the pain is caused by the 'guy ropes' of the uterus softening and stretching may be all that is needed for the woman to 'live with' the discomfort. Warmth, a comfortable bath, or a hot water bottle is soothing, as is gentle stroking massage over the pain. In subsequent pregnancies weakness of the abdominal wall and consequent lack of support anteriorly could be a contributory factor to 'stress' on uterine ligaments.

Disintegrating fibroids

There are many causes of abdominal pain during pregnancy; some are benign, usually attributed to displacement and direct pressure on neighbouring structures; stretching of the abdominal wall and peritoneum can be additional factors. Acute abdominal pain is often associated with obstetric emergencies, although, of course, general abdominal conditions may also affect the woman. Uterine fibroids, benign tumours, tend to increase in size

during pregnancy. This may interfere with their blood supply and lead to 'red degeneration' with accompanying acute abdominal pain. Fibroids are more common in women over 30 and in the Afro-Caribbean population; disintegration tends to occur in the second half of pregnancy.

The author has successfully used TENS for the relief of this incapacitating pain under the direction of a consultant anaesthetist.

Labour

The Biblical explanation for labour pain lays the blame fairly and squarely on Eve for listening to the serpent: 'in sorrow thou shalt bring forth children' (Genesis 3: 16). It has been recognized throughout the ages, and cross-culturally, that labour is painful and this seems to apply to women the world over, notwithstanding their level of sophistication. Women in primitive societies appear to have pain comparable to ours (Freedman and Ferguson, 1950). 'Primitiveness' does not equate with 'painlessness' in childbirth.

The uterus at term (the end of pregnancy) is a large, hollow sack with a strong muscular wall (myometrium). This is composed of smooth muscle fibres set in a collagenous connective-tissue base. The proportion of muscle fibres to connective tissue is greater in the upper part (the body), becoming less lower down (the lower uterine segment). The 'neck' or cervix is 90% fibrous, collagenous connective-tissue, with about 10% muscle fibres. The highly vascular lining of the uterus (endometrium, but called the decidua in pregnancy) is a rich source of prostaglandins. The innervation of the uterus is T10–L1; the lower uterine segment and the cervix being particularly richly supplied.

During labour the cervix, which is softened and 'ripened' by hormonal action, is gradually drawn up over the fetal head by rhythmical contraction of the myometrium. Most research shows that the pain of the first stage of labour is due to the progressive dilatation of the cervix and the lower uterine segment; ischaemia due to strong muscle contraction has also been suggested. In the second stage pressure on pain sensitive structures in the pelvis, stretching of the pelvic outlet, and distension and damage to the soft tissues of the pelvic floor and perineum will be factors in causing discomfort. In 1981, Melzack *et al.* (Figure 23.14) showed that labour pain recorded on the McGill pain questionnaire ranged from 2 to 62. It was

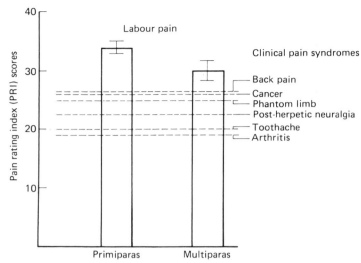

Fig. 23.14   Average total pain rating index (PRI). The intensity of labour pain compared with other clinical pain syndromes. (From Melzack *et al.*, 1981, with permission.)

greater for women having their first babies (primigravidae) than those having second or subsequent babies (multigravidae), labour pain scored higher than pain syndromes such as back, cancer, or phantom limb pain, or post-herpetic neuralgia.

In common with other visceral pain, labour pain is referred to the dermatomes supplied by nerve roots which innervate the uterus and cervix, pelvic organs and pelvic floor, T10–L1 and S2–4. The physiological reactions to labour pain are the same as for other acutely painful conditions, i.e. increased tension of skeletal muscle and an increase in blood pressure, ventilation, cardiac output and oxygen consumption. Preparation for childbirth has always been based on the theory that knowledge will remove fear and instil confidence in the mother, both in her own body and its ability to give birth, and in those caring for her. Many women are apprehensive at the thought of losing control in labour, but at the same time express the hope that they will achieve the birth of their baby 'on their own' without active intervention or analgesia. Melzack *et al.* (1981) showed that primiparae who elected to have prepared childbirth training had significantly lower pain scores than those who did not attend antenatal classes.

The obstetric physiotherapist has much to offer women, both in the relief of their labour pain and the control of their pain behaviour, by teaching techniques that are free of side-effects to mother or baby. These include:

Relaxation

Relaxation was first suggested for use in labour by Minnie Randall (a physiotherapist at St Thomas's Hospital) and Dr Grantley Dick-Read in the 1920s. There are many techniques for achieving relaxation: the **contrast** method (in which the muscles are tensed and then relaxed) and **disassociation** (where one part of the body is relaxed while tightening another). These are two techniques which were frequently taught in antenatal classes together with **imaging** (imagining pleasant and relaxing experiences) and **touch relaxation** (relaxing a part of the body in response to touch). Most obstetric physiotherapists now use the Mitchell method of Physiological Relaxation as a method for reducing stress and tension (Mitchell, 1977). It is suggested that women greet each uterine contraction by relaxing through it in whatever position they find comfortable. In this way it is hoped that the natural physiological pain responses will be modified, the mother will feel calmer and more in control of her body, will require less oxygen, and her metabolic rate will be lower thus decreasing the need for glycogen (which is essential for good uterine activity).

Breathing

Unprepared women frequently hyperventilate during uterine contractions and even those who have attended antenatal classes will find it difficult to maintain a normal rate and depth of respiration. Hypocapnia (a drop in the carbon dioxide concentration in the blood) could result and can be followed by a period of hypoventilation between contractions as a response to the hypocapnia. This could decrease the PaO_2 in the placenta and in the fetus with consequent distress. Breathing into cupped hands or a paper bag can help to prevent and alleviate the effects of hyperventilation.

The breathing techniques in the psychoprophylactic method of preparation for childbirth (Buxton and Buxton, 1966) actually increased the risk of maternal hyperventilation. The most calming, and a safer way for the mother to breathe during contractions, is slowly, easily, deeply and as normally as possible. Starting a contraction with a breath out (and relaxing); pausing momentarily between expiration and inspiration, and quietly allowing as much air into her lungs as she needs effectively helps to increase her relaxation response. Emphasis is always on the outward breath and thus the instruction *breathe in* is never given. Concentrating on breathing and relaxation, 'riding the waves' of labour contractions, greeting each pain as a positive life-giving experience bringing her closer to her unborn baby, helps the mother cope with the intensity of her experience and gives her a feeling of control and increased confidence. Strategies for coping with pain suggest dealing with one spasm at a time. Short-term bursts of willpower and short-term goals make it easier to face a complete pain experience.

As labour progresses the contractions will become stronger, more frequent, and will last longer. It is then helpful to allow the breathing to become shallower and slightly faster (but still calm and quiet) following the body's natural response, air passing in and out through the nose or through relaxed, slightly parted lips. At the end of the first stage of labour the contractions will be very fierce and powerful, and may seem, to the mother, almost continuous. Occasionally the urge to push is felt before the cervix is fully dilatated and while the baby's head is still high in the pelvis. It is then helpful to use breathing techniques which prevent breath holding and bearing down. Sighing '*hoo hoo hah hah*' breaths or saying '*I won't push*' with expiration can help at this difficult time.

Some women find the second stage of labour painful and others find that the urge to push is overwhelming but pain free. Careful preparation antenatally can prevent panic as the pelvic floor stretches around the baby's head. Pushing with the breath held, or while breathing out should both be taught so that the mother can use whichever technique her midwife thinks best at the time. It is suggested that women use a gentle panting breathing as the baby is being born.

Massage

When experiencing discomfort or pain, the instinctive response is to 'rub it better' (p. 54). Labour pain can be relieved by massaging the back or abdomen during contractions. It has been suggested that this stimulates the afferent nerves and gives pain relief by the pain gate control mechanism (see p. 54); massage may also stimulate the production of endorphins, and in labour probably acts as a 'counter-irritant'.

Back massage

This should be deep, slow and painless; enthusiastic partners can inflict more pain than they relieve if not taught properly during antenatal classes! Deep, soothing kneading, one hand placed on the other over the sacrum, or deep slow effleurage over the sacral and lumbar regions with the mother sitting astride a chair and leaning forward, can successfully increase her pain tolerance level (Polden and Mantle, 1990).

Abdominal massage

This is very light, the fingers just brushing the skin over the pain. It can be carried out with one hand stroking from side to side over the pain, or by a double-handed effleurage. It can be done by the woman herself during a contraction in conjunction with relaxation and controlled breathing. Alternatively, it can be performed by her partner or labour companion (Polden and Mantle, 1990).

Movement and positioning

The 'medicalization' of childbirth led to the immobilization of women on a bed, often flat on their backs. Thus, the beneficial effect of gravity helping the fetus descend through the pelvis is lost. The supine position has also been shown to decrease the efficiency of labour contractions (Caldeyro-Barcia, 1979), probably because utero-placental blood perfusion is reduced due to aorto-caval compression by the heavy uterus. As the uterus contracts during the first stage of labour it also anteverts (tips forward), the better to 'drive' the fetus into the pelvis; the supine position would interfere with this action too. Melzack (1991) found that women who adopted vertical positions reported less pain in early labour. About 35% reported less front pain and 50% felt less back pain than when they were lying down on their back or side.

It has been shown that frequent changes of position stimulates more efficient uterine contractions (Roberts *et al.*, 1983) and that women who were encouraged to mobilize and walk during labour required less analgesia and had shorter labours (Flynn *et al.*, 1978). Women who are equipped with this knowledge and who are taught comfortable alternative positions during antenatal classes (incorporating upright or forward leaning postures) could benefit in that the severity and length of their pain will be reduced.

Transcutaneous Electrical Nerve Stimulation (TENS)

In common with other acute pain syndromes, the pain of childbirth may be relieved by the use of TENS (Bundsen *et al.*, 1981; Bundsen and Erickson, 1982; Bundsen *et al.*, 1982; Harrison *et al.*, 1986). Units for use in labour are available from several manufacturers. However, some of these units do not meet standards sufficient to produce the type and intensity of stimulation necessary to relieve the high levels of pain experienced in labour. As well as modifying the response of the spinal cord to noxious stimulation (Woolf, 1989) and stimulating the production of endogenous opiates (Thompson, 1990), which may act on receptors on C-fibre terminals within the spinal cord, the cognitive appreciation of the stimulation (often over the site of pain) is a vital component in achieving satisfactory pain relief in labour. This cerebral component of pain control is of equal, and some would say greater importance than local effects on the nerves (Crothers, 1994). It has also been suggested that in certain circumstances (i.e. labour), TENS may

act to make pain less disturbing without reducing its intensity (Woolf, 1989).

Labour pain is felt in the lower back, abdomen and possibly the thighs (first stage), and in the perineum, vulva, back and abdomen (second stage). It varies in intensity as labour progresses and is felt in the dermatome areas T10–L1 and S2–4 (Polden and Mantle, 1990). Unlike pethidine (Demerol, USA) or entonox (analgesics used during labour), it is preferable for TENS to be applied early rather than for the parturient to wait until she cannot bear her pain any longer. Low frequency, burst mode is used in between contractions as it has been suggested that low frequency, high intensity stimulation activates opioid systems (Thompson, 1990). High frequency, high intensity stimulation is used during a contraction, which probably initiates a neural blockade and also a cognitive appreciation of the stimulus.

Because of the very particular causes, intensity and perception of labour pain, it is essential that an obstetric TENS unit is able to produce suitable stimulation and for it and its accessories to withstand hard wear and usage. It must, therefore, be robust, very easy to apply and simple to operate (i.e. ease of replacing batteries and manipulation of controls, which should not be hidden or small). Manufacturers instructions *must* be accurate and electrodes should be of sufficient size to cover the relevant dermatomes. Unfortunately, suggestions for the size of electrodes and for their placement in at least two so-called 'obstetric' TENS units at the present time are not based on research or current clinical practice.

Important considerations in choosing a TENS unit for labour:

- The unit should be dual channel so that the two pairs of electrodes can be controlled independently. Skin oiliness and fat over the sacral area could lead to higher skin impedence, requiring a greater energy output and, where low back pain is present, a higher intensity of stimulation will be needed on the lower pair.
- It should be possible to alter the frequency so that the woman chooses the most comfortable and effective rate for herself at different points in labour.
- The specifications of the machine must permit it to produce sufficient energy to reduce pain. Physiotherapists should look at these carefully – TENS units are *not* all the same!
- It must be possible to change from the burst,

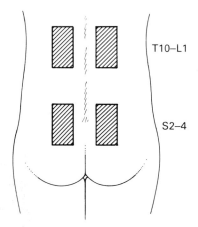

T10–L1

S2–4

Fig. 23.15 Positions for TENS electrode placement during labour.

low frequency mode to the continuous, high frequency mode easily and without the woman having to maintain a continuous pressure on the 'patient control' switch. This must be a 'press/release' mechanism and *not* 'press/hold'.

- It is most desirable for there to be an automatic 10% increase in intensity when the unit is switched from the burst to the continuous mode for a contraction, so that the woman does not have to adjust the controls.
- Guarantees from manufacturers for maintenance and aftercare should be for more than one year.

Electrodes are placed paravertebrally (Figure 23.15), preferably in early labour, over nerve roots T10–L1 and S2–4 (the innervation of the uterus, cervix, vagina, pelvic viscera, vulva and perineum). Intense back pain, often a feature of the first stage of labour, is felt in the sacral region; the lower electrodes are actually over the site of pain (Chapter 14, Fig. 14.4). Lower abdominal pain may also be experienced during the first stage of labour. Some women find that abdominal massage used in conjunction with dorsally placed electrodes is sufficient to help them cope with contractions. Robson (1979) found that suprapubic abdominal electrodes in addition to the electrodes on the back were helpful. Bundsen and Erickson (1982) mention a theoretical possibility that high intensity stimulation with conventional electrodes over the parturient's lower abdomen could, in unfavourable cases, induce irregularities in fetal heart function,

although this did not occur during their trial. They also describe a specially made abdominal electrode which gave shallow stimulation and some pain relief. Occasionally TENS causes interference on the cardiotocograph (fetal head monitor) trace, when a scalp electrode is attached to the baby's head. A filter could eliminate this but has proved too expensive to be manufactured. This problem does not arise with external monitoring.

The major benefit of TENS in labour is that it allows the mother to remain mobile. It has been shown (Mendez-Bauer *et al.*, 1976) that the woman who is able to walk, move freely and change her position at will during the first stage of labour has fewer, stronger, more efficient contractions and requires less analgesic medication. Traditional obstetric analgesia (pethidine, entonox or epidural anaesthesia) is invasive, prevents mobility and affects the baby as well as the mother. TENS may not give sufficient relief for those women experiencing high levels of pain, but it is undoubtedly useful in many cases.

It is essential that women intending to use TENS during labour are properly taught antenatally exactly how to apply the electrodes, adjust the unit's controls and how to deal with problems such as gel drying out under the electrodes or a failing battery. Because so few hospitals have a loan service, many women are renting units direct from manufacturers and are struggling to make sense of instructions without proper guidance. Physiotherapists working with pregnant women have a duty to organize instruction for these women, all of whom should experience TENS stimulation prior to labour. Physiotherapists also have a duty to be aware of which TENS units will be able to relieve labour pain satisfactorily and which should be avoided, and they should advise their clients accordingly.

In 1984, Clifford Woolf wrote in *Textbook of Pain*:

> The ability of a clinician to reduce pain in a patient by exploiting the patient's own in-built neurophysiological control mechanisms must surely rank as one of the great achievements of contemporary medical science.

The analgesic effect of TENS is said to be based on this premise. Its use in labour is comparatively new and much remains to be learnt. The position of the electrodes, the mode of stimulation, the frequency and wave form are all important factors which could usefully be altered so that the woman in labour receives better analgesia. Pain relief in labour is an important area affecting thousands of women. Research by physiotherapists into better ways of using TENS should be encouraged.

After The Baby is Born

The puerperium – first six weeks

In spite of the joy most women feel following the safe delivery of their baby, the immediate postnatal period (puerperium) is frequently uncomfortable to say the least! Perineal, back, or breast pain are physical discomforts widely experienced; and fatigue, anxiety and uncertainty about handling and feeding her baby may lower the woman's pain tolerance level.

Many women dislike taking analgesics while breastfeeding in case small amounts reach their baby via breastmilk. Physiotherapeutic techniques can usefully be applied to relieve the common postnatal 'aches and pains', which are often dismissed as part of 'new motherhood', without affecting the baby. The obstetric physiotherapist who has, hopefully, built up a caring relationship with the woman during antenatal classes, is the ideal person to treat existing problems and prevent many new ones arising by giving advice and information.

Common early pain problems are:

- Perineal pain
- Backache/neck ache
- Caesarean section
- Haemorrhoids
- 'After pains'
- Breast engorgement
- Fatigue
- Diastasis symphysis pubis

Perineal pain

Many mothers recall the perineal pain they felt following the birth of their babies as the worst part of their childbirth experience. Episiotomy (the cut in the vaginal and perineal tissue to enlarge the opening as the baby's head is being delivered) can give rise to intense postpartum pain especially when it is complicated by post-forceps bruising and oedema. Tears are a common occurrence. Physiotherapy techniques normally used for the treatment of soft tissue injury can often give speedy relief and in this way facilitate the development of a happy mother/baby relationship.

Treatment

Ice

Nerve conduction drops with decreasing temperature and this reduces nociceptive impulses from the damaged area (Lehmann and de Lateur, 1984). Ice is commonly used to relieve oedema, which sometimes affects the perineum and labia following delivery. Crushed ice in a disposable plastic glove or bag (frozen peas can be used at home), which is covered with a damp gauze or lint swab, can be applied to the painful area while the mother rests.

Ultrasound

The traumatic oedema and bruising which often develops after a difficult vaginal delivery can be treated with ultrasound in the same way as other acute soft tissue injuries. It is not essential for the site of the affected area to be sterile as the postpartum lochia (bleeding) makes this impossible to achieve, however cleanliness *is* important. Before every treatment it is suggested that the ultrasound head is washed in detergent and carefully dried; afterwards it is washed in detergent again, dried, and then immersed in glutaraldehyde (Asep or Cidex) for 10 min, after which it should be rinsed and carefully dried once more. Physiotherapists using ultrasound for immediate postpartum perineal pain relief should be alert to new directives on hygiene from the Department of Health or their local Infection Control Officer.

The damaged area is gently swabbed clean and the coupling medium applied. Using a pulsed beam a low intensity (0.5 W/cm^2) is applied for 3–5 min depending on the size of the bruise. If the improvement does not occur the intensity of the ultrasound and the length of treatment time can be increased at the next session.

The analgesia produced by ultrasound and the removal of the traumatic exudate enables the mother to gently contract and relax the pelvic floor which further improves her condition. Treatment is continued daily while the woman is in hospital.

Infrared radiation

Many women find that mild infrared irradiation is both soothing and relaxing when applied to their painful perineum. The mother lies on her side, with her knees drawn up, or on her back, legs apart and supported on pillows. Exposure for 10–20 min twice a day is adequate.

Infrared is particularly useful where the wound has broken down or is infected and is an inexpensive method of helping a new mother cope with this unaccustomed discomfort.

Pulsed high frequency energy (pulsed electromagnetic energy, PEME)

Bewley (1986) showed that megapulse treatment of the damaged perineum resulted in rapid healing. Pulse widths of 40–65 μs used in conjunction with low pulse repetition rates were used for 15 min initially. Bruising and oedema resolved and pain was reduced over the 3-day trial period. This form of treatment could beneficially be used for broken down episiotomy wounds.

Pelvic floor exercises

Many women are frightened to do anything which increases perineal discomfort following delivery and are therefore scared to contract their pelvic floor muscles. Pelvic floor exercising is a most valuable 'self-help' method of reducing oedema, and so pain. Gentle muscle contractions will improve perineal circulation and promote absorption of exudate. Women often compain of vaginal 'numbness' and 'sluggish muscles' in the immediate postpartum period and find it difficult to initiate or feel a pelvic floor contraction. Where this is the case, the obstetric physiotherapists should watch for pelvic floor activity while the woman tries to contract her muscles. It is possible for the birthing process to damage the nerve supply to the pelvic floor muscles (Snooks et al., 1984; Allen et al., 1990), resulting in short-, and sometimes long-term muscle weakness and loss of sensation.

Women should be encouraged to gently 'squeeze and relax' their pelvic floor muscles very frequently while their discomfort is acute (ten times every 5 min is not too much). Simple knee-bending movements will relieve stiffness caused by the fear of moving and will increase confidence.

An essential part of the physiotherapy regime to ease perineal pain must be advice about sitting comfortably while feeding the baby. Perching on the edge of a bed or chair will increase pain; the woman should sit well back in her chair (on a soft pillow if necessary), with her back supported. Sometimes sitting on two pillows (with a gap between them for the painful area) will be more suitable. Breastfeeding women should be encouraged to feed lying on their side while their pain is severe.

Back pain

A commonly voiced complaint immediately following the birth is back pain. This can range from coccydynia to sacroiliac, lumbar, thoracic or even cervical discomfort. It may just be a dull, inconveniencing ache or an acute, incapacitating pain that grossly interferes with the new mother's quality of life. Simple postural advice may be all that is needed to relieve some symptoms, but in others a thorough assessment by a physiotherapist should be followed by immediate, appropriate treatment. Causes of early postnatal back pain are varied:

- Coccydynia – the coccyx is forced backwards as the baby is born; this damages ligaments and the coccyx occasionally fractures (Brunskill and Swain, 1987).
- Sacroiliac – this may just be due to the 'opening out' of the pelvic joints; it can be associated with the lithotomy position for forceps deliveries or postpartum suturing, if the woman's legs were not lifted simultaneously.
- Lumbo-sacral/lumbar – awkward positions in the second stage of labour; epidural anaesthesia often results in a sore, 'bruised' sensation; poor feeding, nappy changing and lifting techniques.
- Thoracic – often associated with unsupported feeding positions and constant bending over the baby on a low surface, i.e. nappy changing.
- Cervical – can be acute if enthusiastic 'helpers' forced the woman's head down onto her chest in the second stage of labour.

Treatment

Coccydynia: ice, hot packs, ultrasound. Advice about sitting (well-padded chair or rubber ring); weight on ischial tuberosities and not on coccyx; breastfeeding in a side-lying position; rest in prone-lying position; gluteal contractions can all relieve discomfort. It may take several weeks to resolve. TENS may be useful in this case.

Sacroiliac: 'self-help' movements (Figures 23.11–23.13); support – double-thickness Tubigrip, sizes K or L; small size pregnancy sacroiliac support; specific mobilizations if these suggestions are not successful.

Lumbo-sacral/lumbar; appropriate advice concerning activities with baby; postural advice; hot packs; pelvic tilting exercises in side-lying, crook-lying, sitting and standing positions; Tubigrip supports; mobilizations if indicated.

Thoracic: appropriate advice about feeding positions; hot packs; elbow circling and arm swinging exercises (thoracic pain is frequently aggravated by fatigue and tension); pelvic tilting in sitting position with good back extension; mobilizations; TENS.

Cervical: gentle mobilizations where necessary; often responds to hot packs, massage and gentle neck movements.

Essential back-care advice

Even if backache and its possible causes plus its prevention were discussed in antenatal classes, it must still form part of routine postnatal physiotherapy care – many women will not have attended antenatal classes and many more will have forgotten antenatal discussions! Apart from the usual 'back school' advice with regard to household and other chores and activities, time must be spent discussing and thinking about all the new baby-care routines; it is useful to have pictures of 'Dos' and 'Don'ts':

Feeding

The mother must be shown how to make herself comfortable on a chair by placing a cushion behind her waist. She should raise her baby by using a pillow on her lap and use a low footstool for her feet (Figure 23.16 *b*). If she prefers to feed in bed, then, again, her back must be well supported (Figure 23.17 *a*) or she may be more comfortable lying down (Figure 23.16 *c*). She must be dissuaded from feeding in unsupported positions (Figures 23.16 *a*, 23.17 *b*).

Nappy changing

Any position which involves stooping will lead to or increase back pain – women should think in advance where and how they will be carrying out this constantly repeated task. It should be done at waist level (on a worktop), on the mother's lap while she sits in a chair, or on the floor – but *not* while the mother bends over her baby (Figures 23.18, 23.19).

Baby bathing

The use of baby baths on low stands should be discouraged; apart from the bending and stooping involved there is also the question of filling and emptying the bath! If the mother particularly wants a separate bath for her baby, the type which fits over a standard bath should be recommended (with the mother kneeling alongside instead of stooping). Bathing small, young babies in the bathroom hand basin or a washing up bowl on the kitchen table are good alternatives for better back care.

Cots, prams, buggies and baby slings

Women and their partners should be encouraged to give thought to where their babies will sleep and how they will be transported. Low cots and low-handled prams and buggies are a constant source of back pain. It is important to emphasize the concept of 'bend your knees and not your back' for any lifting, plus 'draw your abdominal muscles in firmly' when picking up weighty objects. Baby slings are ideal for carrying small babies but their straps must be adjusted so that the baby's head is just under the mother's chin; low, dangling babies lead to backache!

Haemorrhoids

These are a very real source of postnatal pain! Haemorrhoids are varicose veins in and around the anus and the anal canal; they often prolapse following delivery and sometimes become thrombosed.

Treatment

Ice packs and pelvic floor exercises are two useful self-help remedies. The woman should avoid prolonged sitting and standing when the pain is severe; prone-lying is helpful. Bewley (1986) found the pain-relieving effect of PEME useful – particularly where the haemorrhoids were thrombosed.

After pains

Murray and Holdcroft (1989) showed that 50% of primiparous (having just had their first baby) and 86% of multiparous (second or subsequent babies) women complained of lower abdominal pain. It ranged between the severity of menstrual and labour pain on the McGill pain questionnaire and must not be discounted! These 'after pains' are often associated with the production of oxytocin, which is released during breastfeeding and also

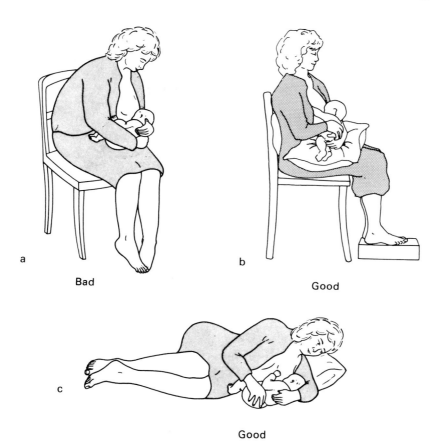

Fig. 23.16   Feeding positions which can cause backache must be avoided. Unless the mother chooses to feed lying down, the back must be well supported.

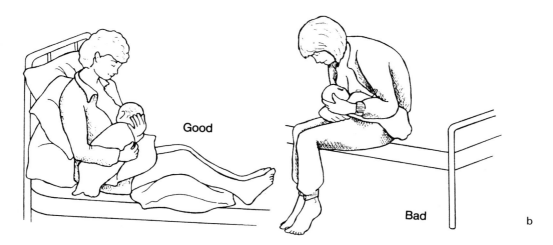

Fig. 23.17   The mother should be well supported and a pillow should be used to raise the baby to prevent stooping.

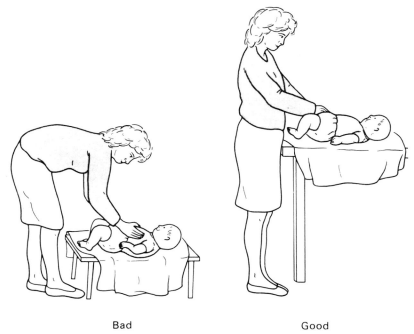

Bad   Good

Fig. 23.18 Changing a nappy on a surface of the correct height.

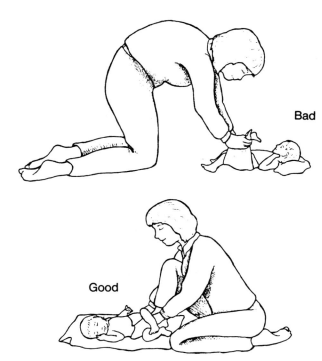

Bad

Good

Fig. 23.19 Changing a nappy at floor level.

causes uterine contractions. 'Physiotherapy exercises' relieved the pain in 40% of the primiparous women but only 10% of multiparous women (these exercises were not defined).

Treatment

'Relaxing and breathing' through the pains (as in labour), hot packs, gentle stroking massage and TENS are all useful therapies where the pain is very severe; plus reassurance and explanation.

Breast engorgement

Although not strictly the province of the obstetric physiotherapist, suggestions for the relief of hard engorged breasts (thankfully less common now that breastfeeding is 'baby-led') are often welcome.

Treatment

Contrast bathing (alternate hot and cold compresses) with gentle massage from the periphery of the breast towards the nipple (Heardman, 1954); gentle elbow-circling can make the mother more

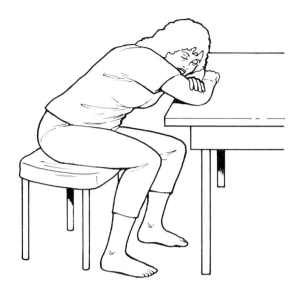

Fig. 23.20   A very useful position for a quick 'cat nap'.

comfortable. Ultrasound can be used to soften the breast and encourage milk flow (Semmler, 1982) and interferential therapy has been suggested for the severe inflammation of mastitis (Maslem, 1982; Collinson, 1986).

Fatigue, Anxiety and Tension

Although not strictly speaking 'painful', tiredness and worry are normal postnatal problems. Encouragement to rest and relax while the baby is sleeping are positive suggestions which should be made to new mothers during the daily postnatal exercise class. The 'blues' and depression are both exacerbated by fatigue. It is useful to teach relaxation in positions other than lying (Figure 23.20) so that the woman can make best use of 'cat naps'. A reminder about slow, calm breathing emphasizing expiration with relaxation could prove beneficial.

Diastasis symphysis pubis

Severe supra-pubic pain occasionally occurs immediately following delivery and weight-bearing can be impossible. The symphisys can be tender and sometimes a gap will be felt.

Treatment

Bed rest will be necessary initially and women will need advice with regard to moving in bed and transferring from bed to a chair. They will also need a walking aid. A trochanteric belt may be helpful but sometimes the problem takes months to resolve (Scriven, 1991) and can even require surgery to stabilize the joint.

Caesarean section

During the past 20 years or so the caesarean section rate in the developed world has increased from 5–7% to 10–15%, with some high risk centres reaching 20–25% (Lomas, 1988). The woman whose baby is delivered in this way has more than her fair share of discomfort and pain to cope with as she adapts to her role as a mother. She is handicapped, and sometimes incapacitated by the pain of her incision, a drip, a drain and, occasionally, a catheter. The procedure may have been carried out as an emergency during the course of labour or it may have been decided upon in advance (elective caesarean section); anaesthesia could have been local (epidural or spinal) or general. Postoperative pain relief medication may 'distance' her from her new baby and she may have very mixed feelings about the inability of her body to give birth vaginally.

In common with other surgical procedures, women who have some prior knowledge as to how they will feel postoperatively and how they can best help themselves cope with the additional burden of acute pain as they care for their baby, will have more confidence and will be less fearful. Every antenatal course of classes should include information about caesarean section and women should be able to discuss ways and means of dealing with discomfort. Women who are to undergo an elective procedure benefit from a preoperative 'briefing' from their obstetric physiotherapist; as well as routine advice with regard to postoperative breathing and leg exercises, it is useful to include instructions on early moving in and out of bed and the most comfortable way to hold the baby.

Postoperatively, comprehensive advice must be given about moving, getting in and out of bed, picking up the baby and feeding positions so that extra pain from carrying out these activities incorrectly is avoided. Where postoperative chest secretions are a problem great care must be taken to help the woman cough comfortably and efficiently.

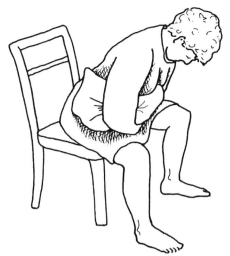

Fig. 23.21   A supported coughing position.

As well as being painful it must be remembered that her abdominal wall is now extremely slack; she must be shown how to support her abdomen as she leans forward to cough (Figure 23.21).

The discomfort of uterine contractions can be eased by relaxation and the breathing techniques used in labour. Abdominal wind, often intensely painful, responds well to physiotherapeutic techniques:

- Deep breathing with abdominal retraction on expiration.
- Crook-lying, gentle pelvic tilting movements mainly using the gluteal muscles.
- Crook-lying, gentle knee rolling from side to side.
- Abdominal massage, single or two-handed effleurage, following the line of the colon (up on the right, transversely from right to left, and then down on the left) can be extremely effective in reducing pain.

Transcutaneous nerve stimulation (TENS) has been used successfully to reduce postoperative pain and may also prove helpful for women who have undergone caesarean section (Hollinger, 1986). The conventional method of applying electrodes on either side of the incison may prove inconvenient if the usual Pfannenstiel (bikini) incision has been used. Electrodes can be placed above the wound (women often experience acute discomfort in one or both iliac fossae). Low frequency, burst

mode could be used most of the time, encouraging endogenous opiate release, with a change to high frequency, continuous stimulation for coughing, moving etc. The Spembly Obstetric Pulsar has the useful addition of a 10% boost in intensity when changed from the burst to continuous mode. Davies (1982) described TENS as being ineffective for women whose caesarean sections were performed under epidural anaesthesia and postulated various possible causes for this: differential block, spinal cord and frequency-dependent effects.

Long term postpartum pain problems

Backache, headache, neck ache, shoulder and arm pain

MacArthur et al (1990) described a powerful association between backache and epidural anaesthesia during labour, but not if this form of anaesthesia has been used for an elective caesarean section. They hypothesized that the backache-producing mechanism is postural, occurring generally during labour, but exacerbated by epidural anaesthesia through loss of muscle tone, inability to move, and inhibition of discomfort-feedback. In *Health After Childbirth* (1991), MacArthur et al. describe musculoskeletal symptoms following an epidural during labour which they propose are related to an epidural-related 'spinal-axis syndrome' and draw attention to the extreme sensitivity of the skeletal/ligamentous system of parturient women.

Carpal tunnel syndrome

While carpal tunnel syndrome often occurs in pregnancy, it has also been reported (Wand, 1989) as occurring for the first time in some women soon after delivery. The suggestion is made that the hormonal effect of lactation may be implicated: symptoms resolved when women ceased breastfeeding.

Dyspareunia (painful intercourse)

Pain from an episiotomy scar or from vaginal scarring sometimes occurs following childbirth. This can give rise to longstanding problems for the couple (Kitzinger and Walters, 1981) if not speedily resolved. Hay-Smith (1993) has investigated postnatal superficial dyspareunia and physiotherapy regimes for its relief.

Ultrasound can be used to soften scars (Dyson,

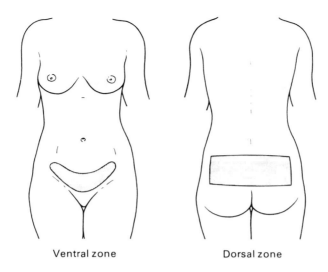

Ventral zone   Dorsal zone

Fig. 23.22   Usual localization of chronic pain of gynaecological origin. (After Renaer, 1984.)

1985) and may be helpful, together with stretching massage carried out by the patient, in the treatment of this extremely distressing problem. Where a painful episiotomy scar is not the cause of dyspareunia, it is possible that it is caused by vaginal atrophy. This can be due to low oestrogen levels in the immediate puerperium, which will continue in lactating women (Wisniewski and Wilkinson, 1991). Oestrogen vaginal cream has been shown to relieve dyspareunia in this case and the woman should be referred to her general practitioner or gynaecologist for this treatment.

The experienced obstetric physiotherapist can beneficially use the treatment time to enable the woman to voice her anxieties about her 'postnatal' body and her sexual difficulties and can suggest to doctors when psychosexual counselling seems appropriate. Obviously, this sort of exchange between patient and physiotherapist cannot take place in a busy department behind curtains; privacy is essential.

Pain of Gynaecological Origin

There is usually no role for physiotherapy in the treatment of pain due to an acute gynaecological pathology. However, there are some conditions of gynaecological origin which produce chronic pain and discomfort which may be amenable to physiotherapy, and the physiotherapist who plays an active role in the team caring for women may receive referrals from obstetricians, gynaecologists and general practitioners. Pain of gynaecological origin is often referred to a ventral lower abdominal zone, a dorsal upper sacrogluteal zone, or to both sites simultaneously. (Figure 23.22).

Although it has been estimated that one-third of women on general practitioners' lists who are over the age of 35 will, when questioned specifically, admit to suffering from backache, in only 10% of these will it be directly attributable to a gynaecological cause (Chamberlain and Dewhurst, 1984). If the backache can be reproduced when the doctor performs a bimanual (simultaneous vaginal and abdominal) examination of the adnexa, uterus and cervix, it is almost certainly of gynaecological origin. Renaer (1984) suggested that lumbar and lumbosacral pain are generally caused by orthopaedic problems.

Gynaecological causes of back pain

(See also Chamberlain and Dewhurst, 1984)

- Dysmenorrhoea.
- Malposition of the uterus.
- Pelvic infection.
- Endometriosis and ovarian blood cysts.
- Pelvic masses.
- Pregnancy and its after effects.

Conditions with gynaecological causes which may be amenable to physiotherapy

Dysmenorrhoea

Pain just before or during menstruation is experienced by many women and, when severe, it can interfere with their quality of life on a regular basis. There are, currently, two classifications:

1. Primary dysmenorrhoea is pain at the time of menstruation for which there is no obvious cause. Secondary dysmenorrhoea is pain due to an underlying pathology.
2. Congestive dysmenorrhoea occurs prior to the onset of menstruation and is relieved by the flow. Spasmodic dysmenorrhoea starts on the first day of the cycle and it is suggested that it may be due to diminished uterine blood flow.

Treatment

Gynaecologists sometimes refer women for pelvic shortwave diathermy in an effort to improve uterine circulation. Superficial heat application to the back or abdomen can also relieve menstrual cramps. Psychological intervention and relaxation training have been shown to be helpful (*Denny and Gerard*, 1981). TENS has also been used successfully in the treatment of dysmenorrhoea. Dawood and Ramos (1990) suggests a technique using three abdominal electrodes. Milsom (1944) have used high intensity TENS in the treatment of primary dysmenorrhoea which induced a prompt relief of pain.

Pelvic Inflammatory Disease (PID)

In the acute phase of PID, which is caused by sexually transmitted organisms such as *Chlamydia trachomatis* and *Neisseria gonorrhoeae*, antibiotic treatment is essential. If correct therapy is not given the woman may be left with pelvic adhesions or salpingitis (chronic inflammation of the fallopian tubes) which can lead to infertility. Her symptoms then may include persistent lower abdominal and sacro-gluteal pain with premenstrual or menstrual exacerbation, heavy periods and deep dyspareunia (pain on intercourse).

Treatment

There is certainly no place for physiotherapeutic techniques in the acute phase of the disease. Short-wave diathermy (continuous or pulsed) is sometimes requested in the chronic phase, although there is no documented evidence as to its success. Mild or 'athermal' doses are indicated and a cross-fire technique can be used.

Some women will receive pain relief from hot packs or a hot water bottle. It is possible that TENS may be helpful.

Genital Prolapse

Prolapse (downward displacement) of the bladder, uterus or rectum can lead to an uncomfortable sensation of pressure or 'dropping out'. Mild cases can respond to an intensive regime of pelvic floor exercises which, by increasing the supportive powers of the pelvic floor muscles, can relieve discomfort (Polden and Mantle, 1990).

Hysterectomy

In common with other surgical procedures, good preoperative physiotherapy assessment and preparation can minimize postoperative discomfort for the patient and make it easier for her to cooperate with her carers. Physiotherapists must be aware of the enormous psychosexual implications to a woman of losing her uterus. Many 'old wives tales' as to the effects of hysterectomy are circulated; the emotional 'pain' of undergoing this and other gynaecological procedures can be relieved if patients fully understand what is going to happen to them, how they will feel immediately after the operation, the effect it will have on their lives, and what they can and cannot do in the early postoperative weeks. A good leaflet to recommend is the one produced by Women's Health Concern (1987).

Carpal tunnel syndrome

Carpal tunnel syndrome is five times more common in women than in men, and outside pregnancy it is found most often in women over 40; it is, therefore, common post-menopausally. Because physiotherapists may be asked to treat this uncomfortable condition, it is interesting to note that there is some evidence that it may respond to hormone replacement therapy (Confino-Cohen, 1991).

Osteoporosis

Although the effects of this common and distressing condition are orthopaedic, strong evidence shows that post-menopausal low oestrogen levels are one of the major factors leading to bone loss.

Exercise has been suggested as a method of building bone mass and decreasing the rate of bone loss and the frequency of falls (Chow *et al.*, 1987; Sinahi, 1989). Physiotherapists interested in preventative health care could, by education, help prevent the acute pain which results from collapsing vertebrae and the crippling effects of hip fractures.

Conclusions

Although the aches and pains of pregnancy, labour and the puerperium, and the conditions giving rise to gynaecological pain, are not normally life-threatening, they can affect the quality of life of thousands of women and should not be ignored. Physiotherapists involved in obstetric and gynaecological care are in a unique position. Their specialized knowledge and access to women during the childbearing years and later enables them to prevent, as well as treat and relieve, some of the physical problems experienced by women of every age.

Obstetric physiotherapy was one of the first special interest groups of the Chartered Society of Physiotherapists (CSP). The Obstetric Association of Chartered Physiotherapists was set up in the 1940s. Later, logically, gynaecology was included and the group became known as the Association of Chartered Physiotherapists in Obstetrics and Gynaecology (ACPOG). Fully qualified members of ACPOG have completed postgraduate training (validated by the CSP). The group will now be known as The Association of Chartered Physiotherapists in Women's Health.

The role of the physiotherapist specializing in obstetrics and gynaecology as part of the team caring for women during the adventure of pregnancy and childbirth and its aftermath, and those experiencing gynaecological life changes consists of much more than the relief of pain. Because many physiotherapists take up this specialty when they have already had their own families, they can bring to their work a depth of knowledge and understanding, sympathy and empathy, which can help patients in a way which pure knowledge and technique cannot. Women of all ages can benefit from the training of an experienced physiotherapist specialising in this field and should be able to have access to such expertise both in hospital and in the community.

References

Abramson, D., Roberts, S.M. and Wilson, P.D. (1934) Relaxation of the pelvic joints in pregnancy. *Surg. Gynecol. Obstet.*, **58**, 595–613

Allen, R.E., Hosker, G.L., Smith, A.R.B. and Warrell, D.W. (1990) Pelvic floor damage and childbirth: a neurophysiological study. *Br. J. Obstet. Gynaecol.*, **97**, 770–9

Berg, G., Hammar, M., Möller-Nielson, J. *et al.* (1988) Low back pain during pregnancy. *J. Obstet. Gynecol.*, **71**, 71–5.

Bewley, E.L. (1986) *The megapulse trial at Bristol*. *J. ACPOG*, **58**, 16

Brunskill, P.J. and Swain, J.W. (1987) Spontaneous fracture of the coccygeal body during the second stage of labour. *Br. J. Obstet. Gynaecol.*, **7**, 270–1

Bullock, J., Jull, G.H. and Bullock, M.I. (1987) The relationship of low back pain to postural changes during pregnancy. *Aust. J. Physio.*, **33**, 10–17

Bundsen, P., Petersen, L.E. and Selstrum, U. (1981) Pain relief in labour by transcutaneous electrical nerve stimulation – a prospective matched study. *Acta Obstet. Gynecol. Scand.*, **60**, 459–68

Bundsen, P. and Ericson, K. (1982) Pain relief in labour by transcutaneous electrical nerve stimulation – safety aspects. *Acta Obstet. Gynecol. Scand.*, **61**, 1–5

Bundsen, P., Ericson, K. Petersen, L.E and Thringer, K. (1982) Pain relief in labour by transcutaneous electrical nerve stimulation – testing of a modified stimulation technique and evaluation of the neurological and biochemical condition of the newborn infant, *Acta Obstet. Gynecol. Scand.*, **61**, 129–36

Buxton, R.S. and Buxton, J. (1966) *Maternal Respiration in Labour*, Newsletter of Obstetric Association of Chartered Physiotherapists, London

Caldeyro-Barcia, R. (1979) Physiological and psychological bases for the modern and humanised management of normal labour. In *Recent Progress in Perinatal Medicine and Prevention* of *Congenital Anomaly*, Ministry of Health and Welfare, Tokyo, pp. 77–96

Calguneri, M., Bird, H.A. and Wright, V. (1982) Changes in joint laxity occurring during pregnancy. *Ann. Rheumat. Dis.*, **41**, 126–8

Chamberlain, G. and Dewhurst, J. (1984) *A Practice of Obstetrics and Gynaecology*, Pitman, London, p. 176

Chow, R., Harrison, J.E. and Notarius, C. (1987) Effect of two randomised exercise programmes on bone mass of healthy postmenopausal women. *Br. Med. J.*, **295**, 1441–4

Collinson, T. (1986) Relative Merits of the Use of Interferential Therapy and Ultrasound in the Treatment of Mastitis. Lecture to the Australian Physiotherapy Association

Confino-Cohen, R., Lishner, M., Savin, H. *et al.* (1991) Response of carpal tunnel syndrome to hormone replacement therapy. *Br. Med. J.*, **303**, 1514

Crothers, E. (1994) Labour pains: A study of pain control mechanisms during labour. *J.ACPOG.* **74**, 4–9

Davies, J.R. (1982) Ineffective transcutaneous nerve stimulation following epidural anaesthesia. *Anaesthesia*, **37**, 453–7

Dawood, Y.M. and Ramos, J. (1990) Transcutaneous electrical nerve stimulation (TENS) for the treatment of primary dysmenorrhoea: a randomised crossover comparison with placebo TENS and ibuprofen. *Obstet. Gynecol.*, **75**(4), 656–60

Denney, D.R. and Gerard, M. (1981) Behavioural treatments of primary dysmenorrhoea. *Behav. Res. and Ther.*, **19**, 303–12

Dyson, M. (1985) Therapeutic applications of ultrasound. In *Clinics in Diagnostic Ultrasound*, vol. 16 (eds W.L. Nyberg and M.C. Ziskin, Churchill Livingstone, Edinburgh

Ekman-Ordeberg, G., Salgeback, S. and Ordeberg, G. (1987) Carpal tunnel syndrome in pregnancy. *Acta Obstet. Gynecol. Scand.*, **66**, 233–5

Fast, A. *et al.* (1987) Low back pain in pregnancy. *Spine*, **12**, 368–71

Fisher, A.P. and Hanna, M. (1987) Transcutaneous electrical nerve stimulation in meralgia paraesthetica of pregnancy. *Br. J. Obstet. Gynaecol.*, **94**, 603–5

Flynn, A.M., Kelly, J., Hollins, G. *et al.* (1978) Ambulation in labour. *Br. Med. J.*, **2**, 591–3

Freedman, L.Z. and Ferguson, US (1950) The question of 'painless childbirth' in primitive culture. *Am. J. Orthopsychiatr.*, **20**, 263–79

Gould, J.S. and Wissinger, H.A. (1978) Carpal tunnel syndrome in pregnancy. *South. Med. J.*, **71**, 144–9

Hagen, R. (1974) Pelvic girdle relaxation from an orthopaedic point of view. *Acta. Orthopaed. Scand.*, **45**, 550–63

Harrison, R., Woods, T., Shore, M. *et al.* (1986) Pain relief in labour using transcutaneous electrical nerve stimulation (TENS). A TENS/TENS placebo controlled study in two parity groups. *Br . J. Obstet. Gynaecol.*, **93**, 739–46

Hay-Smith J. (1993) Postnatal superficial dyspareunia. *Physiotherapy* **79**, 384

Heardman, H. (1954) *A way to Natural Childbirth*. Churchill Livingstone, London

Hollinger, J.L. (1986) Transcutaneous electrical nerve stimulation after caesarean birth. *Phys. Ther.*, **66**, 36–8

Kitzinger, S. and Walters, R. (1981) *Some Women's Experiences of Episiotomy*, National Childbirth Trust, London

Lehmann, J.F. and de Lateur, B.J. (1984) Ultrasound, shortwave diathermy microwave, superficial heat and cold in the treatment of pain. In *Textbook of Pain* (eds P.D. Wall and C. Melzack), Churchill Livingstone, Edinburgh, pp. 717–24

Lomas, J. (1988) Holding back the tide of caseareans. *Br. Med. J.*, **297**, 569–70

MacArthur, C., Lewis, M., Knox, E.G. *et al* (1990) Epidural anaesthesia and long term backache after childbirth. *Br. Med. J.*, **302**, 9–12

MacArthur, C., Lewis, M. and Knox, E.G. (1991) Health after childbirth. *Br. J. Obstet. Gynaecol.*, **98**, 1193–5

Mannheimer, J.S. (1985) TENS – uses and effectiveness. In *Pain, International Perspectives in Physical Therapy* (ed. M.T. Hoskins), Churchill Livingstone, Edinburgh, p. 77

Mantle, M.J., Greenwood, R.M. and Currey, H.L.F. (1977) Backache in pregnancy. *Rheum. Rehab.*, **16**, 95–110

Mantle, M.J., Holmes, and Currey, H.L.F. (1981) Backache in pregnancy II: prophylactic influence of backache classes. *Rheum. Rehab.* **20**, 227–32

Mantle, M.J. (1988) Backache in pregnancy. In *Obstetrics and Gynaecology – International Perspectives in Physical Therapy* (ed. J. McKenna), Churchill Livingstone, Edinburgh, ch. 5

Maslem, J. (1982) Interferential therapy in the treatment of a blocked duct in a lactating breast. *Nat. Obstet. Gynaecol. J. Aust. Physiother. Assoc.*, April

McGuckin, N. (1986) The T4 syndrome In *Modern Manual Therapy of the Vertebral Column* (ed. G. Grieve), Churchill Livingstone, Edinburgh, p. 370

Melvin, J.L., Brunett, C.N. and Johnsson, E.W. (1969) Median nerve conduction in pregnancy. *Arch. Phys. Med.*, **50**, 75–80

Melzack, R., Taenzer, P., Feldman, P. *et al.* (1981) Labour is still painful after prepared childbirth training. *Canad. Med. Assoc. J.*, **125**, 357–63

Melzack, R., Belangar, E. and Lacroix, R. (1991). Labour pain: effect of maternal position on front and back pain. *J. Pain. Sympt. Manag.*, **6**, 476–480

Mendez-Bauer, C. *et al.* (1976) Effects of different maternal positions during labour. In *5th European Congress of Perinatal Medicine, Uppsala, Sweden*), Almqvist and Wiksell, Stockholm, 9–12: 233–7

Milson, I., Headner, N. and Mannheimer, C. (1994) A comparative study of the effect of high intensity transcutaneous nerve stimulation and oral naproxen on intrauterine pressure and menstrual pain in patients with primary dysmenorrhea. *Am. J. Obstet. Gyne. Coll.* **170**, 123–129

Mitchell, L. (1987) *Simple Relaxation*, John Murray, London

Murray, A. and Holdcroft, A. (1989) Incidence and intensity of postpartum lower abdominal pain. *Br. Med. J.*, **187**, 1619

Nwuga, V.E.B. (1982) Pregnancy and back pain among upper class Nigerian women. *Aust. J. Physio.*, **28**(4), 8–11

Polden, M. and Mantle, M.J. (1990) *Physiotherapy in Obstetrics and Gynaecology*, Butterworth Heinemann, Oxford

Renaer, M. (1984) Gynaecological pain. In *Textbook of Pain* (eds P.D. Wall and R. Melzack), Churchill Livingstone, Edinburgh

Roberts, J.E., Mendez-Bauer, C. and Wodell, D.A. 983) The effects of maternal position on uterine contractility and efficiency. *Birth*, **10**, 243–9

Robson, J.E. (1979) Transcutaneous nerve stimulation for relief of pain in labour. *Anaesthesia*, **34**, 357–61

Scriven, M.W., McKnight, I. and Jones, D.A. (1991) Diastasis of the pubic symphysis in pregnancy. *Br. Med. J.* **330**, 56

Semmler, D.M. (1982) The use of ultrasound therapy in the treatment of breast engorgement. *Natil Obstet. Gynaecol. J., Aust. Physiother. Associ.*, July

Sinahi, M. (1989), Exercise and osteoporosis – a review. *Arch. Phys. Med. Rehab.*, **70**, 220–8

Snooks, S.J., Setchall, M., Swash, M. and Henry, M.M. (1984) Injury to innervation of pelvic floor sphincter musculative in childbirth. *Lancet*, **ii** 546–550.

Thompson, J.W. (1990) Pharmacology of transcutaneous electrical nerve stimulation (TENS). *J. ACPOG*, **67**, 7–12

Voitk, A.J., Mueller, J.C., Farlinger, D.E. *et al.* (1983) Carpal tunnel syndrome in pregnancy. *Canad. Med. J.*, **128**, 277–82

Wand, J.S. (1989) The natural history of carpal tunnel syndrome in lactation. *J. R. Soc. Med.*, **82**, 349–50

Wisniewski, P.M. and Wilkinson, E.J. (1991) Postpartum vaginal atrophy. *Am. J. Obstet. Gynecol.*, **185** (4), part 2, 1249–54

Women's Health Concern (1987) *Hysterectomy*, 83 Earl's Court Road, London W8 6EF

Woolf, C.J. (1984) Transcutaneous and implanted nerve stimulation. In *Textbook of Pain* (eds P.D. Wall and R. Melzack), Churchill Livingstone, Edinburgh, p. 679

Woolf, C.J. (1989) Recent advances in the pathophysiology of acute pain. *Br. J. Anaesth.*, **63**, 139–46

24 *Physiotherapy in the management of pain in sport*

DAVID FITZGERALD

Introduction

Increased participation in sport and leisure activities brings with it an increased incidence of musculoskeletal disorders. This, in turn, has brought about a higher public expectation in terms of diagnosis and treatment of soft tissue injuries. This discussion will outline the role of physiotherapy in the control of pain which arises as a result of participation in sport. Gross traumatic events, which present little diagnostic difficulty, are beyond the scope of this discussion. It is not intended to be an exhaustive account of the physiotherapeutic procedures which may be employed in the treatment of sports injuries, but rather an overview of the principles of appropriate patient management supplemented with examples from clinical experiences.

The work of Cyriax (1982) represented a milestone in the development of differential diagnosis and treatment of musculoskeletal disorders. Subsequently, significant contributions have been made by Janda (1983), Maitland (1985), Elvey (1986), Butler (1991), and Edwards (1992), in the field of manual therapy and Grisogono (1985, 1991) and McDonald (1992) in sports physiotherapy. The result of this, together with advances in biomechanical evaluation, has been the evolution of a highly skilled clinical speciality.

Diagnosis

As in all areas of medicine, correct diagnosis forms the cornerstone of effective patient management. The evaluation of musculoskeletal disorders relies heavily on a comprehensive physical examination in conjunction with a detailed subjective history. With this as a basis, diagnostic tools such as radiological evaluation, form a useful adjunct to comprehensive physical examination but not a substitute for it. Other diagnostic aids include the following;

- X-Ray.
- CT scan.
- MRI scan.
- Isotope bone scans.
- Arteriograms.
- Compartment pressure studies.

Generally speaking, X-rays, the most commonly requested investigation due to cost and convenience, are most appropriate for exclusion of more serious or sinister pathology rather than positive assistance in determining the source of pain. However, although there is poor correlation between symptomatology and radiographic appearance (Lawrence et al., 1966; Arnoldi et al., 1975; Dieppe et al., 1986; Dieppe, 1989), the investigation of stress fractures serves to illustrate the relevance of X-ray investigation in sports injuries. Shin pain, commonly referred to as 'shin splints', can result from a number of mechanisms and diverse pathological processes (Kues, 1990), one of which is a stress fracture of the posteromedial cortex of the tibia (Devas, 1958). Radiographically, this appears as new subperiosteal bone formation, but may not become evident for some weeks post injury (Martin, 1983). As there are many pathological possibilities (tendonitis, periostitis, compartment syndromes, entrapment syndromes and Lumbar spine dysfunctions) capable of producing similar clinical features, this diagnosis may only be made in retrospect from radiographic evidence.

Diagnosis or musculoskeletal evaluation?

Treatment of pain resulting from sporting injuries requires a search for the structures at fault. Unlike

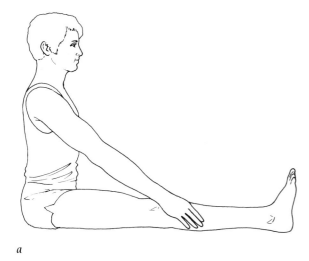

a

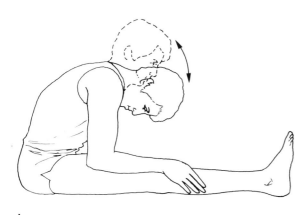

b

Fig. 24.1 *a*, Symptoms are noted in long sitting prior to 'slump'. *b*, Long sitting slump, approximating the shoulders towards the hips to increase the length of the spinal canal. Cervical flexion is added, then subtracted, monitoring the effect on hamstring pain.

visceral or systemic disease where a collection of signs and symptoms are usually attributable to specific pathological processes, the symptoms resulting from soft tissue injury are often multifaceted in origin. Therefore, recognition and thorough understanding of the diversity of pain presentations attributable to each of the anatomical components of the musculoskeletal system, together with a knowledge of associated alterations in function, is fundamental to effective diagnosis. For this reason diagnostic labelling (such as ligament strain or muscle tear) rarely describes the full extent of

pathology and may limit the approach to rehabilitation. Often, disturbance of multiple anatomical structures (ligament, tendon, bone, articular surface, capsule or neural tissues) accounts for the signs and symptoms produced and treatment should address each of the contributing elements. Sound clinical reasoning is of the utmost importance and should form the basis on which a diagnosis of the structures at fault is made. 'Functional disturbance' has been emphasized because it represents adaptation by multiple elements of the musculoskeletal system and, while one structure may be primarily implicated, it is rarely affected in isolation. For example, hamstring pain which is increased by neck flexion – a movement which increases tension in the nervous system (Brieg, 1978) but has no direct effect on hamstring length, is suggestive of an element of neural irritation in the symptomatology (Kornberg and Lew, 1989). Clinically, such neural involvement is commonly seen in association with primary muscle tears in that region. Figure 24.1 illustrates this example.

Predisposing Factors

There are many biomechanical and anthropometric factors which can contribute to the development of pain in sport. There are also many 'extrinsic' influences such as equipment, environment or physical conditioning which may predispose to injury and must be controlled to minimize the risk. These factors are discussed in detail later. Just as certain occupations may be associated with an increased incidence of certain types of disorders (Kelsey and Golden, 1987), there are characteristic injuries which occur with predictable frequency in specific sporting activities (e.g. Achilles tendonitis/ anterior knee pain in runners, low back pain in gymnasts, shoulder impingement syndromes in swimmers). With prior knowledge of the vulnerable regions associated with specific sports, it is increasingly common practice for physiotherapists to perform 'pre-participation screening' for irregularities with the potential to contribute to musculoskeletal pain. This is particularly so in competitive team sports where a pre-season phase precedes competition presenting the opportunity to evaluate joint and muscle flexibility, muscle strength and coordination, together with routine exercise performance tests. Also, because similar pain patterns are commonly seen in non-athletic individuals, the contribution of functional, occupational or ergonomic factors in the aetiology of musculoskeletal dysfunction must be considered and may be just as relevant to the athlete as to the sedentary individual.

Pain-sensitive structures

The commonly considered pain-sensitive structures involved in sports injuries are:

- Muscle.
- Ligament.
- Tendon.
- Bone.
- Neural tissue and its connective tissue coverings.

Nerve tissue involvement may be suspected when typical neurological symptoms such as weakness or paraesthesiae become evident, as in compartment syndromes (Kopell and Thompson, 1963; Weinstein and Herring, 1992). Traditionally, electrodiagnostic investigations have been employed to examine the conductivity of the nervous system implicating the site and degree of conduction block, i.e., entrapment neuropathies. The role of the nervous system in the production of pain has been referred to in previous chapters and has come under greater scrutiny in recent years (Butler, 1991). While impulse conduction is of paramount importance the capacity for neural structures to adapt to motion is a fundamental requirement of normal movement and disturbance of this mobility can create pain and functional impairment. This requirement is most dramatically demonstrated by the painful limitation of straight leg raise caused by dural adhesions in post-laminectomy patients (Yong-Hing *et al.*, 1980; Lee and Alexander, 1984). Of particular importance in this regard is the varied, and often bizarre, nature of the symptoms produced when adverse neural tension (ANT) is present. Clinically, neural tissue showing pathomechanical behaviour has a tendency to mimic the symptoms of localized muscle, ligament or tendon trauma (e.g. groin strains, tennis elbow or shoulder impingement syndromes). The mechanisms of such phenomena are not certain but may relate to the trophic influence of disturbed axoplasmic flow on the respective target tissues (Gunn, 1980; Rydevik *et al.*, 1980; Lundborg, 1988). Clinically, the first signs of such disturbance may be evidenced by an impairment of mobility of the associated neural structures – detectable by appropriate movement/tension tests of the associated nerve. When pain shows a tendency to alter in its distribution, atypical of a primary, localized soft tissue lesion, an exhaustive search for the tissues at fault should subsequently follow in order to determine the nature and extent of pathology – a process described as 'making the features fit' (Maitland, 1985). Neural tissue mobility should be investigated in any situation where there is an inconclusive history of injury or a lack of consistency in the clinical features and should also be examined as a potential secondary source of pain subsequent to a primary soft tissue sporting injury. Because of the diversity of structures which may produce symptoms, it is perhaps more appropriate to talk in terms of an evaluation of the **neuromusculoskeletal system** in disorders of a soft tissue nature.

Injury-related Pain

The mechanisms of pain perception and the physiological response to such stimuli have been discussed in previous chapters. Of significance in relation to sports injuries, and soft tissue dysfunction in general, is the differentiation between so-called 'physiological pain' and 'pathological pain' (Woolf, 1987). Physiological pain can be considered as the response to a noxious stimulus in the absence of tissue trauma or inflammation (such as occurs in a brief thermal or electrical nociceptive stimulus). Pathological pain arises from a stimulus sufficient to initiate an inflammatory response through musculoskeletal trauma or through damage to the nervous system. All recent or 'acute' soft tissue trauma will involve a localized inflammatory response, the size of which is related to the degree of trauma. The concept of a 'fixed' pain pathway system to transmit this information is no longer valid because pathological pain results from changes in the somatosensory system as well as the activation of the spinothalamic and spinoreticular systems (Woolf, 1989). Two concepts which are of importance in understanding the pain response following neuromusculoskeletal trauma such as may occur in sport are highlighted by Woolf (1989):

- Peripheral sensitization of primary afferent neurons.
- Central sensitization of dorsal horn neurons.

Peripheral sensitization refers to the fact that after

peripheral tissue injury the threshold for eliciting pain decreases both within the area of injury (primary hyperalgesia) and in the surrounding uninjured tissue (secondary hyperalgesia) (Cambell *et al.*, 1979.; Thalhammer and LaMotte, 1982; Raja *et al.*, 1988). Many of the biochemicals released directly or indirectly by the damaged tissue (bradykinin, histamine, substance-P and prostaglandins) have the capacity either to excite nociceptors or to increase their sensitivity (Armstrong *et al.*, 1953; Levine *et al.*, 1986; Raja *et al.*, 1988). Thus, peripherally there is a pathophysiological state which produces nocioceptive stimuli and directly influences the severity and nature of the symptoms produced by virtue of the localized 'inflammatory soup' (Woolf, 1991).

Central sensitization refers to the neurophysiological adaptations which occur within the central nervous system. It has been shown that the receptive fields of dorsal horn neurons are not as specialized as the peripheral terminals of the primary afferents with which they synapse (Cook *et al.*, 1987; Ferrington *et al.*, 1987; Guilbaud *et al.*, 1987). Peripheral tissue injury has been shown to alter motorneuron responses by decreasing the threshold of the receptive field and changing the pattern of reflex response from phasic to tonic (Woolf, 1984, 1985; Woolf and McMahon, 1985) or, in other words, from a short, spontaneous activation to a prolonged, sustained response.

The importance of this evidence in relation to sports injuries is to highlight the necessity for a comprehensive examination of the neuromusculoskeletal system and to consider the alterations in function as the manifestation of a complex series of changes. Attention to the site of local pathology is only one of the components of treatment necessary for restoration of normal function. Because of the interactions between the central and peripheral nervous system outlined above and the complex mechanisms of motor regulation, it is unsatisfactory to assume that resolution of the primary site of injury will spontaneously initiate a return to normal function. For example, disturbance of scapulohumeral rhythm, seen in many shoulder and neck presentations, may persist long after the acute lesion has resolved, and the resulting biomechanical alterations predispose the soft tissues to secondary painful irritation. Similarly, inversion injuries of the ankle are one of the most common injuries amongst sportspeople. Functional instability complicates 10–20% of these and has been found to be independent of the severity of the

injury or the degree of mechanical instability (Hansen *et al.*, 1979; Niedermann *et al.*, 1981). Muscle weakness, proprioceptive deficit and nerve damage have all been implicated in this condition (Ryan, 1989), thus highlighting the complex interaction between musculoskeletal function and central nervous system regulation.

Classification of Soft Tissue Injury

Any injury to the soft tissues will initiate an inflammatory response. Because the physiotherapy intervention relates specifically to the pathological processes of injury, it is necessary to categorize injury in relation to the stage of inflammation. These stages are generally referred to as:

- Acute.
- Sub-acute.
- Chronic.

These categories are often loosely applied by referring to the time since onset of symptoms. While this may be generally true, it is important to note that the time scale relates to the cellular and biochemical processes which occur in the inflammatory process. Three phases can be identified (Oakes, 1982).

1. Acute inflammatory phase (up to 72 hours); vascular rupture and cellular infiltration.
2. Repair phase (72 hours up to 6 weeks); collagen deposition.
3. Remodelling phase (3–6 weeks up to 3–6 months).

The detailed cellular events which occur are well described by Evans (1980) and the scientific rationale for therapeutic intervention at each stage is presented in Figure 24.2. The concept of the 'collagen time scale' described within is particularly relevant because good functional recovery is governed by the time constraints of normal physiology and does not necessarily relate to the level of pain. From a rehabilitation perspective the relevance of this lies in the fact that the mechanical properties (maximum failure load, energy absorption capacity, stiffness and compliance) of a tissue are directly related to its collagen content (Noyes *et al.*, 1974). These properties are significantly reduced following immobilization or reduced functional stress (Noyes, 1977) and therefore any modification of functional stress must be evaluated in terms of the risk/benefit ratio. It should also be noted that there are several

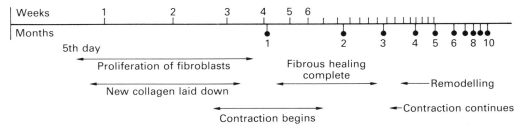

Fig. 24.2 Collagen timescale.

factors which may prolong or interfere with the normal inflammatory reaction and will thus influence the response to treatment, regardless of the time since onset of symptoms. Of primary importance in this regard, is the necessity to reduce oedema thereby minimizing the potential for secondary cell necrosis due to ischaemia. It is more correct to think in terms of a good healing environment as opposed to 'speeding-up' the healing process.

Soft tissue injuries may be classified in terms of aetiology or severity (Oakes, 1982):

Aetiology
1. Direct injuries due to trauma, e.g. contusions, lacerations.
2. Indirect injuries, which may be further subdivided into:
   (a) Acute – occurs with sudden overloading such as muscle tears or ligament ruptures.
   (b) Chronic – due to repeated overload, e.g. tendonitis.
   (c) Acute on chronic – due to sudden rupture of a persistent lesion, e.g., rupture of Achilles tendonitis.

Severity
1. Grade 1 – mild pain at the time of injury or within 24 h of injury, especially when stress is applied to the injury: local tenderness may or may not be present.
2. Grade 2 – pain during activity, usually requiring cessation of activity; pain and local tenderness when the injury is stressed.
3. Grade 3 – complete, or near complete rupture of a portion of ligament or tendon with severe pain and loss of function; a palpable defect may be present but stressing the structure may be paradoxically painless, due to loss of continuity of the tissue.

Injuries to muscle have been graded in a similar fashion, based on a four-tier system according to the degree of anatomical disruption and percentage of fibres torn (Muckle, 1982; Hamer, 1991). The above classifications give useful information with regard to treatment planning and prognosis.

Pain control in acute injury

Whether this trauma results from intrinsic or extrinsic mechanisms (i.e. forces generated from within the body or external to it, respectively) the therapeutic procedures are similar.

The initial task is to evaluate the severity of the injury and decide whether:

1. The injury precludes any further current participation.
2. Continued/modified participation is possible.

This is usually the most difficult, yet crucial, decision to be made as there is often a conflict of interests between player, management and medical personnel. The grading systems previously mentioned relate to the degree of structural disruption following injury. Because this scale is a continuum with overlap between stages, there can be no precise categorization of the extent of injury and an assessment of the degree of functional impairment is the most valid method. All Grade 3 injuries require cessation of activity, as gross structural damage has occurred. In the case of ligament damage this is evidenced by excessive mobility of the involved joint, often associated with a characteristic 'soggy' end-feel to stress testing. It may be relatively painless because loss of continuity means that the traumatized tissues are not stimulated when stretched. In the case of muscle, complete rupture is evidenced by relatively painless weakness on resisted movement and sometimes, visible bulging of the ruptured ends.

The difficulty arises in evaluating Grades 1 and 2 in terms of the degree of structural damage and the implications of further activity. The deciding factor which determines this is the ability to perform the required functional task. This may be sprinting, kicking or, in racket sports, serving a ball. If this causes severe pain it is unlikely that participation can continue. If it is moderate, or severe at the extreme of range, it may be possible to alter the movement using strapping to prevent the traumatized tissues from being stretched to the limits of pain. A more detailed strategy is outlined below.

Treatment if continued participation is indicated

The physiotherapeutic measures to reduce pain and improve function which can be applied immediately 'on site' to permit further activity include the following:

1. Cold therapy – ice / iced water; – spray analgesia.
2. Passive joint mobilization.
3. Compression bandaging.
4. Strapping.

Cold therapy (see also Chapter 16)

The purpose of ice application (cryotherapy) is to provide cooling of the tissues. The efficacy of such intervention has been well documented (Barnes, 1979; Hocutt et al., 1982; Kalenak et al., 1975; Starkey, 1976). The most frequently used methods of application are ice packs (containing crushed ice or chemical substances) and immersion. The degree to which the tissues are cooled is dependent upon:

1. The temperature difference between the coolant and the tissues.
2. The thermal conductivity of the tissues.
3. The period of application.
4. The size of the area (Low and Reed, 1990).

Application of analgesic spray utilizes the principal of 'latent heat of evaporation' to provide its effect. Application of liquefied ethyl chloride or fluorimethane by aerosol spray causes it to evaporate on contact with the skin. The heat energy required to facilitate this response is 'drawn' from the surrounding tissues causing them to cool. Cooling from such sprays can be very rapid but does not last very long (Low and Reed, 1990).

For a detailed discussion of the physiological and therapeutic effects of cold therapy the reader is referred to the review in chapter 16 and Low and Reed (1990, ch. 9). The important elements are summarized below:

1. Vasoconstriction of the cutaneous vessels.
2. Reduced muscle blood flow.
3. Lowered metabolic rate accompanied by reduced oxygen uptake.
4. Alteration in peripheral nervous system conductivity.

Cooling within the first 2 hours of injury will minimize secondary cell necrosis by reducing the metabolic rate (McLean, 1989). Reduction in muscle temperature causes reduction in blood flow by altering blood viscosity and inducing vasoconstriction (Barcroft and Edholm, 1943; Pappenheimer et al., 1948).

Passive mobilization

This constitutes a large and specialized area within physiotherapy but in this context relates to the performance large amplitude, passive physiological movements of the affected limb or area. Following the initial shock of trauma active movement is often inhibited and this reflex inhibition can be overcome by performing repeated passive movements several times and then progressing to active-assisted and full active movements within a few minutes. It is probable that these procedures are effective by virtue of restoring a more normal proprioceptive input from the injured area which may help to reactivate the correct neural control required for normal movement. If full active movement does not return spontaneously within a few minutes of these procedures then more serious injury should be suspected and investigated accordingly. Specific passive movement techniques using physiological and accessory joint motion (Maitland, 1985) are more relevant to the rehabilitation process when participation cannot continue in the short term.

Compression bandaging

Historically and still in widespread use today, the

best-known compression bandage is that of Robert-Jones, and while being effective, it does not allow adequate function for sporting activity. The use of elasticated bandages and composite, pre-shaped supports, on the basis of thermal insulation as well as mechanical support, is now common practice in sporting activities. It is postulated that application of external compression bandaging increases the interstitial fluid pressure which may counter the tendency for extravasation of fluid and proteins which cause oedema. While it is common practice to apply cold therapy with compression there appears to be a scarcity of documented evidence vindicating the role of compression. Apart from the advantages of reducing oedema to improve healing time (Evans, 1983) the mechanisms in reducing pain may relate to:

1. Reduction in mechanical distortion of the tissues which could potentially stimulate sensitized mechanoreceptors in the vicinity.
2. Reduced inflammatory exudate which contains pain producing substances such as histamine, bradykinin, substance-P and prostaglandins (Armstrong *et al.*, 1953, Levine *et al.*, 1986).

Strapping

There are several authoritative books on strapping/taping techniques both for prophylaxis and treatment of sports injuries (Klafs and Arnheim, 1981: McDonald, 1992). The purpose of strapping is:

1. To provide external structural support.
2. To control the range of motion.
3. To minimize oedema.

The application of external strapping for support has been applied to many regions of the body with the aim of reinforcing the structure to allow it to sustain the applied loads. In the ankle the efficacy of such procedures has been extensively investigated by attempting to quantify the degree of mechanical support afforded (Kimura *et al.*, 1987; Vaes *et al.*, 1985; Capasso *et al.*, 1989), the functional adaptations following application (Greene and Roland, 1989; Hamill and Knutzen., 1986; Hamill *et al.*, 1988), and the period of effectiveness (Laughman *et al.*, 1980; Myburg *et al.*, 1984; Green and Hillman, 1990).

In contrast to strapping of joints, it is questionable whether a muscle can be additionally supported by the application of strapping. As a contractile

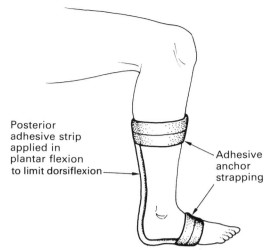

Posterior adhesive strip applied in plantar flexion to limit dorsiflexion

Adhesive anchor strapping

Fig. 24.3   Taping to limit tension in the tendo Achillis.

structure consisting of bundles of interdigitating fibres which slide relative to each other, it is not realistic to consider that strapping applied comfortably to the skin can create significant compression to alter this relative movement. However, the vast majority of strapping procedures involve techniques which cross one or more joints and by so doing will alter the length/tension relationships within the muscle. It is this mechanism of reduction in tension through damaged fibres which is more likely to reduce pain. The taping procedures for calf or Achilles tendon strain illustrate this principle (Figure 24.3). The mechanics of muscular activity can be altered by changing either its length of action or its line of action through controlling its tendon, thereby altering the point of force application. For example, anterior knee pain resulting from a dysfunction in the extensor mechanism may be altered by taping to control the line of quadriceps pull through the patellar tendon (Figure 24.4).

Strapping for prophylaxis is now widespread, particularly in contact sports. The regions usually involved are the ankle, wrist and fingers. Indeed some professional sports such as basketball and gridiron football will not allow participation unless such measures are taken. However, consideration should be given to the fact that most strapping techniques will in some way alter joint function and that this alteration may have secondary mechanical influences anywhere along the kinematic chain, particularly in the lower limb. These biomechani-

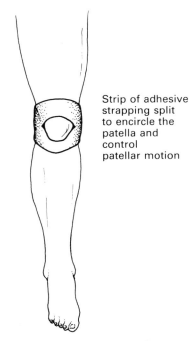

Strip of adhesive
strapping split
to encircle the
patella and
control
patellar motion

Fig. 24.4 Taping to control anterior knee pain.

cal alterations may subsequently be responsible
for the development of secondary musculoskeletal
pain at some other site. For example, in the case
of the medial collateral ligament of the knee, the
position of minimal tension is approximately 30°
flexion (Evans, 1986). With further extension the
ligament tension increases (MacConaill, 1964).
The purpose of strapping the knee is to prevent full
extension but in so doing creating a functional
short leg. This may produce alterations in the
mechanics of all structures associated with the
functional activity and put them at greater risk of
injury.

Treatment if participation is contraindicated

In determining whether participation must cease it
is important that a thorough examination be carried out immediately. Often, by observing the
mechanism of injury, an educated guess as to the
structures involved in the injury can be made. The
level of pain, the degree of swelling and its speed of
onset also indicate the severity of injury. When an
individual is in pain it is tempting to perform a
cursory examination only, but in doing so the
opportunity to detect serious disruption may be
missed because the ensuing haemarthrosis/inflam-
matory response may in itself restrict motion, e.g.
anterior cruciate ligament injury.

If the severity of the injury is such that the
activity must cease then the well-described first aid
measures of: **rest, ice, compression** and **elevation
(RICE)** are appropriate (O'Connell, 1981).

Electrotherapy

There are many electrotherapeutic modalities employed in the treatment of joint and soft tissue
injuries, many of which have been discussed in
other chapters. The indications, applications and
therapeutic effects of the various forms of electrotherapy in the treatment of acute and chronic
injuries are also discussed.

The role of rest

Of particular significance in this regard is the 'rest'
component which should really be considered as
'relative rest'. A large body of scientific evidence
has now accumulated documenting the physiological, biomechanical and functional benefits of early
controlled tissue mobilization as opposed to absolute
rest by splinting immobilization (Tipton et al. 1970;
Salter et al., 1975; Vailas et al., 1981; Leach,
1982; Zarins, 1982; Frank et al., 1983; Salter,
1989).

It has been shown that the use of continuous
passive motion assists the nutritional support of
synovial joint components, especially articular cartilage, ligaments and synovium (Woo and Akeson,
1987). It has also been shown to have a significant
effect on the clearance of haemarthrosis (O'Driscoll,
1983). Whether these effects can be achieved with
manual, intermittent, passive motion is not certain
but clinical experience suggests that motion of any
description, as opposed to immobilization, is more
likely to produce the desired physiological effect.
Passive mobilization of the neuromusculoskeletal
system should be an integral part of treatment
from initial presentation. The many varied treatment techniques to address each component of the
neuromusculoskeletal system are discussed in
Chapter 17 on manipulation. Techniques which
move into the functionally restricted range, showing
respect for the symptoms produced, may also be
employed. This might, for example, involve the use
of a passive straight leg raise procedure when
neural tissue has been involved in a lumbar facet
joint strain and is a component limiting lumbar

movement. Passive mobilization refers to movement of all the tissues which require mobility, i.e. joint, muscle, ligament, tendon and neural tissue, and it can be applied selectively to emphasize each of the component elements. Controlled movement of the tissues within the region of trauma can be imparted by movement of structures proximal or distal to the affected area. For example, pain at the lateral epicondyle of the elbow (commonly referred to as 'tennis elbow') may involve several structures, including the superficial radial nerve (Butler, 1991). Selective motion of this structure can be achieved by extending and pronating the elbow with the wrist extended – thus placing the common extensor tendon under tension, and then applying contralateral-lateral flexion of the cervical spine to impart relative motion between the neural structures and the interfacing tissue.

In association with early passive mobilization, active, or active-assisted movement must also start as soon as pain allows. In the case of primary muscle injury this may commence from 48 hours (Herring, 1990), but sub-maximal isometric contractions, incremented through range, may be acceptable earlier. The progression is then made to low intensity, small range motion, paying particular attention to both the eccentric and concentric phases of muscle activity (Belka, 1968; Costil *et al.*, 1971; Steadman, 1979; Hakkinen and Komi, 1981). As active movement imparts motion to both the contractile and inert structures, these principles can be employed in the treatment of both.

Clinical evidence suggests that functional movement, modified as required, should be incorporated as early as possible (Vasey and Crozier, 1980; Oakes, 1982; Ihara and Nakayama, 1986;). This is required to facilitate optimal recovery of proprioception and return to normal movement patterns. This is the principle on which proprioceptive neuromuscular facilitation (PNF) (Knott and Voss, 1956) is based as are several other schools of thought (Klein-Vogelbach, 1990; Sahrmann, 1990). Of particular importance in the axial skeleton and lower limbs is the degree of weight bearing involved in the functional activity. This is largely determined by the reaction of the individual joint structures to injury (Hettinga, 1979a, 1979b, 1980) and the associated level of pain. If structures normally function under load of body weight, then the closest approximation to this should be instituted as early as possible in rehabilitation. For example, performing a quarter range squat with controlled weight bearing through the upper limbs is more desirable for inner range quadriceps work than using a weighted boot. Some research suggests that the stresses involved in a non-weight bearing, knee extension exercise are more likely to cause excessive shearing forces on the anterior cruciate ligament than controlled, modified, functional weight bearing exercises (Grood *et al.*, 1984). The progression can then be made from relatively static loads to more dynamic weight-bearing activity using body weight, and finally through to explosive jump or sprint work depending on the rate of progression.

Evaluation and Treatment of chronic/ recurrent injuries

The previously mentioned injury classification 'acute on chronic' is a particularly useful term to describe this category of pathology. It describes pain resulting from an acute inflammatory response at a site of previous pathology, indicating a failure of the tissues to withstand the applied stress. Frequently, there may be some suspicion of dysfunction indicated by increased tightness, fatiguability or subtle uncoordination and such symptoms may be indicators of imminent failure. Conversely, examination of an apparently 'acute onset' injury often reveals evidence of previous sub-clinical trauma such as tissue thickening, adaptive shortening, or restriction of joint range. Therefore, the significant difference between this patient group and the 'initial acute onset' injury is that there may be residual soft tissue changes or functional disturbance from previous episodes. In the evaluation and treatment of pain related to chronic injuries the critical question to ask is 'Why has this problem occurred?'. Is it related to environmental or some other extrinsic factors, such as running surface, footwear, racket size or equipment? If this is so, will adaptations or modifications allow the individual to continue with the chosen activity? If the source of the problem relates to intrinsic factors, specific to the individual, can these be treated or modified to allow continuation?

Extrinsic factors

The extrinsic contributory factors to recurrent and/or overuse injuries relate to those factors external to the body but which can exert a direct influence on the way in which it functions. These may include general environmental factors such as temperature or playing surface, or relate more specifically to the type of equipment used such as the style of running shoe, the length of cleat/stud (Cook *et al.*, 1990) or the size of racket in racket sports. One often sees the individual who's old training shoes have lost all their shock absorbing capacity or who's football boots are held together with adhesive tape! While the implications of faulty equipment are obvious to the professional it must be remembered that the vast majority of sports-people compete at a social level and are thus not exposed to the scrutiny associated with elite competitors.

If it is considered that extrinsic factors are contributing to the injury then they should be adjusted as appropriate. This may involve, for example, change in grip size for racket sports or shoe type for runners (Cook *et al.*, 1990). The level or grade of participation is an important consideration in all age groups and particularly so in contact sports. In adolescence it is mandatory to participate on an equal basis in terms of age or size because the unnecessary risk of injury to immature growing tissue during development is unacceptable. Likewise, it is important to match the intensity, frequency and duration of training, and the type of equipment used, to the stage of skeletal maturity. Abnormal or excessive force applied to an immature skeleton may not only produce pain at the time of insult but also induce structural alterations which may be pain-provoking in later life (e.g. asymmetrical activities such as rowing or tennis).

Intrinsic factors

The intrinsic factors which may contribute to an increased risk of injury in sport are closely related to general anthropometrical considerations. While experience suggests that there is a certain 'self selection' process in relation to chosen activity (e.g. unsuitability of a tall individual as a front row rugby player!), none the less, clinically one often sees the individual who has decided to 'take up' a sport for which they are neither physically nor mechanically suited. This particularly relates to the episodic fun runner, squash or tennis player or those who partake in physical contact sports in which a prerequisite degree of learned skill is essential, e.g; rugby, soccer, martial arts. The physical attributes which facilitate safe participation in

sport relate not only to size and strength but also to the individual's co-ordination and the degree of muscular control.

Greater understanding of the mechanisms of neuromuscular control (Basmajian and Delucia, 1985) has resulted in improved rehabilitation which, in the past, has been dominated by an emphasis on development of strength. We know that absolute measures of muscle strength are only part of the spectrum of muscle physiology and cannot be used in isolation as a measure of appropriate muscle function. Clinically, the important relationship between agonist/antagonist muscle activity has been long recognized (Sherrington, 1906) and has more recently been refined by the concept of 'muscular imbalance' (Janda, 1983). Detection of the muscular imbalances which may produce pain or functional alteration may not be evident on routine static muscle tests (Kendall and McCreary, 1983). More specific evaluation of functional movement in terms of the patterns of muscle recruitment and degree of muscle work involved is necessary, as it is thought that alterations in muscle synergies produce a pathomechanical situation which can become a potential source of pain due to repeated microtrauma (Janda, 1983). Such imbalances may manifest themselves as muscle or tendon damage due to hyperactivity/overuse of a particular muscle group, or as damage to articular structures due to abnormal stress transmission through joint surfaces and periarticular tissues. This is often seen in the neck/shoulder complex with athletes who perform repeated overhead moments.

Clinical observation of the abnormal state would suggest that certain preventative measures could be employed by way of prophylaxis. Another important component of muscle function, together with strength and coordination, is the flexibility of the musculotendinous unit. The validity of warm-up in the prevention of muscle injury has been a source of great academic debate but among the benefits attributed to it are an increased range of motion and a reduction in stiffness due to increased muscle temperature (O'Neil, 1976; Moller *et al.*; 1978; Ekstrand and Gillquist, 1982; Ciullo and Zarins, 1983). Safran *et al.* (1988) have shown that greater force and increase in length are needed to tear an isometrically preconditioned (warmed) muscle. In the case of chronic Achilles tendonitis it is considered that lack of flexibility is a significant aetiological factor (Reynolds and Worrell, 1991) in the development of this condition. When the resting length of the musculotendinous unit is increased (as by stretching), there is an associated decrease in the deformational strain induced through a particular range of motion (Curwin and Stanish, 1984), thus reducing the potential for injury due to mechanical disruption. On balance it would appear that the beneficial effects of flexibility extend not only to the improvement of neuromusculoskeletal function, but also to minimize the potential for injury. In summary, the clinical subgroupings of soft tissue injury as defined by Maitland (1991) offer useful guidelines in terms of aetiology, treatment and prognosis in neuromusculoskeletal dysfunctions. These are:

- New use.
- Misuse.
- Overuse.
- Abuse.
- Disuse.

These classifications relate to 'the type and vigour of an activity being performed, the state of the structures being used and their ability to accept the use' (Maitland, 1991: 55). In determining whether there is a significant intrinsic aetiological component, two aspects should be considered:

1. Structural anomalies.
2. Acquired anomalies.

Structural factors refer to osseous anomalies such as genu valgum, patella alta or scoliosis. Acquired factors refer to the connective tissue changes which may develop secondarily to abnormal biomechanics such as shortening of hyperactive muscle groups (hamstrings, psoas) or tightening of fascial structures (lliotibial band). Here it is important to remember the point made at the beginning of this chapter regarding the similarity of many soft tissue injuries incurred outside the sporting arena as opposed to in it. Tissues have a finite capacity to sustain applied load and the forces produced during sport merely represent another variable in the pattern of functional stress. The acquisition of soft tissue changes may, or may not, necessarily be as a direct result of sport but it may be that sport is the critical factor responsible for symptom production. For example, a study on cyclists (Richardson and Sims, 1991) concluded that the significant reduction in hip extensor activity observed was related to the dominant hip flexor activity in cycling, resulting in inhibition of the hip extensor muscles. It has also been reported that the hip extensors play an important role in

assisting the lumbar spine during heavy lifting (Macintosh and Bogduk, 1987). The frequent clinical observation of hip extensor inhibition in lumbar spine disorders (Janda, 1983) highlights a potential predisposition to musculoskeletal pain secondary to functional use.

Evaluation of structural anomalies

Because effective evaluation of the neuromusculoskeletal system relies heavily on the ability to assess the intrinsic components of dysfunction, it is these which will be considered in greater detail here.

Initially, the general management of 'acute on chronic' injuries follows the same principles as mentioned for the acute situation but should also address the contributing intrinsic factors which are evident at this stage if possible. The range of structural anomalies which may occur is extensive and the existence of an anomaly does not in itself dictate that dysfunction will follow. For example, Chao et al., (1983) report that during the gait cycle, slight asymmetries between homologous body segments are considered normal while (Charnley and Pusso, 1986) suggest that consistent departures from symmetry are considered abnormal. In relation to the effects of asymmetries during running it has been demonstrated in asymptomatic individuals that the lower limbs of distance runners possess a multifaceted asymmetry for touchdown and foot contact as well as for the entire phase of foot support of the running stride (Vagenas and Hoshizaki, 1992). Thus, deciding on the significance of asymmetries is a complex decision which depends on addressing the most evident abnormalities first, but may ultimately depend on hard-earned clinical experience. The body's adaptability may be extremely variable and the mechanisms of compensation for structural faults are not fully understood. Structural anomalies in one region may manifest themselves as painful dysfunctions at some distant point in the kinematic chain leaving intervening regions apparently unaffected (e.g. excessive pronation of the foot associated with pain in the lumbar spine). Conversely, structures immediately above or below the offending area may become symptomatic.

Treatment of structural anomalies

Obviously, conservative treatment cannot hope to alter structure but it can provide adequate functional compensation to allow pain-free motion. An example of the patello-femoral joint will serve to illustrate. Historically, pain in the anterior knee region has proved to be particularly resistant to physiotherapy. Most anterior knee pain in adolescence was diagnosed as chondromalacia patella (Goodfellow et al., 1976) and when conservative treatment of rest and physiotherapy failed, various surgical procedures were undertaken (Install et al., 1976; Install, 1979; Bentley and Dowd, 1984). However, the success rate of surgical intervention was not consistent and an alternative conservative approach was pioneered by McConnell (1986) addressing some of the many variables known to influence patello-femoral joint mechanics (Laurin et al., 1978; Marks and Bentley, 1978; Sikorski et al., 1979; Gerrard, 1987). The result of this approach has been a significant improvement in treatment of anterior knee pain and a reduction in surgical intervention.

In situations where no amount of joint and soft tissue mobilization or muscle strengthening can provide adequate, pain-free function, then external compensation for structural faults should be considered. In the lower limb this may involve a shoe raise to compensate for leg length discrepancy or a more sophisticated form of orthotic appliance (Wooden, 1990) to modify foot function. In the upper limb, pain from tennis elbow may be controlled with an epicondylitis clasp used to reduce maximal muscle contraction and alter the angle of pull of the common extensor tendon (Fromson, 1971). Electromyography has shown that this reduces activity in the forearm extensor muscles (Groppel and Hirschl, 1986) and increases the pain-free grip strength (Burton, 1985).

Treatment of acquired anomalies

Changes in joint and soft tissue develop secondarily to the functional demands placed upon them. That this is so is verified by the well-documented deleterious effects of immobilization (Tipton et al., 1970; Salter et al., 1975; Vailas et al., 1981; Leach, 1982; Zarins, 1982; Frank et al., 1983; Salter, 1989). Indeed, there is ample evidence documenting structural adaptations to imposed functional demands (Poss, 1984; Marks, 1991; Cameron et al., 1992). Patterns of functional use and disuse, both in athletic activity and routine daily living, are commonly observed clinically. This habitual use may not only place the inert structures under

constant, repetitive load but initiates a tendency for dominant muscles groups to become overused, or hypertonic (Jull and Janda, 1987; Janda, 1988). Subsequently, the result of this is a tendency for the hyperactive muscle groups to become shortened, in association with a lengthening of the antagonistic muscle groups due to reciprocal inhibition. The implications on movement are such that the normal synergies of muscle activation may become disturbed. These alterations should not be viewed as due to an isolated muscle weakness which must be strengthened, but in terms of a disturbance in the complex mechanisms of neuromuscular control (Janda, 1978). Poor motor regulation will subject other elements of the musculoskeletal system to potentially harmful stresses which may result in repeated microtrauma and eventually pain.

The treatment of acquired faults varies according to the structures implicated, which may be:

- Muscle.
- Tendon.
- Fascia/aponeurosis.
- Joint capsule/ligament.
- Neural tissue.

If muscle is considered at fault then restoration to normal length is the objective of treatment and lengthening of shortened muscle groups is the priority. There are several methods of lengthening muscle and the technique chosen will depend on whether the shortening is due to hypertonus, a neurophysiological mechanism, or connective tissue changes. The techniques include:

- PNF.
- Muscle energy techniques.
- Post-isometric relaxation.
- Manual stretching.

Improving the length–tension relationship of the shortened muscle groups has the effect of disinhibiting their antagonists. Subsequently, re-establishment of normal movement patterns then requires conscious activation of normal synergies with further progression to increasingly demanding, spontaneous activities. Frequently, an apparent lack of strength in a particular muscle group improves immediately following appropriate stimulation in a functional pattern. Stretching of tight fascia and aponeurosis requires direct lengthening procedures applying tension parallel to the fibre orientation. This may be in the form of connective tissue manipulation (Ebner, 1985), or deep friction massage (Cyriax, 1982). An example of acquired changes secondary to functional demands is illustrated by the iliotibial band friction syndrome. This condition is commonly seen in runners (Noble, 1980) and is characterized by pain on the lateral aspect of the femur with a positive Ober's sign (Lindenberg *et al.*, 1984). The postulated mode of onset relates to the observation that the involved leg tends to be on the low side of the camber. Biomechanical evaluation of this situation suggests that the low-side leg would be limited in pronation, thereby prolonging external tibial rotation and promoting genu varum. This results in increased tension through the iliotibial band which may then become irritated by the repeated flexion/extension action of the knee. The methods of passive joint mobilization are numerous (Grieve, 1986) and are discussed in other chapters, but all techniques have the common purpose of attempting to restore normal joint mechanics. They may employ both accessory movements using 'joint play' (Gray, 1989) and through range physiological movements of varying amplitude and force. It is important to strive for normalization of all joint signs as any persisting pain may cause reflex inhibition of muscular control (Spencer et al., 1984; Stokes and Young, 1984; Ihara and Nakayama, 1986; Patterson and Steinmetz, 1986; Thabe, 1986; Arena *et al.*, 1989).

This reflex inhibition is commonly interpreted as muscle weakness but detailed examination of the articular structures will usually reveal an abnormality sufficient to cause pain inhibition of the associated musculature. This situation is commonly seen in relation to an extension lag at the knee (Maitland, 1991: 105). A further example of the interdependence of elements of the musculoskeletal system is illustrated in the case of the hip/lumbar spine complex. Reduction in the range of hip extension may cause a compensatory increase in lumbar lordosis and a possibility of painful irritation of any of the structures in the lumbar region (Terry and DeYoung, 1979; Offierski and Macnab, 1983)). An L2/3 segment dysfunction also has the potential to refer pain to the hip, often mimicking a primary hip disorder. Thus, adequate differentiation and appropriate restoration of normal function is essential for successful rehabilitation.

Rehabilitation

Rehabilitation is commonly classified in a somewhat arbitrary three-stage system – early, middle and late – but is in fact a continuum, graded according to the applied work load. The vast spectrum of potential rehabilitation procedures is beyond the scope of this discussion, but in general terms, progression can be made by manipulation of the following variables with attention to quality of task execution and the associated pain response prior to further progression:

1. Degree of weight bearing.
2. Range of joint motion.
3. Type of muscle contraction.
4. Force of muscle contraction.
5. Speed of contraction.
6. Level of static / dynamic load.

Careful monitoring of the tissue response following each progression should be undertaken on an ongoing basis and any sign of increased irritation dictates caution, if not a reduction in the rate of progression.

Equipment

The use of standard exercise equipment such as weights, medicine balls, benches, balance boards, pulleys etc. remains fundamental to effective rehabilitation. The role of therapeutic exercise is sometimes overlooked in favour of more sophisticated training regimes but such practice may produce inadequacies in total rehabilitation. Recent technological innovations have been numerous and the past 20 years has seen a great expansion in the use of isokinetic equipment to evaluate muscle function, perhaps to the detriment of more proven techniques. **Isokinetics** refers to the ability of the muscle to develop torque at a constant speed through a specified range of motion (Hageman and Sorensen, 1991). It can provide information on characteristics of muscle function such as;

1. Force production.
2. Agonist–antagonist force ratios.
3. Force-velocity characteristics.
4. Force-length characteristics.
5. Eccentric-concentric force ratios.

An excellent text by Albert (1991), which discusses aspects of isokinetic training and rehabilitation should be consulted for further information.

While all research in this regard is to be applauded it must be stated that there is a significant lack of normative isokinetic data from which valid clinical judgements can be made and the relevance of the wide number of parameters which can be monitored is the subject of much debate (Nosse, 1982). There are many factors which influence reliability such as: machine calibration, alignment of joint axis to be tested, joint stabilization, positioning and testing protocols, therapist's commands and methods, subject cooperation and fatigue (Hageman and Sorensen, 1991). It should also be noted that the physical constraints of such testing procedures are quite different from the dynamics of normal movement and such testing appears to have limited use in predicting injury or functional capacity (Lamb, 1985; Lankhorst, 1985). One of the advantages of this type of equipment is the control which can be achieved during rehabilitation. Precise control of force production, range of motion and speed of contraction can be achieved.

However, the rapid technological advancement in this area together with other tools of evaluation such as force platforms, pedobarographs and high-speed cinematography provide the physiotherapist with invaluable assistance in evaluating potential factors contributing to the development of musculoskeletal pain occuring in sport. Prior to resumption of sport, joints should have a full, painless range of motion and muscle strength and co-ordination should be normal. This will ultimately require testing of the specific skill and strength components required for the sport and must be undertaken prior to return to competition. This may include such activities as kicking a football, analysis of bowling action, changes of direction at speed, or physical impacts simulating contact sports.

This fundamental requirement for return to normal, pain-free, *functional* status has been strongly emphasized in this chapter and forms the cornerstone of correct management of neuromusculoskeletal conditions which occur in sport. The necessity to examine and treat all the structures which may be involved in injury has been highlighted together with an outline of the principles of complete rehabilitation. While the relief of pain – the overwhelming symptom in the majority of patients – is of primary importance, in the field of sports physiotherapy the demands of participation dictate that restoration of normal function is the ultimate treatment objective.

References

Albert, M. (1991) *Eccentric Muscle Training*, Churchill Livingstone, Edinburgh

Arena, J.G., Sherman, R.A., Bruno, G.M. and Young, T.R. (1989) Electromyographic recordings of 5 types of low back pain subjects and non-pain controls in different positions. *Pain*, **37**, 57–65

Armstrong, D., Dry, R.M.L., Keele, C.A. and Markham, J.W. (1953) Observations on chemical excitants of cutaneous pain in man. *J. Physiol. (Lond.)*, **120**, 326–51

Arnoldi, C.C., Lempberg, R.K. and Linderholm, H. (1975). Intraosseous hypertension and pain in the knee. *J. Bone Joint Surg*, **57B**, 360–3

Barcroft, H. and Edholm, K. (1943) The effects of temperature on blood flow and deep temperature on the human forearm. *J. Physiol*, **102**, 5–20

Barnes, L. (1979) Cryotherapy – putting injury in ice. *Phys. Sports Med.*, pp. 130–6

Basmajian, J.V. and Delucia, C.J. (1985) *Muscles Alive*, 5th edn, Williams and Wilkins, Baltimore, Md

Belka, D. (1968) Comparison of dynamic, static and combination training on dominant wrist flexor muscles. *Res. Q.*, **39**, 244

Bentley, G. and Dowd, G. (1984) Current concepts of etiology and treatment of Chondromalacia Patellae. *Clini. Orthop. Rel. Res.*, **189**, 209–27

Breig, A. (1978) *Adverse Mechanical Tension in the Central Nervous System*, Almqvist and Wiksell, Stockholm

Burton, A.K. (1985) Grip strength and forearm straps in tennis elbow. *Br. J. Sports Med.*, **19**, 37–8

Butler, D.S. (1991) *Mobilisation of the Nervous System*, Churchill Livingstone, London

Cambell, J.N., Meyer, R.A. and LaMotte, R.H. (1979) Sensitisation of myelinated nociceptive afferents that innervate monkey hand. *J. Neurophysiol.*, **42**, 1669–79

Cameron, K.R., Wark, J.D. and Telford, R.D. (1992) Stress fracture and bone loss – the skeletal cost of intense athleticism. *Excel*, **8**, 39–55

Capasso, G., Maffulli, N. and Testa, V. (1989) Ankle taping: support given by different materials. *Brit. J. Sports Med.*, **23**(4), 239–40

Chao, E.Y., Laughman, R.K., Schneider, E. and Stauffer, R.N. (1983) Normative data of knee joint motion and ground reaction forces in adult level walking. *J. Biomech.*, **16**, 219–33

Charnley, J. and Pusso, R. (1986) The recording and the analysis of gait in relation to the surgery of the hip joint. *Clin. Orthop. Rel. Res.*, **58**, 153–64

Ciullo, J.V. and Zarins, B. (1983) Biomechanics of the musculotendinous unit: relation to athletic performance and injury. *Clin. Sports Med.*, 71–86

Cook, A.J., Woolf, C.J., Wall, P.D. and McMahon, S.B. (1987) Dynamic receptive field plasticity in rat spinal dorsal horn following C-primary afferent input. *Nature (Lond.)*, **325**, 15 1–3

Cook, S.D., Brinker, M.R. and Poche, M. (1990) Running shoes – their relationship to running injuries. *Sports Med*, **10**(1), 1–8

Costill, D.L., Fink, W.J. and Habansky, A.J. (1971) Muscle rehabilitation after knee surgery. *Phys. and Sports Med.*, **5**, 71

Curwin, S. and Stanish, W.D. (1984) *Tendinitis: Its Etiology and Treatment*, Collamore Press, D.C. Health and Co., Lexington, Mass.

Cyriax, J. (1982) *Textbook of Orthopaedic Medicine*, Bailliere Tindall, London

Devas, M.B. (1958) Stress fractures of the tibia or 'shin soreness'. *J. of Bone Joint Surg.*, **40** B, 227–139

Dieppe, P.A. (1989) Why is there such a poor relationship between radiographic joint damage and both symptoms and functional impairment in osteoarthritis? *Br. J. Rheumatol.*, **28**, 242

Dieppe, P.A. Hutton, C. and Campion, G. (1986) Osteoarthritis: progressive or controllable. *Pharmalibri*, Monographs in Medicine.

Ebner, M. (1985) *Connective Tissue Manipulations, 2nd edn*, Publisher: Robert E. Krieger, Malabar, 19a

Edwards, B.C. (1992) *Manual of Combined Movements*, Churchill Livingstone, Edinburgh

Ekstrand, J. and Gillquist, J. (1982) The frequency of muscle tightness and injuries in soccer players. *Am. J. Sports Med.*, **10**, 75–8

Elvey, R.L. (1986) Treatment of arm pain associated with abnormal brachial plexus tension. *Aust. J. Physiother.*, **32**, 225–30

Evans, P. (1980) The healing process at cellular level: a review. *Physiotherapy*, **66**(8), 256–9

Evans, P. (1986) *The Knee Joint: a clinical guide*, Churchill Livingstone, Edinburgh

Ferrington, D.G., Sorkin, L.S. and Willis, W.D. (1987) Responses of spinothalamic tract cells in the superficial dorsal horn of the primate lumbar spinal cord. *J. Physiol*, **388**, 681–703

Frank, G., Woo, S.L.-Y., Amiel, O. *et al.* (1983) Medial collateral ligament healing. A multi-disciplinary assessment in rabbits. *Am. J. Sports Med.*, **11**, 379–89

Fromson, A. 1. (1971) Treatment of tennis elbow with forearm support band. *J. Bone Joint Surg.*, **53A**, 183–4

Gerrard, B. (1987) The McConnell technique – applied science or applied persuasion. In *Manipulative Therapists Association of Australia – Fifth Biennial Conference*, Manipulative Therapists Association of Australia, Melbourne

Guilbaud, G., Benoist, J.M., Neil, A. *et al.* (1987) Neuronal response thresholds to and encoding of thermal stimuli during carrageenin-hyperalgesic inflammation in the ventrobasal thalmus of the rat. *Experi. Brain Res.*, **66**, 421–31

Goodfellow, J., Hungerford, D.S. and Zindel, M. (1976a). Patello-femoral joint mechanics and pathology; 1. Functional anatomy of the patello-femoral joint. *J. Bone Joint Surg.*, **58B**, 287–90

Goodfellow, J., Hungerford, D.S. and Zindel, M. (1976b) Patello-femoral joint mechanics and pathology: 2 Chondromalacia patellae. *J. Bone Joint Surg.*, **58B**, 291–9

Gray (1989) Arthrology. In *Gray's Anatomy* (eds P.L. Williams, R. Warwick, M. Dyson and L. Bannister), *Gray's Anatomy*, Churchill Livingstone, London

Green, T.A. (1990) Comparison of support provided by a semirigid orthosis and adhesive ankle taping before, during and after exercise. *Am. J. Sports Med.*, **18**(5), 498–506

Greene, T.A. and Roland, C. (1989) A comparative isokinetic evaluation of a functional ankle orthosis on talocalcaneal function. *J. Orthop. Sports Phys. Ther.*, **11**.

Greenfield, B. (1990) *The Biomechanics of the Foot and Ankle*, F.A. Davis, Philadelphia

Grieve, G.P. (1986) *Modern Manual Therapy of the Vertebral Column*, Churchill Livingstone, London

Grisigono, V. (1985) *Sports Injuries: A Self Help Guide*, John Murray, London

Grisigono, V. (1991) *Sports Injuries*, Butterworths, London

Grood, E.S., Suntay, W.J., Noyes, F.R. and Butler, D.L. (1984) Biomechanics of the knee-extension exercise. *J. Bone Joint Surg.*, **66A**, 725–33

Gunn, C.C. (1980) Prespondylosis and some pain syndromes following denervation supersensitivity. *Spine*, **5**, 185–92

Hageman, P.A. and Sorensen, T.A. (1991) Eccentric isokinetics. In *Eccentric Muscle Training* (ed. M. Albert), Churchill Livingstone, New York, pp. 99–105

Hakkinen, K. and Komi, P.V. (1981) Effect of different combined concentric and eccentric muscle work regimes on maximal strength development. *J. Human Movement Studies*, **7**, 33

Hamer, P. (1991) Classification of injuries. In *Postgraduate Sports Physiotherapy Resource Manual* (ed. D. Hooper), Curtin University, Perth

Hamill, J. and Knutzen, K.M. (1986) Evaluation of two ankle appliances using ground reaction force data. *J. Orthop. Sports Phys. Thera.*, **7**(5), 244–9

Hamill, J., Morin, G., Clarkson, P.M. and Andres, R.O. (1988) Exercise moderation of foot function during walking with a re-usable semirigid ankle orthosis. *Clin. Biomech.*, **3**, 153–8

Hansen, H., Damholt, V. and Termansen, N.B. (1979) Clinical and social status following injury to the lateral ligaments of the ankle. *Acta Orthop. Scand.*, **50**, 699–704

Herring, S.A. (1990) Rehabilitation of muscle injuries. *Med. Sci. Sport Exercise*, **22**(4), 453–6

Hettinga, D.L. (1979a) 1 Normal joint structures and their reaction to injury. *J. Orthop. Sports Phys. Ther.*, **1**(1), 16–21

Hettinga, D.L. (1979b) 2 Normal joint structures and their reaction to injury. *J. Orthop. Sports Phys. Ther.*, **1**(2), 83–8

Hettinga, D.L. (1980) 3 Normal joint structures and their reaction to injury. *J. Orthop. Sports Phys. Ther.*, **1**(3), 178–85

Hocutt, J.E., Jaffe, R., Rylander, C.R. and Beebe, J.K. (1982) Cryotherapy in ankle sprains. *Am. J. Sports Med.*, **10**, 316–19

Ihara, H. and Nakayama, A. (1986) Dynamic joint control training for knee ligament injuries. *Am. J. Sports Med.*, **14**(4), 309–14

Install, J. (1979) Chondromalacia patellae: Patellar malalignment syndrome. *Orthop. Clin. North Am.*, **10**(1), 117–27

Install, J., Falvo, K.A. and Wise, D. (1976) Chondromalacia Patellae. *J. Bone Joint Surg.*, **58A**, 1–8

Janda, V. (1978) *Muscles, Motor Regulation and Back Problems*, Plenum, New York

Janda, V. (1983) *Muscle Function Testing*, Butterworths, London

Janda, V. (1983) On the concept of postural muscles and posture in man. *Aust. J. Physiother.*, **29**(3), 83–4

Janda, V. (1988) Muscles and cervicogenic pain syndromes. In *Physical Therapy of the Cervical and Thoracic Spine* (ed. R. Grant), Churchill Livingstone, New York

Jull, G.A. and Janda, V. (1987) Muscles and motor control in low back pain: assessment and management. In *Physical Therapy of the Low Back* eds J.R. Taylor and L.T. Twomey), Churchill Livingstone, New York, pp. 253–78

Kalenak, A., Medlar, C.E., Fleagle, S.B. and Hotchberg, W.J. (1975) Athletic injuries; heat vs cold. *Am. Family Phys.*, **12**, 131–4

Kellett, J. (1986) Acute soft tissue injuries – a review of the literature. *Med. Sci. Sport Exercise*, **18**(5), 489–500

Kendall, F.P. and McCreary, E.K. (1983) *Muscles: Testing and Function*, 3rd edn, Williams and Wilkins, Baltimore, Md

Kelsey, J.L. and Golden, S.L. (1987) Occupational and workplace factors associated with low back pain. In *Occupational Back Pain* (ed. R.A. Deyo), Hanley and Belfus, Philadelphia

Kimura, I.F., Nawoczenski, D.A., Epler, M. and Owen, M.G. (1987) Effect of the airstirrup in controlling ankle inversion stress. *J. Orthop. Sports Phys. Ther.*, (S), 190–3

Klafs, C. and Arnheim, D.D. (1981) *Modern Principles of Athletic Training*, C.V. Mosby, St Louis

Klein-Vogelbach, S. (1990) *Functional Kinetics: Observing, Analysing and Teaching Human Movement*, Springer Verlag, Heidelberg

Knott, M. and Voss, D.E. (1956) *Proprioceptive Neuromuscular Facilitation*, Hoeber Harper, New York

Kopell, H.P. and Thompson, W.A.L. (1963) *Peripheral Entrapment Neuropathies*, Williams and Wilkins, Baltimore, Md

Kornberg, C. and Lew, P. (1989) The effect of stretching neural structures on grade one hamstring injuries. *J. Orthop. Sports Phys. Ther.*, (June), 481–7

Kues, J. (1990) The pathology of shin splints. *J. Orthop. Sports Phys. Ther.*, **12**(3), 115–21

Lamb, R.L. (1985) *Manual Muscle Testing*, Churchill Livingstone, New York

Lankhorst, G.J., Van de Stadt, R.J. and Van der Korst, J.K. (1985) The relationships of functional capacity, pain, isometric and isokinetic torque in osteoarthrosis of the knee. *Scand. J. Rehabil. Med.*, **17**, 167

Laughman, R.K., Carr, T.A., Chao, E.Y. *et al.* (1980) Three-dimensional kinematics of the taped ankle before and after exercise. *Am. J. Sports Med.*, **8**(6), 425–31

Laurin, C.A., Levesque, H.P., Desalt, R. *et al.* (1978) The abnormal lateral patello-femoral angle. *J. Bone Joint Surg.*, **60A**, 55–60

Lawrence, J.S., Bremner, J.M. and Bier, F. (1966) Osteoarthrosis. Prevalence in the population and relationship between symptoms and X-ray changes. *Ann. Rheum. Dis.*, **25**, 1–24

Leach, R.E. (1982) The prevention and rehabilitation of soft tissue injuries. *Int. J. Sports Med.* (Supp.), **3**, 18–20

Lee, C.K. and Alexander, H. (1984) Prevention of post laminectomy scar formation. *Spine*, **9**(3), 305–12.

Levine, J.D., Lam, D., Taiwo, Y.O. *et al.* (1986) Hyperalgesic properties of 15-lipoxygenase products of arachidonic acid. *Proc. Nat. Acad. Sci.*, **83**, 5331–4

Lewit, K. (1991) *Manipulative Therapy in Rehabilitation of the Locomotor System*, 2nd edn, Butterworth-Heinemann, Oxford

Lindenberg, G., Pinshaw, R. and Noakes, T.D. (1984) Iliotibial band friction syndrome in runners. *Phys. Sports Med.*, **12**, 118

Low, J. and Reed, A. (1990) *Electrotherapy Explained*, Butterworth-Heinemann, Oxford

Lundborg, G. (1988) *Nerve Injury and Repair*, Churchill Livingstone, Edinburgh

MacConaill, M.A. (1964) Joint movement. *Physiotherapy*, **50**(11), 359–67

Maitland, G.D. (1985) *Vertebral Manipulation*, Butterworth, London

Maitland, G.D. (1991) *Peripheral Manipulation*, 3rd edn, Butterworth-Heinemann, London

Marks, K.E. and Bentley, G. (1978) Patella alta and chondromalacia. *J. Bone Joint Surg.*, **60B**, 71–3

Marks, R. (1991) Effect of altered functional demand on the structural and functional properties of articular cartilage. *NZ J. Physiother.*, April, pp. 31–4

Martin, P. (1983) Bone scintigraphy in diagnosis and management of traumatic injury. *Semin. Nucl. Med.*, **13**, 104–22

Mayhew, T.P. and Rothstein, J.M. (1985) *Measurement of Muscle Performance with Instruments*, Churchill Livingstone, New York

McConnell (1986) The management of chondromalacia patellae: a long term solution. *Aust. J. Physiother.*, **32**(4), 215–23

McDonald, R. (1992) *Taping Techniques*, Churchill Livingstone, London

McLean, D.A. (1989) The use of cold and superficial heat in the treatment of soft tissue injuries. *Bri. J. Sports Med.*, **23**, 53–4

Moller, M.H.L., Oberg, B.E. and Ekstrand, J. (1978) Effects of warm up, massage and stretching on range of motion and muscle length in the lower extremity. *Am. J. Sports Med.*, **11**, 249–52

Muckle, D.S. (1982) Injuries in sport. *R. Soc. Hlth J.*, **102**, 93–4

Myburg, K.H., Vaughan, C.L. and Isaacs, S.K. (1984) The effects of ankle guards and taping on joint motion before, during and after a squash match. *Am. J. Sports Med.*, **12**(6), 441–6

Niedermann, B., Andersen, A., Funder, V. *et al.* (1981) Rupture of the lateral ligaments of the ankle: operation or plaster cast? *Acta Orthop. Scand.*, **52**, 579–87

Nirschl, R.P. and Pettrone, F.A. (1986) Tennis elbow: the surgical treatment of lateral epicondylitis. *J. Bone Joint Surg.*, **61A**, 832–9

Noble, C.A. (1980) Iliotibial band friction syndrome in runners. *Am. J. Sports Med.*, **8**, 232

Nosse, L.J. (1982) Assessment of selected reports on the strength relationship of the knee musculature. *J. Orthop. Sports Phys. Ther.*, **78**

Noyes, F.R. (1977) Functional properties of knee ligaments and alterations induced by immobilization. *Clin. Orthop. Rel. Res.*, **123**, 210–42

Noyes, F.R., Torvik, P.J., Hyde, W.B. and DeLucal, J.L. (1974) Biomechanics of ligament failure. *J. Bone Joint Surg.*, **56A**, 1406–17

Oakes, B.W. (1982) Acute soft tissue injuries; nature and management. *Aust. Family Physi.* (Suppl.), **10**, 3–16

O'Connell, T.C.J. (1981) *The Ice Treatment of Muscle Injuries*, 2nd edn, Irish Rugby Football Union, Dublin

O'Driscoll, S.W., Kumar, A. and Salter, R.B. (1983) The effect of continuous passive motion on the clearance of a haemarthrosis. *Clin. Orthop. Rel. Res.*, **176**, 305–11

Offierski, C.M., and Macnab, 1. (1983) Hip-spine syndrome. *Spine* **8**(3), 316–21.

O'Neil, R. (1976) Prevention of hamstring and groin strain. *Athletic Trainer*, **11**, 27–31

Pappenheimer, S.L., Eversol, S.L. and Soto-Rivera, A. (1948) Vascular responses to temperature in the isolated perfused hindlimb of the cat (abstract). *Am., J. Physiol*, **155**, 458

Patterson, M.M. and Steinmetz, J.E. (1986) Long-lasting alterations of spinal reflexes: a potential basis for somatic dysfunction. *Man. Med.*, 38–42

Poss, R. (1984) Functional adaptation of the locomotor system to normal and abnormal loading patterns. *Calcified Tissue International*, **36** (Suppl.) 155–61

Raja, S., Meyer, J.N. and Meyer, R.A. (1988) Peripheral mechanisms of somatic pain. *Anesthesiology*, **68**, 571–90

Reynolds, N.L. and Worrell, T.W. (1991) Chronic Achilles peritendinitis: etiology, pathophysiology and treatment. *J. Orthop. Sports Phys. Ther.* **14**(4), 171–76

Richardson, C.A. and Sims, K. (1991) An inner range holding contraction: an objective measure of stabilising function of an antigravity muscle. In *Proceedings of the 11th International Congress of the World Confederation for Physical Therapy*, London; pp. 829–31

Ryan, L.G. (1989) Functional instability of the ankle. In *Sixth Biennial Conference Proceedings* (eds H.M. Jones, M.A. Jones and M.R. Milde), Manipulative Therapists Association of Australia, Adelaide

Rydevik, B. (1980) Blockage of axonal transport induced by acute graded compression in the rabbit vagus nerve. *J. Neurol. Neurosurg. Psychiatr.*, **43**, 690–8

Safran, M.R., Garrett, W.E., Seaber, A.V. *et al.* (1988) The role of warm up in muscular injury prevention. *Am. J. Sports Med.*, **16**(2), 123–8

Sahrmann, S. (1990) *Diagnosis and Treatment of Muscle Imbalances associated with Regional Pain Syndromes* (Course notes), Washington University, School of Medicine, Physical Therapy Department, Washington, DC

Salter, R.B. (1989) The biologic concept of continuous passive motion of synovial joints: the first 18 years of basic research and its clinical application. *Clin. Orthop.*, **242**, 12–25

Salter, R.B., Simmond, D.F., Makolm, E.J. *et al.* (1975) The effect of continuous passive motion on the healing of articular cartilage defects. *J. Bone Joint Surg.*, **57A**, 570–1

Sherrington, C.S. (1906) *The Integrative Action of the Nervous System*, Scribner, New York

Sikorski, J.M., Peters, J. and Watt, 1. (1979) The importance of femoral rotation in chondromalacia patellae as shown by serial radiograph. *J. Bone Joint Surg.*, **61B**, 435–42

Spencer, J.D., Hayes, K.C. and Alexander, I.J. (1984) Knee joint effusion and quadriceps reflex inhibition in man. *Arch. Phys. Med. Rehab.*, **56** (April), 171–7

Starkey, J.A. (1976) The treatment of ankle sprains by the simultaneous use of intermittent compression and ice packs. *Am. J. Sports Med.*, 147–9

Steadman, J.R. (1979) Rehabilitation of athletic injury. *Am. J. Sports Med.*, 147.

Stokes, M. and Young, A. (1984) Investigations of quadriceps inhibition: implications for clinical practice. *Physiotherapy*, **70**(11), 425–8

Terry, A.F. and DeYoung, R. (1979) Hip disease mimicking low back disorders. *Orthop. Rev.*, **3**, 95–104

Thabe, H. (1986) Electromyography as a tool to document diagnostic findings and therapeutic results associated with somatic dysfunctions in the upper cervical spinal joints and sacroiliac joints. *Man. Med.*, **2**, 53–8

Thalhammer, J.G. and LaMotte, R.H. (1982) Spatial properties of nociceptor sensitisation following heat injury to the skin. *Brain Res.*, **231**, 257–65

Tipton, C.M., James, S.L., Mergner, W. and Tcheng, T. (1970) Influence of exercise on strength of medial collateral knee ligaments of dogs. *Am. J. Physiol.*, **218**, 894–902

Vaes, P., De Boek, H., Handelberg, F. and Opdecam, P. (1985) Comparative radiological study of the influence of ankle joint bandages on ankle stability. *Am. J. Sports Med.*, **13**(1), 46–50

Vagenas, G. and Hoshizaki, B. (1992) A multivariate analysis of lower extremity kinematic asymmetry in running. *Int. J. Sports Biomech.*, **8**, 11–29.

Vailas, A.C., Tipton, C.M., Matthews, R.D. and Gart, M. (1981) Influence of physical activity on the repair process of medial collateral ligaments in rats. *Conn. Tissue Res.*, 25–31

Vasey, J.R. and Crozier, L.W. (1980) A neuromuscular approach to knee joint problems. *Physiotherapy*, **66**(6), 193–4

Weinstein, S.M. and Herring, S.A. (1992) Nerve problems and compartment syndromes in the hand, wrist and forearm. *Clin. Sports Med.*, **11** (1), 161–88

Woo, S.L.-Y and Akeson, W.H. (1987) Response of tendons and ligaments to joint loading and movements. In *Joint Loading* (eds H.J. Helminen, I. Kiviranta, M. Tammi), Wright, Bristol

Wooden, M.J. (1990) Biomechanical evaluation for functional orthotics. In *The Biomechanics of the Foot and Ankle* (ed. R. Donatelli), F.A. Davis, Philadelphia, pp. 131–47

Woolf, C.J. (1983) Evidence for a central component of post injury pain hypersensitivity. *Nature (Lond.)*, **308**, 686–8

Woolf, C.J. (1984) Long term alterations in the excitability of the flexion reflex produced by peripheral tissue injury in the chronic decerebrate rat. *Pain*, **18**, 325–43

Woolf, C.J. (1987) Physiological, inflammatory and neuropathic pain. *Adv. Tech. Stand. Neurosurg.*, **15**, 209–14

Woolf, C.J. (1989) Recent advances in the pathophysiology of acute pain. *Bri. J. Anaesthiol.*, **63**, 139–46

Woolf, C. (1991) *Generation of Acute Pain: Central Mechanisms*, Churchill Livingstone, London

Woolf, C.J. and McMahon, S.B. (1985) Injury induced plasticity of the flexor reflex in chronic decerebrate rats. *Neuroscience*, **16**, 395–404

Worth, D.H. (1969) The hamstring injury in Australian rules football. *Austr. J. Physiother.*, **15**(3), 111–13

Yong-Hing, K., Reilly, J., de Korompay, V. and Kirkaldy-Willis, W.H. (1980) Prevention of nerve root adhesions after laminectomy. *Spine*, **5**(1), 59–64

Zarins, B. (1982) Soft tissue injury and repair-biochemical aspects. *Int. J. Sports Med. (Suppl. 1)*, **3**, 9–11

Index